Neurorehabilitation for the Physical Therapist Assistant

Darcy Umphred, PT, PhD, FAPTA

Emeritus Professor

University of the Pacific

Stockton, California

Constance Carlson, PT, MS Ed

Mount St. Mary's College

Los Angeles, California

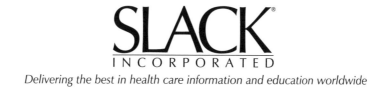

SLACK®

INCORPORATED

Delivering the best in health care information and education worldwide

ISBN 13: 978-1-55642-645-2

The procedures and practices described in this book should be implemented in a manner consistent with the professional standards set for the circumstances that apply in each specific situation. Every effort has been made to confirm the accuracy of the information presented and to correctly relate generally accepted practices. The author, editor, and publisher cannot accept responsibility for errors or exclusions or for the outcome of the application of the material presented herein. There is no expressed or implied warranty of this book or information imparted by it.

The work SLACK publishes is peer reviewed. Prior to publication, recognized leaders in the field, educators, and clinicians provide important feedback on the concepts and content that we publish. We welcome feedback on this work.

Printed in the United States of America

Library of Congress Cataloging-in-Publication Data

Neurorehabilitation for the physical therapist assistant / edited by Darcy Umphred, Constance Carlson.
     p. ; cm.
Includes bibliographical references and index.
ISBN-13: 978-1-55642-645-2 (alk. paper)
ISBN-10: 1-55642-645-3 (alk. paper)
1. Nervous system--Diseases--Physical therapy. 2. Nervous system--Diseases--Patients--Rehabilitation. 3. Physical therapy assistants.
  [DNLM: 1. Nervous System Diseases--rehabilitation. 2. Physical Therapy Modalities. 3. Rehabilitation--methods. WL 140 N49403 2006] I. Umphred, Darcy Ann. II. Carlson, Constance, PT.

RC350.P48N55 2006
616.8'046--dc22

                                                       2005034476

Published by: SLACK Incorporated
                 6900 Grove Road
                 Thorofare, NJ 08086 USA
                 Telephone: 856-848-1000
                 Fax: 856-853-5991
                 www.slackbooks.com

Contact SLACK Incorporated for more information about other books in this field or about the availability of our books from distributors outside the United States.

Last digit is print number: 10 9 8 7 6 5 4 3 2

DEDICATION

"To my immediate and extended family, who have always supported and encouraged me in any commitment I have accepted. To my friends and colleagues who have deepened my belief in the importance of empowerment of individuals who also are in need of health care services."

~Darcy

"To my husband for his unconditional love and support, to my parents for their endless love and encouragement, and to Lynn Lippert for being a role model for physical therapist assistant educators."

~Connie

CONTENTS

ACKNOWLEDGMENTS

The editors of this text want to acknowledge and recognize all those individuals that have laid the foundation for the formulation of this text. First, we need to thank our teachers and mentors along our journey. All the patients that have taught us clinical skills and reinforced our reasons for becoming physical therapists have played a significant role in our development. Of course, all the colleagues that have made this text a reality need to be acknowledged and thanked. The time and commitment needed to write chapters with the quality and depth of those within this text shows not only professional expertise but also a desire by each author to help future colleagues learn and grow and the respect they have for the PTA. Great appreciation needs to be given to John Bond and Carrie Kotlar for the gentle shoves and encouragement they have always had as the book progressed from an idea into a copy of a text. Of course, all the individuals at Slack that have worked hard to transition the manuscripts into what you are holding today need recognition. Lastly, we want to thank our families for supporting our efforts. Without that support, the time and energy needed to complete this project would have arrested its development.

ABOUT THE EDITORS

Dr. Darcy Umphred graduated from the University of Washington with a BS in Physical Therapy, from Boston University with a MS in Allied Health Education, and from Syracuse University with a PhD in Teacher Education and Theories of Learning. She has taught in both Physical and Occupational Therapy Programs throughout the United States. Over the course of her career, she frequently has taught educational programs both within and outside the northern hemisphere. Her love for clinical practice has driven her to question the "why's" behind movement function and dysfunction. She is the editor of the textbook *Neurological Rehabilitation* that is in its 5th reediting process and is translated into a large number of languages. She has received numerous awards locally, within her state, and APTA sections, as well as being made a Catherine Worthingham Fellow in 2003. In 2004, she retired as chair and professor of the Department of Physical Therapy at the University of Pacific in Stockton, California and is now an Emeritus Professor. Her respect for the Profession of Physical Therapy and the two educated professionals, the physical therapist and the physical therapist assistant, has been demonstrated by her commitment to the responsibilities and services both professionals play in the delivery of physical therapy services throughout the world.

Ms. Constance "Connie" Carlson graduated from the University of Evansville with an AS in Physical Therapist Assistance and a BS in Psychology. She later returned to the University of Evansville and graduated with a BS in Physical Therapy. She received her MS in Education from Mount St. Mary's College. She was the Director of the Physical Therapist Assistant Program at Mount St. Mary's College for 12 years and has taught in the college's baccalaureate, master's, and doctoral entry-level Physical Therapy Programs. She has been an advocate for the education and role of the physical therapist assistant throughout her career on a local, state, and national level, serving as a member of state government task forces and committees related to the physical therapist assistant. She has served as the Chair of the Education Section's Physical Therapist Assistant Educators Special Interest Group and provides presentations on the appropriate use and supervision of the PTA on a local and state level. Her current professional focus is working with people with neurological disorders in community-based and wellness programs with an emphasis on enablement. Her love and respect for the physical therapy profession and the physical therapist assistant drives her commitment to enhancing the general public's understanding of who we are and what services the physical therapist and physical therapist assistant provide to all of our patients and clients.

Contributing Authors

Claire E. Beekman, PT, MS, NCS
Retired Physical Therapy Manager
Spinal Injury Service
Rancho Los Amigos National Rehabilitation
  Center
Downey, CA

Gordon U. Burton, OT, PhD
Professor Emeritus
San Jose State University
Past Chair and Professor
Department of Occupational Therapy
Consultant, Practitioner, International Lecturer
Partners in Learning Clinic
Sacramento, CA

Constance "Connie" Carlson, PT, MS Ed
Consultant, Practitioner
The Carlson Group
Culver City, CA
Former Director, PTA Program
Mount St. Mary's College
Los Angeles, CA

Kristine N. Corn, PT, MS, DPT
Owner and Clinician
Sierra Pediatrics
Granit Bay, CA

Carol Davis, PT, EdD, MS, FAPTA
Professor
Division of Physical Therapy
University of Miami School of Medicine
Miami, FL

Dennis W. Klima, PT, MS, GCS, NCS
Faculty-Department of Physical Therapy
University of Maryland-Eastern Shore
Princess Anne, MD
Former Director, PTA Program
Baltimore City Community College
Baltimore, MD

Rolando T. Lazaro, PT, MS, DPT, GCS
Assistant Professor
Department of Physical Therapy
Samuel Merritt College
Oakland, CA

Becky S. McKnight, PT, MS
Program Coordinator, PTA Program
Ozarks Technical Community College
Springfield, MO

Dale Scalise-Smith, PT, PhD
Chair and Professor
Department of Physical Therapy
Health and Human Studies Division
Utica College
Syracuse University
Utica, NY

Eunice Shen, PT, DPT, MS, PCS
Therapy Manager
California Children's Services
County of Los Angeles
El Monte, CA

James M. Smith, PT, MA
Assistant Professor of Physical Therapy
Utica College
Utica, NY
Former Director, PTA Program
Connecticut Community Colleges
Waterbury, CT

Darcy Umphred, PT, PhD, FAPTA
Emeritus Professor
University of the Pacific
Retired Chair and Professor
Department of Physical Therapy
Consultant, Practitioner, International Lecturer
Partners in Learning Clinic
Sacramento, CA

Christine R. Wilson, PT, PhD
Assistant Professor
Department of Physical Therapy
University of the Pacific
Stockton, CA

INTRODUCTION

The conceptualization of this text originated from all the controversy that has arisen within the physical therapy profession regarding the roles and expectations of both the physical therapist (PT) and the physical therapist assistant (PTA). Both individuals are critical to the optimal delivery of physical therapy to consumers in need of that service. How to identify appropriate roles within the health care setting has been a focus within each chapter of this text. Although the patient population encompasses individuals who have had or do have pathologies/diseases/traumas within the human nervous system, the process of delineation and delegation of responsibilities is not specific to neurologic rehabilitation. PTs are responsible for the evaluation of patients and the design of a treatment plan and intervention program. PTAs certainly have the skill to participate in the examination process and carry out many aspects of the designed treatment plan. Similarly, many patients just need practice, which can be assisted by family members and does not require the presence of either the PT or the PTA. The PTA is an educated individual and plays a critical role in patient interaction and observation of patient changes. The PTA's eyes, ears, and kinesthetic systems are collecting data on a moment-to-moment basis when interacting with the patient. That information needs to be shared with and analyzed by the PT in a collaborative manner in order to determine changes in intervention management and to determine patient problems that fall outside of the scope of practice of physical therapy.

The first six chapters of the text encompass foundation concepts and areas in which the PTA must develop cognitive, motor, and psychosocial competencies before trying to apply that information to specific clinical problems within the area of neurologic rehabilitation. These chapters also focus upon general examination and intervention concepts and the roles the PTA may assume when participating in either area. Discussion within a general arena of appropriate and inappropriate delegation practices by the PT has been included in order to better define specific roles. When the PTA is asked to perform some examination or intervention procedure that has not been learned or the PTA feels is outside his or her scope of practice, that information needs to be communicated to the PT. This concept is stressed throughout the text along with all the complex procedures that are within the scope of the PTA practice.

The next six chapters focus upon general categories of pathologies that create specific movement dysfunctions that are referred to physical therapy. Although many of these pathologies/diseases or traumatic events may be age-related, the examinations and interventions discussed have a much broader framework and can be intertwined with all the other chapters within this section. The final two chapters of the text incorporate additional ideas and areas that can affect patient outcomes and offer additional resources and intervention suggestions that the PTA might want to or be expected to consider as part of the PTA's role.

The roles of the PT and PTA are evolving as the profession becomes more autonomous and assumes a more proactive role as movement specialists. The PT and PTA must remember that as professionals, we evaluate and treat movement dysfunction that affects an individual's ability to succeed at normal activities of daily living (ADLs) and to participate in life. Many daily living movement limitations have resulted from neurologic disease and trauma, but PTs and PTAs do not treat those diseases or traumas; that is the role of the physicians and other health care practitioners. We do treat the movement dysfunctions by identifying impairments within systems and subsystems of the human body that affect movement. PTs identify and document problems with ADLs and determine impairment problems causing those limitations. Similarly, patient goals and past participation in ADLs play a critical role in intervention selection and outcome. The PT should determine which functional activities and which impairments need to be addressed as part of the intervention plan, but the PTA interacts with the patient and ensures that the movement focus has meaning to the patient. The role of PTA in this interaction and motivation is critical to the success of any physical therapy intervention. As previously stated, the profession of physical therapy includes PTs and PTAs, and the successful interaction of these practitioners depends upon mutual respect and understanding of the roles and expectations each have within the health care delivery system as a whole.

Chapter

1

INTRODUCTION TO NEUROREHABILITATION FOR THE PHYSICAL THERAPIST ASSISTANT

Darcy Umphred, PT, PhD, FAPTA
Constance Carlson, PT, MS Ed

KEY WORDS

disablement
enablement
neurorehabilitation
physical therapist assistant (PTA)
physical therapy diagnosis
prognosis
systems model

CHAPTER OBJECTIVES

- Discuss the difference between a disablement model and enablement model.

- Discuss the difference between the medical model and the diagnostic model used by physical therapists (PTs).

- Discuss the factors involved when a PT determines which tests, measures, and interventions are appropriate to be delegated to a physical therapist assistant.

INTRODUCTION

The magnitude of the topic referred to as *neurorehabilitation* encompasses all the neurosciences, behavioral sciences, and social sciences; an understanding of development across the lifespan; and the pathologies or diseases relating to the nervous system. The causations and treatments for all known neuropathologies or diseases fall within the domain of medical practice. Physical therapists (PTs) and *physical therapist assistants* (PTAs) do not treat those diseases, although understanding the pathologies is important in selecting examination tools, goal expectations, parameters for interventions, limitations on motor control, motor learning, and neuroplasticity. The impairments or functional limitations that lead to the development of a pathology are classified under a health and wellness model and fall within the scope of practice of most therapists. Similarly, those impairments and functional limitations that developed from a combination of the pathology or disease of the nervous system and the preexisting health status of the individual come under the scope of physical therapy, as well. Traditionally, this postpathology or disease scope of practice, regarding the peripheral and central nervous system (CNS), is considered *neurorehabilitation*. Generally, those patients with CNS problems are sent to the PT through a referral process. The focus of this text will be on this traditional scope of practice and the role of the PT and PTA when a referral has been made.

Differentiation of the roles of a PTA within a neurorehabilitation setting is often hazy because PTAs start their clinical practice as novices upon leaving the educational environment. However, following those degrees should come a lifetime of learning and the addition of intervention skills. Most PTAs continue their learning through continuing education courses, in-service education, formal academic degree programs, and certification or licensure in other areas of health care delivery. For this reason, a PT may delegate certain interventions and reassessments of specific basic impairments to a novice PTA while, to a more experienced PTA, the PT delegates more complex interventions, reassessment of functional skills and more complex impairments, and a role in discharge planning.

Conceptual understanding of various topics lays the foundation for general discussion of the specific neurological clinical problems presented within the text. These specific clinical problems, crossing a lifespan of development, will also play a role in determining what should and should not be delegated. The PTA must always remember that although a specific age population may be the focus of a pathology topic, many clinical problems can occur at any age. Obviously, those problems that occur in utero, at birth, or with a genetic link will set the stage for alternative paths to development. Yet, these children can develop any of the other clinical problems discussed in this text. That is, someone with an early medical diagnosis of cerebral palsy (CP) can later have a stroke, a spinal injury, a head injury, or can develop some demyelinating disease as an adult. Thus, those interventions presented within the clinical problem chapters are within the scope of a PTA and might be delegated as part of the treatment plan for an individual on a PTA's caseload.

DISABLEMENT/ENABLEMENT MODELS

Physical therapy, like many health professions throughout the world, analyzes and implements theoretical models that may explain the sequential progression from an acute disease or pathology, through the onset of specific and general life problems that may result from the disease, and may explain how these residual problems can affect that individual's life. In 1980, The World Health Organization (WHO) developed the first widely accepted *disablement* model, known as the International Classification of Impairments, Disabilities, and Handicaps (ICIDH).[1] This model helps classify diseases so that doctors around the world

have a common classification system. Similarly, the WHO model has a classification for specific system problems, identified as impairments. The third classification within the WHO model is disability, and this area deals with everyday life activities that an individual can no longer perform. Both the impairment and disability groups are identified by the health care practitioner. The last category is labeled handicap, and the patient identifies these problems. This model remains widely accepted by other countries and has allowed for communication across cultures and hemispheres.

Another disablement model was developed by a sociologist in 1965[2] and follows a very similar sequence to the first WHO model. This model, known as the Nagi model, also begins with disease or pathology, followed by impairments. Unlike the WHO model, the third category is labeled functional limitations and directly correlates with the activities of daily living (ADLs) that the patient can no longer perform. The fourth postdisease category is called disability. The American Physical Therapy Association has embraced the Nagi model and has incorporated it into the *Guide to Physical Therapist Practice*.[3]

In the later half of the 1990s, the WHO developed a new model based on the *enablement* of the individual, known as the ICIDH-2.[4] The past disease category became the health condition category. Impairments became body functions or structures and disabilities became activities. The last category is labeled enablement and focuses upon participation in those ADLs the patient can still do versus those ADLs no longer available. Table 1-1 identifies the three models displaying their commonalities and differences.

The Nagi model will be consistently used throughout this text because the *Guide to Physical Therapist Practice*[3] is the only guide available to PTs. Both PTs and PTAs need to become aware of the differences between the two WHO models and the Nagi model in order to be able to accurately communicate with other professionals who may not be familiar with the model used by the physical therapy profession. Many PTs are currently developing wellness clinics, which encourage empowerment of individuals regarding the responsibility of maintaining health whenever possible. The concept of enablement and health maintenance is hard to translate into a model of practice that is based on disease. As the physical therapy profession embraces predisease (health, wellness, and disease prevention) and postdisease (empowerment of the patient regarding quality of life issues), models will change to better reflect the relationship between the PT or PTA and the individual in need of services. These models have been, and will continue to be, used in the diagnostic process of PTs.

Table 1-1
Disablement/Enablement Models Widely Accepted Throughout the World

Identified Model	Medical Condition	Subsystem Category	Activities of Daily Living	Social Level of Function
World Health Organization Disablement Model (ICIDH)	Disease/Pathology	Impairments	Disabilities	Handicaps
Nagi Disablement Model	Disease/Pathology	Impairments	Functional Limitations	Disabilities
World Health Organization Enablement Model(ICIDH-2)	Health Condition	Body Functions and Structure	Activities	Participation or Enablement

GUIDE TO PHYSICAL THERAPIST PRACTICE

This text will incorporate the terminology and definitions of terms utilized in the *Guide to Physical Therapist Practice* (the *Guide*), published by the American Physical Therapy Association.[3] The reader is encouraged to refer to the *Guide*[3] for detailed explanations of terms and the presented patient/client management model in order to more fully comprehend those terms and the role of the PTA in relationship to the *Guide* and patient/client management.

The PT performs examinations and evaluations that identify the specific functional activity problems and determine the impairments of systems and subsystems causing the patient to have functional loss. The *physical therapy diagnosis* identifies functional limitations and the impairments that have caused those limitations.[3] The *prognosis* identifies the predicted optimal improvement in function and the time parameters needed to change the existing limitations into functional activities the patient will be able to perform. The prognosis also includes the plan of care established by the PT, which specifies the patient/client management and incorporates goals, outcomes, and the specific interventions to be used, including the frequency and duration of each.[3] The interventions delegated to PTAs are classified under both impairment training, such as strength training or range of motion (ROM) exercises, and functional limitations training, such as coming to stand, walking, sitting, or golfing.

SYSTEMS MODEL

In order for the PT to differentiate the possible physical causations of the various impairments and the resulting functional limitations, that individual must understand how certain body system functions relate to motor performance or control. The *Guide*[3] identifies four large system practice patterns on which PTs commonly focus their practice. Those areas are as follows: integumentary (skin), cardiopulmonary (heart, lung, and circulation), musculoskeletal (muscles, joints, and boney structure), and neuromuscular (sensory and motor peripheral nerves and CNS processing, including somatic and autonomic). This book will focus upon the clinical problems that develop out of the fourth practice pattern, neuromuscular. The reader must be aware that patients may have difficulty in more than one practice area, and the interactions may be significant. For that reason, a chapter on cardiopulmonary problems in patients with CNS deficits has been included (see Chapter 13) and should help the PTA understand primary and secondary system interactions.

Although the *Guide*[3] clearly identifies the four practice patterns used by PTs, there are additional systems that can play a role in habilitation or rehabilitation of those individuals referred to physical therapy. Organ systems can play a critical role in the effectiveness of the PT interventions. The gastrointestinal system plays a primary role in nutrition intake and elimination of toxic waste. The liver, kidney, and bladder organ systems play a vital role in filtering out unwanted or unneeded chemical waste and excess fluid. The lymphatic system helps the vascular system with fluid elimination. Any one of these other systems can dramatically affect the cardiac, smooth, and striated muscles' metabolism and function. Similarly, a system such as the neuromuscular one can affect an organ system's function and a patient's willingness to participate in or adhere to home programs. For example, an individual may be referred to physical therapy with the medical diagnosis of Parkinson's disease. The patient may complain of constipation but has been told by the doctor that Parkinson's disease does not cause constipation. The PT should be able to diagnoses the neuromusculoskeletal interactions between the disease causing rigidity in the abdomen and the lack of motility of the colon. Knowing that trunk rotation modifies the rigidity of the abdominal muscles caused by the disease, a treatment recommendation might be to perform some rotational patterns in sitting a few minutes before that individual's usual time to have a bowel movement; decreasing the rigidity should allow for more normal peristaltic movement of waste in the colon. Decreasing rigidity will simultaneously assist in diaphragmatic breathing and, thus, may decrease cardiopulmonary problems in the future. The objective set by the PT may not be related to gastrointestinal problems, but certainly, the outcome will affect the patient's needs and empower that individual to have additional control over bodily function.

ROLE OF THE PHYSICAL THERAPIST AND PHYSICAL THERAPIST ASSISTANT

Although the role of the PTA within a clinical setting is dictated by the licensing board of the state, the specific types of delegation fall under the responsibilities of the PT and should directly relate to the needs of the patient. The PTA is the physical therapist *assistant* and should never practice autonomously or without supervision of a PT. The PT is, and will always be, legally responsible for the physical therapy provided the patient regardless of the fact that it may be delivered by a PTA.

Theoretical Framework

The authors have chosen a theoretical framework to assist the reader in understanding the role of the PTA in working with patients/clients with neurologic conditions. The theoretical framework outlining interventions performed by the PTA is aligned with key components of the Nagi Disablement Model, the Patient/Client Management model, and effective delegation principles (Figure 1-1).

As noted above, looking at neurologic diseases from the Nagi model perspective, the resultant pathologies may yield impairments such as muscle weakness, motor control problems, lack of range, and possible cognitive deficits.[2] These impairments may ultimately lead to functional limitations in bed mobility, transfers, gait performance, and aerobic capacity. Therefore, related disabilities will emerge when patients are unable to perform functional tasks in the community

environment. Designated interventions for patients recovering from neurologic pathologies are directed at improving the patient's functional status through comprehensive interventions at the impairment, functional limitation, and disability levels. In addition, the PTA must employ effective strategies to address the cognitive, musculoskeletal, and neuromuscular needs of the patient.

In the Patient/Client Management model continuum, the PTA will ultimately be delegated select interventions.[3] As discussed above, the determination of these interventions follows a thorough examination by the PT. The PT will summarize findings of the examination in the evaluation and will formulate a diagnosis and prognosis based upon these findings. Designated interventions will then be indicated in the plan of care, and the PTA will perform select intervention activities in conjunction with ongoing communication with the supervising PT.

Effective delegation strategies were presented to our profession within a few years of the development of the PTA in an article by Nancy Watts in 1972.[5] The PT's responsibility for determination of the tasks, including interventions, that can be delegated to a PTA is a complex issue. Watts proposed a method for making such decisions that includes analyzing the physical therapy tasks involved in the interventions under consideration to determine the degree to which it represents *decision-making* versus *doing* and the degree to which the elements are separable. She suggests that both components interact and both are necessary to quality care. The *decision-making* aspect of care requires evaluation and treatment planning skills. These skills require complex problem solving, up-to-date knowledge of the science of physical therapy, and a sophisticated ability to analyze and synthesize information from various sources in order to rationally choose the best alternative. The *doing* aspect of care requires excellence in skill, the knowledge of various therapeutic interventions, the capacity to recall correct treatment sequences, the artful manipulation of one's hands and body, and the ability to be sensitive to patient response moment to moment. Watts maintains that, in general, "decision-making skills involve dealing with data, while doing skills require dealing with people and things."[5] But she hastens to add, "the distinction drawn in this model between these two categories of skill should not be misconstrued as implying any hierarchy of importance nor any lack of interdependence between activities in the two realms."[5]

Watts also identifies **five factors** that are present in treatment, which more adequately characterize the continuum that flows between deciding and doing. These factors are discussed briefly following:

- **Predictability of consequences:** How uncertain is the situation? How confident can the

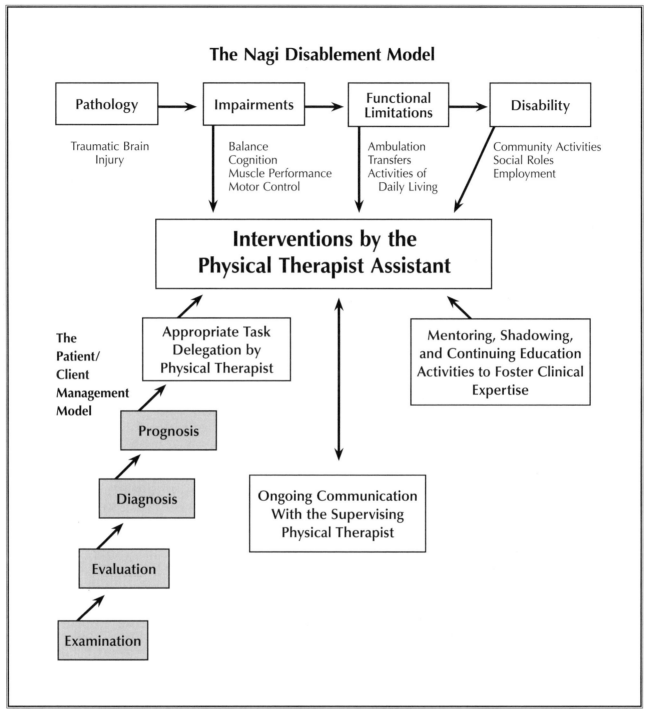

Figure 1-1. Theoretical framework for interventions provided by the PTA.

decision-maker be in the predictions about the consequences of action? For example, a gait-training program for a sprained ankle with no other medical conditions versus a gait-training program for a person with a recent lower extremity (LE) amputation, uncontrolled diabetes, and a new prosthesis.[5]

- **Stability of the situation:** How much and how quickly is change likely to occur in the factors upon which decisions are made? For example, a mat exercise program for someone with a complete spinal cord injury (SCI) will change relatively little compared to a mat program for an individual with an incomplete SCI. The person with the incomplete SCI may vary greatly in his or her ability within a short period of time.[5]

- **Observability of basic indicators:** How difficult is it to elicit the phenomena on which decisions are based? How easy are these phenomena to perceive or observe? For example, an obligatory reflex may be easy to elicit and observe whereas a maximal voluntary contraction requires full patient participation and may be more difficult to elicit.[5]

- **Ambiguity of basic indicators:** How difficult are the key phenomena to interpret? How easily might they be confused with other phenomena? For example, possible signs of an extension of a cerebral vascular accident (CVA) would be more difficult to interpret than interpreting if a muscle substitution was used in a manual muscle test.[5]

- **Criticality of results:** How serious are the consequences of a poor choice of method? For example, a wrong choice in a facilitation method that resulted in no response of the muscle would be of less consequence than the wrong choice in the amount of exercise without rest to be given to a patient with cardiac compromise.[5]

These five factors are present to varying degrees in all treatment situations. In deciding which interventions to delegate to the PTA, the PT must clearly differentiate between the deciding and doing aspects of the intervention and then, using the factors listed previously, determine the extent to which these two aspects of care can be separated. These components will guide a PT regarding when to delegate select interventions for a client with CNS damage to a PTA. If the patient needs constant guarding and guidance in order to carry out a specific functional task and the amount of guarding and guidance varies from moment to moment, delegation of that activity to a PTA seems inappropriate. On the other hand, if the patient is able to run a motor program, such as moving from sit to stand, but needs guidance to stay within a parameter of range of limits of stability (LOS) or balance, delegation of the intervention to a PTA is very appropriate. If the patient does not need guidance and only needs practice in order to overcome functional limitations, usually a family member or aide can assist, and this may not be an appropriate use of the PTA. Although there are many overlapping variables that might determine when a PT versus a PTA should be responsible for the intervention, having time to provide a service should not be a reason. If the PTA is being asked to treat someone because he or she has time and not because the PTA is the best provider given the needs of the patient, then that delegation is inappropriate and is a misuse of the PTA within a clinical setting.

Effective delegation strategies are enhanced by ongoing communication with the supervising PT to optimize interventions performed by the PTA in the trajectory of care. If an intervention is delegated to a PTA and the skill is outside of what the PTA has learned, it is always appropriate for the PTA to ask the PT for help or guidance. If what was delegated seems to contradict what the PTA has learned as contraindications, the PTA should always ask the PT for clarification before beginning treatment.

When looking at the clinical interactions between a PT and PTA from a business model, roles may change. One scenario that has developed is the PTA owning a physical therapy practice within which PTs and PTAs are employed. Most state physical therapy licensing boards have identified the practice relationship of this business model. If the PTA owns the practice, then that individual cannot function as a PTA within that setting. The conflict of interest between the role of a boss to the PT and being the assistant to the same individual is self-explanatory and legally controlled by most state regulations governing the practice of physical therapy.

Another role the PTA may assume in a clinical setting is that of receiving certification or licensure in a complementary approach, such as being a Feldenkrais practitioner, a Rolfer, or a craniosacral therapist (refer to Chapter 14 for additional information). In these cases, the PTA may develop intervention skills outside the skills of the PT. Hopefully, open communication exists between the PT and PTA that encourages implementation of all interventions that can benefit the patient, but again, the PTA must remember that the PT is responsible for deciding which interventions are to be used and which interventions will be delegated to the PTA. The PTA should always make the PT aware of intervention strategies that may be helpful but are not already provided within the plan of care.

If the PTA is practicing as a complementary therapist independently of a physical therapy practice setting and outside the supervision of a PT, then she or he must remember that she or he is not practicing as a PTA and that what is offered is not physical therapy and cannot be billed as such. PTAs who have additional certification should also be aware of the legal and liability issues that may apply to them as licensed PTAs practicing as complementary therapists. Discussion of these issues is beyond the scope of this text.

FUTURE ROLES

Physical therapy is a profession that has been evolving since its conception. The roles of the PT and PTA will change in the future, as they have changed over previous decades. Yet, the interactions should remain as two clinicians whose responsibility it is to help guide patients toward functional recovery and higher quality of life. As PTs develop more wellness clinics and disease prevention programs, the roles of PTAs will enlarge in these practice areas, as well. As the aging population deals with chronic diseases and the loss of life-altering functional skills, maintaining quality of life versus regaining function will become part of an ever-expanding scope of practice. The role of the PTA certainly has the potential of enlarging both in intervention strategies and responsibilities for patient care. As these roles change, so will the educational requirements for entry-level practitioners, as can be seen by the rapid movement of the physical therapy educational community toward a professional doctorate as the terminal degree for a PT. There certainly is the possibility that PTA educational requirements will also change in the future. PTAs of today may well be facing the same dilemma as PTs that graduated with bachelors degrees in the past. Those younger graduates may have a degree higher than the one a current practitioner has. This only means that the younger therapist may have knowledge to teach the seasoned clinician, just as the clinician has skills to teach the novice. The key to not being caught with limitations in practice parameters is to continue with one's learning no matter the degree received that opened the door to entry into this profession. It is hoped that this text will provide a background to the PTA that will not only help during study as a student but also provide insight and help once the student moves into an exciting practice arena as a PTA.

ACKNOWLEDGMENTS

The authors would like to thank Dennis Klima, PT, MS, GCS, NCS, for his contributions to this chapter in the section on Theoretical Framework and for the development of the theoretical framework presented in Figure 1-1.

REFERENCES

1. *International Classification of Functioning, Disability, and Health.* Geneva, Switzerland: World Health Organization; 2001.

2. Nagi S: *Disability Concepts Revisited: Implication for Prevention.* Washington, DC: National Academy Press; 1991.

3. *Guide to Physical Therapist Practice.* 2nd ed. Alexandria, Va: American Physical Therapy Association; 2001.

4. Wood, PH. Application of the international classification of diseases. *World Health Statistics Quarterly.* 1990;43(4):263-268.

5. Watts NA. Task analysis and division of responsibility in physical therapy. *Journal of Physical Therapy.* 1972;51(1):23-35.

Chapter

2

NORMAL MOVEMENT DEVELOPMENT ACROSS THE LIFESPAN

Dale Scalise-Smith, PT, PhD

KEY WORDS

cognition
development
dynamic systems theory
innate motor behaviors
locomotion
motor development

CHAPTER OBJECTIVES

- Recognize the interaction among multiple systems in performance of motor behaviors.

- Explain motor changes that occur across the lifespan and variability of motor performance amongst individuals.

- Examine the impact of health and fitness (physical activity) sustained over the lifespan on motor skill performance.

- Discuss the impact of age and age-related changes in exercise and training programs.

INTRODUCTION

Effective clinicians recognize the processes of motor development across the lifespan. The human motor system comprises over 700 muscles and the nerves that supply them. Motor behaviors require coordinated efforts among these and other bodily systems to produce movements.

Until the late 1960s, research in motor development focused on infants and children. In the 1970s, it became evident that changes in motor behaviors did not end in adolescence, leading to the recognition that motor development is a continuous process throughout the lifespan. Thus, models of motor development have expanded to include changes that occur throughout the lifespan. Consequently, lifespan motor development now examines movement from early infancy through older adulthood. Motor development is characterized by acquisition of motor skills during infancy (birth to 1 year) and childhood (1 to 10 years), followed by a period of stability from adolescence (10 to 19 years) through early and middle adulthood (20 to 59 years) and finally, a decline in execution of movements during late adulthood (60 years to death).

This chapter provides an overview of motor development to help the reader (1) recognize typical and atypical changes in motor behaviors across the lifespan, (2) appreciate factors that influence motor development, and (3) apply knowledge of motor development to intervention strategies.

Lifespan motor development reflects motor behaviors observed from the prenatal period through older adulthood. The acquisition and retention of motor skills is not confined to any one part of the lifespan. During early infancy, acquisition of postural control and grasping are primary foci. Later in infancy, mobility and object manipulation become primary objectives. During childhood, the skills acquired earlier are refined and coalesce to produce complex motor behaviors. Throughout adolescence and adulthood, opportunities to practice motor behaviors in different environmental contexts expand, and motor skills mature. As individuals grow old, the ability to perform motor skills declines. Whether this decline is due to aging, disuse, or a combination of both along with disease is open to debate. Within this context of motor development, the impact of various bodily systems on motor skills will be considered both individually and collectively.

THEORIES OF DEVELOPMENT

Development is defined as "the changes that occur in one's life from conception to death."[1] Many aspects of human behavior change over time, including cognitive, motor, language, social-emotional, and physical characteristics.

Early studies of motor development were based upon maturational models of CNS organization.[2,3] These studies provided elegant descriptions of posture acquisition and a time line for skill development. Most research development has focused on the emergence of cognitive and affective behaviors and neglected the processes and mechanisms involved in learning motor tasks.[4] Development was thought to occur in a fixed sequence, and behaviors observed were a direct reflection of the maturation of intrinsic mechanisms.[5]

This traditional model of development relied on motor milestones to evaluate ability levels in infants and children. While motor milestones provided an assessment of actual motor skills a child performed, they failed to provide information about the process of attaining motor skills.

Researchers have proposed theories on motor development that emphasize the forces behind behavioral changes. Some scientists[2,3] theorized that developmental changes arise from internal factors (genetics and/or maturation), while others associated changes with external variables (environmental, experience, and/or learning).[6,7] While sufficient evidence exists to support the idea that some predetermined processes occur at relatively similar points in development, not all motor behaviors emerge at the same biological,

chronological, or psychological age in every individual. The traditional theories on development and maturation fail to adequately address the variation inherent in human motor development.

Researchers that have focused on developing new models for motor skill acquisition in infants and young children include Heriza, Thelan, and Zelazo et al.[8-10] Rather than using traditional methods to measure changes in motor development and assess the outcomes, these researchers examined the process of motor skill acquisition.[11,12] These contemporary developmentalists support an interactive model of motor development in which both intrinsic and extrinsic variables impact the development and acquisition of motor skills (Figure 2-1). The primary foundation for this model is dynamic systems theory.

Dynamic systems theory states that an individual uses all possible strategies to accomplish a task, and as physiological systems are modified, the motor behavior changes.[13] Systems theorists purport that modifications in motor behaviors are the result of dynamic interactions between and among the musculoskeletal, neuromuscular, cardiovascular, pulmonary, and cognitive systems. Communicative and social-emotional aspects are equally considered. Interactive, multidimensional systems are susceptible to changes in organizational and behavioral capabilities as one ages.[14] As an individual acquires a skill, the organization of the behavior may change, thereby allowing the person to identify the most efficient strategy for effective functioning.

It is clear that a small change in any subsystem may result in a change in a motor behavior. For example, Thelan and colleagues examined stepping in infants 8 weeks of age.[13] During the baseline phase of this study, the infants' feet were placed on a treadmill with trunk support in an upright position. When the treadmill was turned on, the infants stepped. Immediately afterward, weights were applied to each leg, and the infants were again placed on the treadmill. The treadmill was turned on, but no infant stepped. The authors concluded that small changes in one subsystem, in this case, the musculoskeletal system, resulted in a change in the whole behavior, stepping. This evidence supported the premise that modifying one aspect of a multi-component system, especially during a critical period, results in a change in behavior.

As one ages, organizational changes of bodily systems increase the complexity of the collective system, allowing for greater adaptability and more efficient functioning. Scott defined periods of rapid differentiation or change during development when an organism is most easily altered or modified as *critical periods*.[14] These periods are when physiological systems are most vulnerable and may be seriously impacted by both

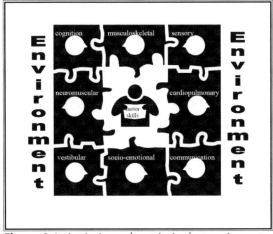

Figure 2-1. Intrinsic and extrinsic factors in motor development.

intrinsic and extrinsic factors acting upon the system (Figure 2-1). These periods occur at different times for different systems throughout the body.

Understanding systems theory and the concept of critical periods is crucial to all aspects of motor development. These theories illustrate the complexity of development and the difficulty in identifying the variables that influence performance of motor behaviors across the lifespan and in identifying the most effective treatments to use when a motor skill is compromised.

AGING

Just as changes to physiological systems early in development impact movement, aging also affects motor performance. Age is defined in terms of *chronological age* and *biological age.*[15] *Chronological age* is the period of time that a person has been alive, beginning at birth. In infants, it is measured in days, weeks, or months, while in adults, it is expressed in terms of years.

Unlike chronological age, biological age is not measured according to the calendar. Instead, *biological age* measures functional age in different body systems in relation to chronological age.[16] For example, an individual who competes in marathons may have biologically younger cardiovascular and pulmonary systems than same age peers who are not runners. As another example, a female may go through menopause prematurely. A postmenopausal woman experiences a decrease in estrogen levels that, in turn, negatively affects bone strength as measured by bone density. This woman has less dense bones than her same age peers, who will experience menopause later. No consistent method has been established for measuring biological age, but there is general agreement that a wide variability of biological aging exists among individuals.

Some changes are thought to be age-dependent and others thought to be age-related. Age-dependent behaviors are changes observed in all individuals at a similar age, whereas age-related behaviors are observed in many but not all individuals at a similar chronological age. One reason why behaviors may be designated as age-related rather than age-dependent is that individuals of the same chronological age may not be the same biological age. From a genetic perspective, structural and functional changes in general are thought to be a consequence of aging and are, therefore, predictable and consistent across physiological systems. Affecting the genetic potential for longevity are the strong effects of environmental factors, such as toxins, radiation, and oxygen-free radicals – highly reactive molecules produced as cells turn food and oxygen into energy.[17] Consequently, using biological age rather than chronological age may be a more accurate reflection of changes in a biological system.

Researchers are unsure how much of the decline in motor behaviors in older adults is due to a decline in physiological systems or to decreased practice and/or conditioning.[18] Rowe and Kahn found that "with advancing age, the relative contribution of genetic factors decreases and the nongenetic factors increases."[18] These age-related factors, including elements of lifestyle, are changeable and may be used to identify individuals who may or may not age successfully. Nongenetic risk factors can be identified through screening and addressed through clinical intervention and patient education. Lifestyle choices, including diet, physical activity, and other health habits, as well as behavioral and social factors have a potent effect on aging processes.

PHYSIOLOGICAL CHANGES IN BODY SYSTEMS ACROSS THE LIFESPAN

Following dynamic systems theory, researchers and clinicians who examine motor behaviors across the lifespan know that many biological systems are involved in the execution of motor skills and their associated behaviors. This discussion will be limited to the influence of the musculoskeletal, cardiovascular, pulmonary, neuromuscular, and cognitive systems on motor behaviors across the lifespan.

Musculoskeletal System

The musculoskeletal system is comprised of muscles, bones, cartilage, tendons, and ligaments. The roles of the musculoskeletal system are to provide a structural framework for the body to move and to protect internal organs.

Development of the muscular system initiates in utero and continues into young adulthood as a direct result of growth in both the number and size of the fibers. Between 5 and 8 fetal weeks is a period of rapid development for the musculoskeletal system.[19] In fact, most development of the muscular system occurs before birth.

Muscles grow at a rate two times faster than bones from 5 months to 3 years of age.[20] Throughout development of the musculoskeletal system, changes occur in muscle length, width, and girth, but the overall outward appearance remains unchanged. There is considerable variation in this growth. The structural and functional capabilities of an infant's muscular system are different from those of an adult. One example of a structural difference between the infant and adult is in muscle fiber type. A high prevalence of Type I muscle fibers are present in infant muscles compared to adult muscles that contain both Type I and Type II fibers. Functionally, the impact of infants' predominance of Type I fibers is that they are more readily able to produce high-speed muscle contraction than long-duration contractions, whereas adults are able to produce both types of muscle contractions.

As individuals age, the size of the fibers, muscle fiber recruitment, and quantity of fast-twitch fibers decreases.[21] After age 50, the cross-sectional area of muscles begins to decrease, deteriorating up to 40% by age 80.[22] These structural changes in muscle result in loss of strength. Initially, this was thought to be age-dependent because many individuals over 60 had similar loss of fast-twitch fibers and decreased fiber size. Current evidence supports the idea that changes in the muscular system may be attributed to decreased motor activity levels rather than age.[21] Thus, keeping physically active while progressing into older adulthood may be a primary key to maintaining functional independence.

Differences exist in the chronological ages at which musculoskeletal changes occur in males and females. Males exhibit rapid periods of differentiation in muscular development from birth to 2 years of age and then, between 10 and 16 years, demonstrate doubling in the number of muscle fibers.[23] Conversely, females exhibit a more gradual increase in fiber size from 3.5 to 10 years of age. Another difference is that overall fiber size increase is 14-fold in males between 2 months and 16 years of age while the female increase is 10-fold. Muscle fibers continue to increase, while at a slower pace, in both males and females into middle adulthood.

The skeletal system follows a similar path of growth, stability, and degeneration as the muscular system. The primary difference between the child and adult skeletal systems is the presence of the growth plate complex in children. Ossification centers appear from birth through skeletal maturity.[24] Primary ossification begins in utero and is complete by birth, whereas secondary ossification centers in the epiphysis remain cartilaginous. By the time the epiphyseal plate is ossified, bone growth in length is complete. Bone growth in length is complete when a child reaches skeletal maturity, generally at 14 years in girls and 16 years in boys.

Even after bone length is complete, bones continue to grow on the surface. This is termed *appositional growth* and continues throughout most of life. During childhood and adolescence, new bone growth exceeds bone resorption, and bone density increases. Until age 30, bone density increases in most individuals, and bone growth and resorption remain stable through middle adulthood. Later in adulthood, resorption exceeds new bone growth, and bone density declines.[25] Women exhibit more loss of bone mass than men. Decreased bone density in women is generally attributed to differences in the type and level of hormones present. While the difference is most significant during menopause, premenopausal women still lose bone density at a higher rate than their male peers do. Progressive loss of bone density, observed into older adulthood, is commonly identified as *osteoporosis.* Osteoporosis is more common in women than in men and is a major cause of fractures and postural changes in both sexes.[26]

Overall, much of the growth in the musculoskeletal system relates to demands placed on the system. Typically and atypically developing children have many intrinsic and extrinsic forces exerted upon their individual musculoskeletal systems. Movement patterns differ in children characterized as typically developing from those identified as atypical in motor development. The outcome is that the musculoskeletal system develops differently. Age-related changes in older adulthood might be related to decreased activity levels. An older adult who maintains a more active lifestyle and places greater demands on the musculoskeletal system has a better outcome, with improved bone density and muscle mass, than do his or her peers who are not as active.

Strength and flexibility are two areas of the musculoskeletal system that PTs examine. Strength is defined as the ability of a muscle to generate force against a specific resistance or produce torque at a joint.[25] Flexibility is the ability to bend.

Strength increases because of higher levels of resistance applied gradually during a muscular contraction. As the cross-sectional area of the muscle fibers hypertrophy, the ability to produce force increases. Consequently, changes in the cross-sectional area of muscles directly influence the force production of a given muscle. Conversely, as the cross-section of muscles diminishes, the ability to produce force decreases. As an individual ages, the number and size of the muscle fibers decrease, resulting in a reduction in strength.[26] While strength is critical to musculoskeletal function, flexibility is equally as important.

According to Dutton, flexibility incorporates joint motion and the extensibility of the tissues that cross the joint.[25] Changes in flexibility occur across the lifespan.[7] Early in postnatal life, infants exhibit limited flexibility due to the environmental constraints of the uterine environment. As the infant ages, flexibility increases in direct relation to increased joint play and extensibility of surrounding tissues. Flexibility increases in both males and females through early childhood. By 10 years of age for boys and 12 years for girls, flexibility begins to decrease. However, this may not be true of athletes, dancers, and other individuals involved in activities that incorporate flexibility training.

As activity levels decrease, so does flexibility. Flexibility is directly related to the amount, frequency, and variability of motor activities performed. Individuals often exhibit decreased levels of motor activity as they age. The result is that as individuals age, strength and flexibility decrease. While this appears to be age-dependent, it may be more likely that it is age-related.[21] Regularly performing motor activities (exercise) directed towards improving strength and/or flexibility can reverse the effects of inactivity for most individuals, even those older than 90 years of age.[21] While it may take longer for older individuals to regain strength and/or flexibility than young adults or children, musculoskeletal tissue is modifiable. Modifying strength and flexibility of an older adult requires that other systems are capable of modifying performance levels to meet the increased needs of the musculoskeletal system. Both training and system analyses are the primary roles of a PT. Delegation to the PTA for the training is very appropriate. The cardiovascular and pulmonary systems' physiologic response to exercise is directly related to the age of the individual. Physiologic response to exercise declines in the older adult. Conversely, physiologic performance of the cardiovascular and pulmonary systems of infants and children improve in response to growth and development.

Cardiovascular and Pulmonary Systems

The cardiovascular system is composed of the heart and vascular complex. The pulmonary system is comprised of the lungs and structures that connect to the external environment. The cardiovascular and pulmonary systems are responsible for delivering oxygen and nutrients throughout the body in addition to removing waste products. Oxygen is delivered to the blood through the pulmonary system. Transport of nutrients and oxygen to the tissues and waste product removal from the tissues is managed by the vascular system.

Development of the cardiovascular system begins during week 3 of prenatal life, with the heart structure formed by week 8. All other structures of the cardiovascular system are fully developed and functional shortly after birth. At birth, the left and right ventricles are of similar size, but by 2 months of age, the muscle wall of the left ventricle is thicker than the right ventricle. The significance of difference in thickness between the muscular wall of the left and right ventricles is related to function. The left ventricle is responsible for pumping blood to the whole body, while the right ventricle is responsible for pumping blood only to the lungs.

The heart doubles in size by an infant's first birthday and increases four-fold by age 5. Much of the cardiac growth occurs during childhood. As the size of the heart increases, the heartbeat decreases, and blood pressure (BP) increases. Heart rate in a newborn may be 120 to 140 beats per minute (bpm), 80 bpm by age 6, and 70 bpm by age 10. *Systolic blood pressure* (defined as maximal pressure on the artery during left ventricular contraction or systole) increases from 40 to 75 millimeters of mercury (mm Hg) in the newborn to 95 mm Hg by age 5. BP continues to rise into adolescence. The capacity to maintain exercise for longer periods and greater intensities increases throughout early childhood. Children as young as 5 years of age that have not had opportunities for adequate aerobic exercise and nutritional intake may show signs of or be at risk for cardiovascular disease.[27]

Much of the development of the respiratory system occurs during later fetal development and into infancy. The weight of the lungs triples by 1 year of age. As the size of the lungs continues to grow, the capacity and efficiency of the lungs increase, and respiratory rate decreases. The vital capacity of a 5-year-old is one-fifth that of an adult, but this is not usually a limiting factor during exercise. Overall, aerobic capacity increases during childhood and is slightly higher in males than females. The overall work capacity of children increases most dramatically from 6 to 12 years of age.[28] Peak oxygen consumption is achieved early in adulthood and changes in direct relation to activity levels.

As activity decreases in older adulthood, so do the structural and functional capacities of the cardiovascular and pulmonary systems. Many of these changes are due to decreased elasticity of the tissues, decreased efficiency of the structures, and decreased ability to increase workload. Functional changes include a decrease in the overall maximum heart rate from 200+ bpm through young adulthood to 170 bpm by age 65. Older adults have less elastic vessels, and resistance to blood volume increases. Consequently, older adults reach peak cardiac output at lower levels than younger individuals do. These cardiovascular changes may be compounded by high levels of inactivity, and the result may be decreased capacity to perform activities that raise metabolic demands and increase the requirement for oxygen transport.[29] However, these normal aging responses can be reduced through aerobic activities.

Throughout life, performance of motor activities and ADLs is highly dependent upon the integrity of an individual's cardiopulmonary and cardiovascular systems. Introduction of aerobic activities during early childhood has implications for improved health and wellness across the lifespan. While aging affects the performance and efficiency of the cardiopulmonary and cardiovascular systems, aerobic exercise can improve the capacity and efficiency of the cardiovascular and cardiopulmonary systems. All of these changes in the cardiovascular and pulmonary systems have a significant impact on other systems and, consequently, on overall body function. Information from the cardiovascular and pulmonary systems (eg, BP and oxygen saturation rates) is communicated through the nervous system. The nervous system, in turn, regulates responses of the cardiovascular and pulmonary systems through the autonomic nervous system.

Neurological System

The nervous system is comprised of the central and peripheral nervous systems. The CNS includes the brain and spinal cord and directs all bodily functions. The peripheral nervous system includes both the autonomic and somatic nerves and is responsible for transporting impulses to and from the CNS.

Development begins during the third week of fetal life and continues throughout prenatal development. The most critical period in CNS development is the first year of postnatal life, when the infant's brain develops from one-fourth to one-half the size of the adult brain. Much of the growth during this period is related to increases (1) in the number of glial cells, (2) in myelin in the brain, and (3) in the size of neurons. During this period, the cerebral cortex undergoes rapid growth. These structural changes observed in the brain are directly related to motor behaviors and cognitive development observed during the first few years of life. Growth in the CNS slows after 2 years of age, but it continues into adulthood. As the nervous system matures, the complexity of the gross and fine motor skills and cognitive processes increases. By adolescence, the brain has reached adult size, but myelination and differentiation continue into adulthood.

Decline of the nervous system generally begins after age 30. Decline is noted in the death of thousands of neurons and in decreased weight of the brain. Loss of neurons in the centers controlling sensory information, long-term memory, abstract reasoning, and coordination of sensorimotor information negatively affect function. For some individuals, this may not have significant implications. For others, CNS changes have serious implications. Alterations in the CNS may play a role in postural instability and impaired sensation, and these changes can result in falls.[30]

As with other systems, the CNS has the capacity to compensate for some changes related to aging. Repetition of motor activities may stimulate activation of new growth in dendrites located proximal to neurons previously lost. Activation of new pathways may or may not result in improved functional ability. (See Chapter 3, specifically motor learning and neuroplasticity.)

Implicit in performance of many functional activities is cognition. If changes in cognition coexist with changes in other systems, it may be difficult to accurately interpret the underlying causes.

Cognitive System

The cognitive system uses the five senses (sight, smell, sound, touch, and taste) to process, interpret, store, and retrieve information. *Cognition* is directly related to problem solving and information processing. Often, cognition is not measured directly but rather is inferred.

One of the most important skills that infants learn early in life is to differentiate familiar and unfamiliar people. The infant's ability to act on the environment improves as comprehension of cause-effect improves. Early in development, infants and young children are unable to recognize relevant cues when processing information and cannot chunk information for storage. Consequently, infants and young children may not use or interpret the information as efficiently as older children. An example may be a parent giving instructions to a young child. If the young child is given more than one instruction, he or she may be delayed in processing or may not accurately process the information. Consequently, the child produces an inaccurate response.

During childhood, higher-level cognitive processing skills emerge as the ability to accurately identify relevant cues, filter irrelevant information, and process information faster. Optimal processing occurs throughout adolescence and into middle adulthood.

As an individual grows older, information is processed more slowly, and the time necessary to perform motor skills increases. Additionally, while learning may occur more slowly with age, once a behavior is learned, retention is no different than for a younger individual. While the time necessary to perform the task may increase, older adults are able to execute many tasks without incident. Other motor tasks may be altered because of processing. One example is driving a motor vehicle. Delayed processing in individuals over 70 years of age may significantly delay execution of the task and pose a danger to the driver, passengers, pedestrians, and individuals driving in other vehicles. While driving may be a longstanding activity of an older adult, impaired cognitive and/or motor abilities may make driving a vehicle unsafe. The associated risks of injury to self and others may outweigh the individual's desire to maintain community independence.[31]

Throughout the life span, physical growth and development of many systems affect the acquisition and performance of motor skills. Changes in one system and the interactive effects on all other systems can lead to deleterious changes in motor performance as a whole.

MOTOR DEVELOPMENT

Haywood referred to *motor development* as the gradual process of refining skills and integrating biomechanical principles of movement so that the result is a motor behavior that is consistent and efficient.[7] Efficiency is attained through practice of a behavior to reduce intra-individual variability and improve stability of performance.

Traditional developmental researchers regarded infants as passive beings that were acted upon (stimulated) by external forces in the environment, more often reactive to external stimuli than actively producing purposeful movements. Infants were thought to produce responses that were stereotypic in nature and referred to as primitive and postural reflexes.

Contemporary research refutes the premise that infants are passive beings. Rather, infants are seen as competent beings capable of complex interactive behaviors beginning at birth.[32,33] One example of the infant's ability to produce purposeful interactions at birth is observed when the infant turns his or her head to his or her mother's voice.[34]

Primitive reflexes represent an example of infant behaviors that classify infants as passive beings. These reflexes, now referred to as *innate motor behaviors*, are based on traditional models of CNS organization and motor development theories. More recently, researchers have produced evidence that these behaviors are not solely dependent upon the CNS but are the result of interactions and interdependence of intrinsic and extrinsic factors.[34] One example of an innate motor behavior is sucking. Infants will generally suck if a stimulus is placed strategically in the infant's mouth. However, the stimulus may not produce a similar response if an infant has recently been fed and is satiated. Innate motor behaviors, present at birth, are modifiable and represent functional behaviors observed in very young infants.

The extensive literature on motor development indicates that not all individuals acquire the same motor skills at the same chronological age, nor will every individual exhibit motor behaviors in a fixed sequence of activities.[5,33] Additionally, while most children acquire skills in a somewhat fixed order, the sequence in which motor behaviors emerge may also vary and does not impact functional independence later in life.

Changes in motor performance, measured both qualitatively and quantitatively, are evident throughout life. These changes are not thought to be purely age-dependent, but rather age-related. Practice of skills through repetition improves motor performance. Similarly, decreased frequency in performing activities as an individual ages may be the factor that most contributes to a decline in motor skills. Acquisition of motor skills is multi-factorial, interweaving maturation and experience. Declines in motor skills may be attributable to changes that occur as part of the aging process. Changes in these behaviors do not occur at exactly the same time for any two individuals.

Aging is a process seen in all species on earth, and it varies within and among individuals. This variability is dependent upon intrinsic factors such as maturation of physiological systems and extrinsic factors such as environment. Motor development, seen as changes in motor behaviors, can be recognized across the lifespan (Table 2-1).

Prenatal (0 to 40 Weeks Gestation)

During prenatal development, fetuses have been observed reaching, grasping, thumb sucking, and kicking in utero. These complex behaviors lend evidence to the theory that at birth, infants are competent beings. Postnatally, the extra-uterine environment is quite different for the newborn infant. Behaviors observed in utero, through ultrasound, may not be observed immediately after birth, as the newborn must adapt to this new environment and modify movements given the new forces imposed by gravity. Consequently, the newborn must learn to perform these tasks under different environmental constraints.

Infancy (Birth to 12 Months)

Emergence of motor behaviors is more rapid during the first year of life than at any other time. At birth, the infant is an interactive, competent organism capable of purposeful movements. Brazelton reported that, even at birth, infants turn toward the sound of their mother's voice and visually focus on and track objects 8 to 12 inches from their faces.[32]

During the first 3 months of life, infant motor behaviors focus on acquisition of head control in all planes of movement. Gaining head control enables the infant to visually track people and objects and coordinate eye-hand activities during reaching activities. Manipulative skills acquired during this period include

Table 2-1
Motor Development

Age	Prone	Supine	Sitting	Locomotion	Hand
0 to 1 months	Lifts head. Turns to side.	Head turns side-to-side. Tracks objects. Prefers head to one side.	Head upright 1 to 2 seconds. Slumped in supported sitting.	Makes crawling movements.	Arm movements jerky.
2 to 3 months	Lifts head to 90 degrees. Chest elevated. Weight-bearing on arms. May begin rolling.	Hand to foot play.	Head upright bobs. Head lags in pull to sit. Requires support to sit. Rounded back.	Pivots 30 degrees prone.	Briefly holds toy placed in hand. Hand to mouth. Bats at bright objects. Hands to midline.
4 to 6 months	Reaches in prone. Pushes up onto extended arms.	Begins rolling supine to sidelying.	Propped to independent sitting (Figure 2-2).	Pivots in prone.	Retrieves object within reach. Holds two objects. Holds object with two hands. Brings toy to mouth.
7 to 10 months	Rocks on hands and knees. Moves into sitting.	Lifts head as in sit-up.	Moves from sitting to prone or quadrupled. Rotates in sitting to retrieve object.	Moves forward on belly. Pushes up to hands and knees. Pulls to standing. Briefly stands independently.	Grasp progresses from radial to inferior to lateral pattern. Spontaneously releases objects.
11 to 12 months	Prone to standing (Figure 2-3).		Side-sits.	Walks - one hand held. Stands alone. Moves stand to sit.	Begins to use objects as tools.
13 to 14 months	Moves to standing using half-kneel.			Walks without support. Stoops to retrieve objects, regains standing. Walks backward. Assists with feeding.	Holds two cubes in same hand. Grasps with thumb and first two fingers. Pats pictures in book.
15 to 18 months	Creeps up stairs. Walks up stairs with support.			Carries objects while walking. Walks sideways. Running immature.	Builds three-cube tower. Propels ball. Pokes with finger.
19 to 22 months				Stoops and retrieves objects (Figure 2-4). Ascends stairs with step-to pattern.	Builds five- to six-cube tower.
24 months				Kicks ball. Throws ball forward. Jumps off low step.	
30 months				One foot leads jumping off step. Climbs on tricycle.	Eight-cube tower. Imitates circular and horizontal strokes with crayon.

Table 2-1 (continued)
Motor Development

Age	Prone	Supine	Sitting	Locomotion	Hand
3 to 3.5 years				Propels self on tricycle. Balances one foot momentarily. Arms reciprocate in running. Independent on tricycle activities. Balances one foot >3 sec.	Nine-cube tower. Unbuttons and buttons. Attempts cutting. Dominant hand emerging. Builds bridge with blocks. Strings large beads.
4 to 4.5 years				Hops 2 to 3 times. Walks on tiptoes. Runs with arm swing. Catches large ball. Throws ball 8 to 12 inches. Jumps both feet 2 to 3 inches.	Tripod pencil grasp. Attempts to trace line. Hand preference established. Places raisins in jar. Cuts shapes from paper.
5 to 8 years				Jumps forward and sideways. Jumps over 6- to 8-inch object. Skips, gallops, bounces large ball, and jumps.	Draws letters, shapes, and numbers. Places small pegs in pegboard. Prints well. Buttons small buttons.
9 to 12 years				Mature patterns in running, jumping, and throwing.	Handwriting develops. Learns to draw.

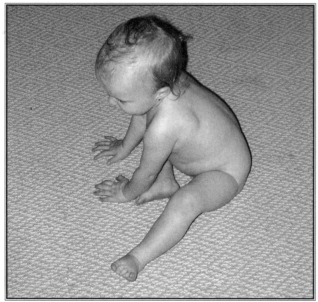

Figure 2-2. Infant in sitting.

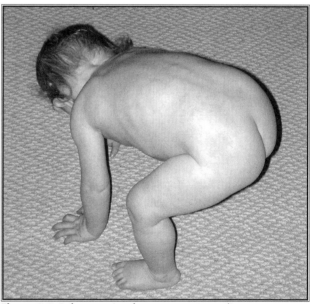

Figure 2-3. Infant moving from prone to standing.

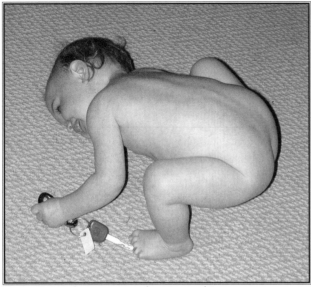

Figure 2-4. Infant stoops and retrieves object.

reaching for objects held 6 to 8 inches away and grasping an object placed in the infant's hand. Initially, both grasping and reaching are inefficient, but with practice, efficiency and accuracy improve.

At 4 to 6 months of age, infants begin to maintain an upright posture during supported sitting and, soon after, begin to prop sit and then sit independently (see Figure 2-2). When in the prone position, infants prop on elbows and are able to roll. These motor behaviors represent the emergence of postural programming integrated with the power and range to maintain gravitational demand during upright holding and movement patterns (see Figure 2-3).

Sitting is an important behavior critical to the performance of most ADLs and a requirement for most occupational and leisure activities. As infants' independent sitting improves, so does their perspective of the world. These motor behaviors not only require postural programming but now integrate balance strategies as well. Manipulative skills that emerge from 4 to 6 months include retrieving objects if placed within reach (see Figure 2-4), holding two objects (one in each hand), using two hands to hold an object (bottle), and holding a toy in one hand while retrieving another toy with the free hand.

By 6 months to 1 year of age, the primary focus is on mobility, as seen in rolling, belly crawling, creeping on all fours, cruising, and independent ambulation. Balance and posture, as part of mobility tasks, incorporates sensory input and motor actions, including visual, vestibular, and somatosensory systems.

Infants use visual input to modulate reaching and grasping in order to accurately retrieve objects as manipulative skills by 8 months of age. By 9 months

of age, an infant can grasp a spoon and bang it on the high chair tray but is not yet able to feed himself with the spoon. These patterns illustrate the development of trunk and axial posture and mobility control but still need to link the fine motor, corticospinal system to accomplish intentional fine-motor activities.

Early Childhood (1 to 5 Years)

At the onset of the second year of life, independent ambulation emerges and the primary focus is dynamic balance in an upright bipedal posture. As infants develop independence in ambulation, they exhibit wide-based gait patterns with little rotation of the pelvis and little reciprocal movement of the upper extremities (UEs). While upright, infants begin to independently move sideways and backward in addition to moving forward. This allows them to maintain their center of gravity (COG) within a given base of support (BOS) as well as lateral hip control. Manipulative skills observed during this period include banging two blocks together, retrieving small objects using a rake, finger-thumb or pincer grasp, and placing objects into a container.

Motor activities that emerge during this period include running, climbing, and jumping. Toddlers find particular pleasure in throwing, kicking, and catching balls. Additionally, toddlers begin to propel themselves on ride-on toys. The focus on this period for toddlers is independence.

Fine motor skills emerging during this period include eating with a utensil (spoon usually), with fewer spills than before. Additionally, infants build small block towers, color with crayons, button large buttons, turn doorknobs, and open and close small jars. These fine motor skills have been integrated in axial and trunk gross motor patterns as well as the cognitive spatial ability and limbic desire to move.

Postural control continues to improve during this period.[35] Preschool age children ambulate using a narrow BOS. They begin to demonstrate a more mature gait pattern, including reciprocal arm swing with a heel-to-toe gait pattern. The child mimics a true run but continues to have difficulty starting and stopping efficiently. In addition, receipt and propulsion of balls of all shapes and sizes improves qualitatively.

Fine motor skills expand significantly during this period, as children begin to cut with scissors, copy circles or crosses, copy a crayon on a circle, match colors, and may demonstrate hand preference. These specific skills reflect innate ability, environmental demands, repetition, and motivation to succeed by the child.

Childhood (5 to 10 Years)

School-age children, 5 to 8 years of age, experience rapid increases in muscle growth that accounts for much of the weight gained during this period. Girls continue to be physically more mature than boys are.

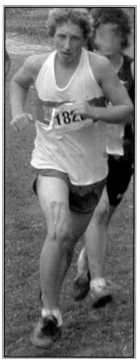

Figure 2-5. Adolescent athlete performing high level motor skills.

Children at this age are extremely flexible predominantly because of the fact that muscle and ligamentous structures are not firmly attached to bones. One must always remember that development of these skills is directly related to practice and demand. A child who skis 6 months out of the year is developing different programs than a child who surfs daily.

Skills that emerge during this period include: galloping, hopping on one foot for up to 10 hops (hopscotch), jumping rope, kicking a ball with improved control (soccer), and bouncing a large ball (basketball). Mobility, balance, and fine-motor skills improve dramatically. Girls and boys exhibit similar abilities in speed up to age 7, but by age 8, boys begin to outperform girls.

Qualitative changes are observed in coordination, balance, speed, and strength while performing previously acquired skills. These qualitative improvements of motor skills may be due to children's limbs growing faster than the trunk. Consequently, they exhibit better leverage. Existing motor skills become more refined, more controlled, more efficient, and more complex.[36] Motor skills have strong influence in social domains, as boys and girls begin to perform in organized sports teams in school and the community. Competition within sports becomes a powerful force in motivating children to practice motor skills or directing children away from organized sports. Children with poorly developed motor skills, due either to genetics or opportunity, may be excluded from team activities and experience social isolation.[36]

Between 5 and 8 years of age, manipulative skills increase exponentially. Hand preference is confirmed by this age. Children acquire and practice many manipulative and fine-motor skills as part of their academic experience. Manipulative skills that improve dramatically include dressing self, particularly buttoning and unbuttoning clothing items; building with blocks; coloring with crayons; and handwriting and printing. As children move towards preadolescence (9 to 12 years of age), manipulative skills improve qualitatively. Children now progress to cursive handwriting and more complex drawings.

Adolescence (11 to 19 Years)

In early adolescence, motor skills are refined and, for most individuals, considered mature. Balance skills, coordination, eye-hand coordination, and endurance may plateau. Exceptions may be elite athletes who continue to improve motor skills into adulthood.

Motor skills continue to develop until 12 years of age. By then, individuals have achieved 90% of mobility and the reaction times of adults. While most motor skills are acquired throughout childhood, proficiency continues into adolescence consistent with musculoskeletal growth, leading to increased strength, endurance, and coordination. Previously acquired skills, like running, jumping, and throwing, progress quantitatively with respect to speed, distance, accuracy, and power. In adolescence, motor performance during competitive sports requires that basic skills are integrated and performed in more dynamic environments (Figure 2-5). During this period, children who may be genetically predisposed to performing high-level motor activities stand apart from their peers, as do children who are less competent in motor abilities. Always remember that practice and motivation to succeed also play a significant role in performance outcome. Similarly, environmental restraints also influence motor behavior. For example, a child who has the genetic predisposition for downhill skiing but lives in a warm climate may never ski and, thus, never actualize that ability.

By adolescence, manipulative skills are complex and resemble skills observed in adults. Greater dexterity of the fingers for more complex tasks including art, sewing, crafts, knitting, and musical performance enables adolescents to perform these motor tasks with greater precision and proficiency.

Adulthood (20 to 39 Years)

Motor performance in adulthood is directed at either leisure activities or high-level athletic competition. Exercise is probably one of the most easily modifiable behaviors affecting an individual's health and wellness. Adults perform various types of exercise to remain physically fit and to decrease the risk of

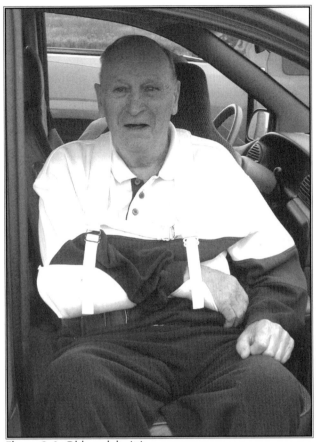

Figure 2-6. Older adult sitting.

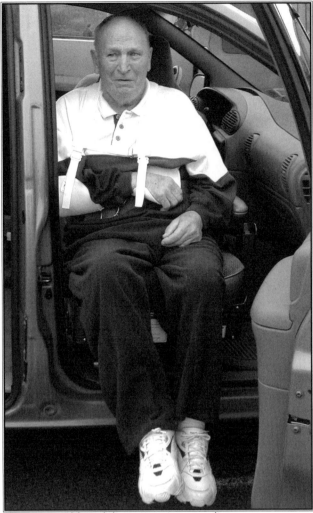

Figure 2-7. Older adult moving sit to standing.

degenerative diseases. For those who do not routinely exercise, obesity and associated syndromes emerge as primary health problems. For the many young adults who integrate fitness training as part of their leisure activities, fitness continues as a way of life.

The peak of muscular strength occurs between 25 and 30 years of age in both males and females. After that period, muscle strength decreases as result of reduction in the number and size of the muscle fibers.[37] Loss is related to genetic factors, nutritional intake, exercise regimen, and daily activities.

Middle Adulthood (40 to 59 Years)

With aging comes changes in the neuromuscular, musculoskeletal, cardiovascular, and pulmonary systems. Changes in these systems greatly affect motor performance, although the degree of the impact is individually specific. Between 30 and 70 years of age, strength loss is thought to be moderate with about 10% to 20% of total strength lost, which is, for most activities, insignificant and undetectable by the individual.[30,37] Mechanisms to counter muscle atrophy and assist in muscle strengthening include exercise regimes that emphasize aerobic and strengthening activities.

Older Adulthood (60+ Years)

Most older adults function reasonably well until an acute illness, a traumatic event such as a fall, or a compounding of small incidents results in an alteration of a motor skill or associated skills[30] (Figures 2-6 and 2-7).

While some effects are age-associated and may be reduced with regular exercise and increased motor activity, not all are modifiable. Timing appears to impact performance of motor skills. As individuals age, they appear less able to modulate timing of muscles during contraction and relaxation phases. The outcome is that motor skills are performed more slowly, and agonist-antagonist movement is more poorly coordinated than earlier in adulthood. Besides being less efficient in movement production, variability in performance of motor skills increases. These age-related changes have serious implications for older adults because these changes put them at increased risk for falls.

Thirty percent of individuals over the age of 65 experience at least one fall each year.[38] Factors thought to be associated with falls include impaired balance, muscle weakness, and medication. The risks associated with falls increase with age and the number of associated risk factors. The most significant intrinsic alterations in the older adult with implications for performance of motor skills occur when functions of the neuromuscular, musculoskeletal, cardiovascular, pulmonary, and sensory systems deteriorate.

Jette et al[39] examined manipulative skills in older adults. They found that changes in hand function associated with muscle weakness and decreased ROM negatively impacted performance of ADLs.

Age-related changes may be attributed to compensations in the neural mechanisms in response to changes between and within the different systems involved in motor skill performance.[40] The integrated effects may include slowing in movement production and increased activation of agonist-antagonist muscle groups. An example of agonist-antagonist activation is during dynamic balance activities.[41] After 70, most individuals are said to incur losses in muscle strength of up to 30% over the next 10 years. Overall, the loss of muscle strength through adulthood may be as much as 40 to 50% by the time an individual reaches 80 years of age.[30] Again, the percentage will correlate with the demand by the individual for repetition of the movements. For example, if the individual continues to play tennis daily, run, play golf, or downhill ski, the percentage of loss may be significantly less.

Promoting Motor Skill Development in a Therapeutic Environment

Motor skills such as *locomotion*, reaching, grasping, and maintaining upright posture allow infants, children, and adults of all ages to acquire, refine, and retain skills to interact in their environment due to continual everyday practice. Before intervening with clients or patients, clinicians must recognize motor behaviors that typically occur from infancy to older adulthood and factors that affect the performance of these behaviors. A comprehensive approach that considers the individual is the optimal strategy for intervention. The best practice integrates the combined perspectives and unique contributions of each professional involved with the patient. Interventions are directed toward motor learning and organized around activities that challenge individuals and motivate them to practice tasks. Activities must be functional and appropriate to age and ability level. Movement and activity should be the emphasis of the program. Practice is critical to acquisition and refinement of motor skills (see Chapter 3). The dilemma associated with this fact is

that with practice comes repetition and boredom and this may lead to decreased motivation. It is critical to vary tasks by frequently altering the environmental context to keep a child's or an adult's interest while practicing and refining a task. The PT should suggest strategies to the PTA that will incorporate the target motor skills into the patient's daily life. Both the PT and PTA should encourage physical fitness as a lifelong activity to promote health and wellness of the body and spirit. During each treatment session, the PTA should seek feedback from the patient (verbal, visual, and/or kinesthetic) and modify his or her feedback to the patient or client according to the responses of the patient.

Initially, the professional provides feedback to the individual about results and performance. The goal is for the individual to develop the ability to detect and correct errors in movement without the clinician present. Visual feedback in the form of mirrors and videotape provide information about motor performance. Auditory feedback may be provided through verbal feedback or auditory switches. The PT may guide the PTA according to the specific perceptual skills and disabilities of the patient or client.

Play as Therapy

Children perceive play time as an opportunity to engage in an enjoyable activity of their own choosing without any specific goal. Adults perceive play as a child-directed activity used to achieve a desired outcome. Both children and adults use play as a social context to promote acquisition of motor skills. As infants and children grow older, techniques for utilizing play must be modified consistently with the child's cognitive and motor skill performance and social skills. Adults must be careful not to direct play specific to a child's particular sex. Examples of play directed at a child of a particular sex include playing house only with females and truck games only with boys. While some genetic differences exist in play preferences between males and females, gender-neutral activities should be encouraged during play sessions whether play has been delegated to the PTA or the family. All sessions should be directed to the developmental ability and interest of the child with activities that motivate the child to practice motor skills by varying the task and the environment. In this way, the child remains motivated and dedicated to accomplishing new motor skills. Play positively reinforces development of motor skills in a non-competitive environment. Adults are generally working on ADL skills. Allowing choice, self-motivation, and error correction within the activity will lead to better ADL skills.

CONCLUSION

Development of motor skills occurs out of a need to solve specific motor problems in the environment. Effective practitioners work cooperatively with patients or clients to identify the motor problems and develop strategies that solve the problems and promote functional interaction in the environment. While genetic and environmental factors play a role in acquisition of motor skills, the relative importance of these factors changes across the lifespan. During early acquisition of motor behaviors, genetics has a greater role. Later in life, environmental factors are stronger.

Systems theory provides a model for why individuals exhibit motor skills at different biological ages and why the quality of motor behavior varies.[42] It is the PT's responsibility to examine the influence of sensory, musculoskeletal, neuromuscular, vestibular, and cognitive systems on motor development in order to provide an understanding of how different systems exert influence at different points in development. Delegation of specific interventions is certainly within the role of the PTA. The human organism is complex and is comprised of interactive and interdependent systems. The underlying theoretical constructs of systems theory may more fully explain development than traditional theories. Human systems do not function unidirectionally but collaboratively across the lifespan. Just as not all individuals exhibit motor behaviors such as sitting, creeping, or walking at the same time, not all individuals lose their ability to perform certain tasks (eg, driving a car or independently performing personal care) at the same biological, chronological, or even psychological age.

No one theory explains the development of complex motor behaviors completely, and none encompass the essence of inter- and intra-individual variability in aging. Aspects of theories provide evidence that an integrative perspective may be a more accurate reflection of aging. Lifestyle choices, including diets, physical activity, and other health habits, and behavioral and social factors have potent effects on aging processes.

An integrated approach to intervention addresses the complex nature of motor behaviors observed throughout life. All systems discussed here play significant roles in the acquisition, refinement, and retention of motor behaviors. Careful consideration of each system individually and the interactive effects among systems is important to understanding motor behaviors. Remember, if a child, adult, or elderly individual repetitively practices a stereotypic movement limited in function, that will become the program used by the individual. Thus, intervention can both limit and expand the functional skill of the patient or client.

CHAPTER QUESTIONS

1. Explain why an exercise program would be different for a child than for an adult.

2. Explain the role of cognition in motor development.

3. Explain how older adults may differ from younger adults in musculoskeletal parameter.

4. Discuss how balance training would differ for a young child not yet walking and an older adult with a history of falls.

5. Identify cardiopulmonary changes with normal aging. Discuss how these cardiopulmonary changes affect intervention.

Suggested author answers are available at www.slackbooks.com/neuroquestions.

REFERENCES

1. Short-DeGraf M. *Human Development*. New York, NY: John Wiley; 1988.

2. Gesell A. *The First Five Years of Life*. New York, NY: Harper and Brothers Publishers; 1940.

3. McGraw MB. *Neuromuscular Maturation of the Human Infant*. 2nd ed. New York, NY: Hafner; 1943.

4. Singer RN. The readiness to learn skills necessary for participation in sport. In: Magill RA, Ash MJ, Smoll FL, eds. *Children in Sport: A Contemporary Anthology*. Champaign, Ill: Human Kinetics; 1978.

5. Smith LB, Thelan E. *A Dynamic Systems Approach to Development*. Cambridge, Mass: MIT Press; 1993.

6. Gibson JJ. *The Ecological Approach to Visual Perception*. Boston, Mass: Houghton Mifflin; 1979.

7. Haywood KM. *Lifespan Motor Development*. Champaign, Ill: Human Kinetics; 1986.

8. Heriza CB. Motor development: traditional and contemporary theories. In: MJ Lister, ed. *Contemporary Management of Motor Control Problems*. Alexandria, Va: Foundation for Physical Therapy; 1991.

9. Thelan E. Developmental origins of motor coordination: leg movements in human infants. *Dev Psychobiol*. 1985;18:1-22.

10. Zelazo PR, Weiss MJ, Leonard EL. The development of unaided walking: the acquisition of higher order control. In: Zelazo PR, Barr R, eds. *Challenges to Developmental Paradigms: Implications for Theory Assessment*. Hillsdale, NJ: Erlbaum Associates Incorporated; 1976.

11. Bradley, NS. Animal models offer the opportunity to acquire a new perspective on motor development. *Phys Ther*. 1990;70:776-787.

12. Thelan E. The role of motor development in developmental psychology: a view of the past and an agenda for the future. In: Lockman J, Hazen N, eds. *Action in Social Context: Perspectives in Early Development.* New York, NY: Plenum; 1990.

13. Thelan E. The (re) discovery of motor development: learning new things from an old field. *Dev Psych.* 1989;25:946-949.

14. Scott JP. Critical periods in organizational processes. In: Faulkner F, Tanner JM, eds. *Human Growth.* New York, NY: Plenum Press; 1986:181-196.

15. Chodzko-Zajko WJ. Biological theories of aging: implications for functional performance. In: Bonder BR, Wagner MB, eds. *Functional Performance in Older Adults.* 2nd ed. Philadelphia, Pa: FA Davis; 2001:28-41.

16. Karasik D, Hannan MT, Cupples AL, Feslon DT, Kiel DP. Genetic contributions to biological aging: the Framingham study. *J Gerontol: Series A: Biological Sciences and Medical Sciences.* 2004;59A:218-226.

17. Goldstein S, Gallo JJ, Reichel W. Biologic theories of aging. *Am Fam Physician.* 1989;40:195-200.

18. Rowe JW, Kahn RL. Successful aging. *T Gerontol.* 1997;37:433-450.

19. Sadler TW. *Langeman's Medical Embryology.* Baltimore: Williams and Wilkins; 1984.

20. Ashburn SS. Biophysical development during infancy. In: Schuster CS, Ashburn SS. *The Process of Human Development: A Holistic Life-span Approach.* Philadelphia, Pa: Lippincott; 1992:118-140.

21. Lieber RL. *Skeletal Muscle Structure, Function, and Plasticity: The Physiological Basis of Rehabilitation.* Philadelphia, Pa: Lippincott, Williams and Wilkins; 2002.

22. Thompson LV. Physiological changes associated with aging. In: Guccione AA, ed. *Geriatric Physical Therapy.* 2nd ed. St Louis, Mo: Mosby; 2000:28-55.

23. Wilder PA. Muscle development and function. In: Cech D, Martin S, eds. *Functional Movement Development Across the Lifespan.* Philadelphia, Pa: Saunders; 1995:137-157.

24. Sullivan JA. Introduction to the musculoskeletal system. In: Sullivan JA, Anderson SJ, eds. *Care of the Young Athlete.* American Academy of Orthopedic Surgeons and American Academy of Pediatrics; 2000:242-258.

25. Dutton M. *Orthopedic Examination, Evaluation, and, Intervention.* New York, NY: McGraw-Hill; 2004.

26. Lewis CB, Kellems S. Musculoskeletal changes with age: clinical implications. In: Lewis CB, ed. *Aging The Health-Care Challenge.* 4th ed. Philadelphia, Pa: FA Davis; 2002:104-126.

27. Overbay JD, Purath J. Self-concept and health status in elementary-school-aged children. *Issues in Comprehensive Nursing.* 1997;20:89-101.

28. Stout J. Physical fitness during childhood and adolescence. In: Campbell S, ed. *Physical Therapy for Children.* 2nd ed. Philadelphia, Pa: Saunders; 2000:141-169.

29. Dean E. Cardiopulmonary development. In: Bonder BR, Wagner MB, eds. *Functional Performance in Older Adults.* 2nd ed. Philadelphia, Pa: FA Davis; 2001:86-120.

30. Wagner MB, Kaufman TL. Mobility. In: Bonder BR, Wagner MB, eds. *Functional Performance in Older Adults.* 2nd ed. Philadelphia, Pa: FA Davis; 2001:61-85.

31. Ekelman BA, Mitchell S, O'Dell-Rossi P. Driving and older adults. In: Bonder BR, Wagner MB, eds. *Functional Performance in Older Adults.* 2nd ed. Philadelphia, Pa: FA Davis; 2001:448-477.

32. Brazelton TB. *Neonatal Behavioral Assessment Scale.* London, England: Blackwell Scientific Publications, Ltd; 1984.

33. VanSant AF. Motor control, motor learning and motor development. In: Montgomery PC, Connolly BH, eds. *Clinical Applications for Motor Control.* Thorofare, NJ: Slack Incorporated; 2003:26-50.

34. Montgomery P, Connolly B. *Clinical Applications for Motor Control.* Thorofare, NJ: SLACK Incorporated; 2003.

35. Shumway-Cook A, Woollacott MH. *Motor Control: Theory and Practical Applications.* Philadelphia, Pa: Lippincott, Williams, and Wilkins; 2001.

36. Owens KB. *Child and Adolescent Development: An Integrated Approach.* Belmont, Calif: Wadsworth; 2002.

37. Ashburn SS. Biophysical development during early adulthood. In: Schuster CS, Ashburn SS. *The Process of Human Development: A Holistic Life-span Approach.* Philadelphia, Pa: Lippincott; 1992:556-577.

38. Tinnetti ME, Baker DI, McAvay G, et al. A multifactorial intervention to reduce the risk of falling among elderly people living in the community. *N Engl J Med.* 1994;331:821-827.

39. Jette AM, Branch LG, Berlin J. Musculoskeletal impairments and physical disablement among the aged. *J Gerontol.* 1990;45:M203.

40. Patten C, Craik RL. Sensorimotor changes and adaptation in the older adult. In: Guiccone AA, ed. *Geriatric Physical Therapy.* 2nd ed. St Louis, Mo: Mosby; 2000:78-109.

41. Benjuva N, Melzer I, Kaplanski J. Aging-induced shifts from a reliance on sensory input to muscle cocontraction during balanced standing. *J Gerontol. Series A: Biological Sciences and Medical Sciences.* 2004;59A:166-171.

42. Adolph KE. Babies' steps make giant strides toward a science of development. *J Infant Beh and Dev.* 2002;25:86-90.

Chapter
3

MOTOR LEARNING, MOTOR CONTROL, AND NEUROPLASTICITY

Darcy Umphred, PT, PhD, FAPTA

KEY WORDS

extrinsic feedback
intrinsic feedback
motor learning
motor control
neuromechanisms
neuroplasticity
practice context
practice schedule
stages of motor learning

CHAPTER OBJECTIVES

- Identify the differences among motor learning, motor control, and neuroplasticity.

- Differentiate between context practice and practice schedule.

- Discuss the stages of motor learning and the relationships those stages have to the need for practice and the degree of external feedback.

- Discuss the differences between external and internal feedback, and identify which feedback schedule is appropriate for a patient's stage of motor learning.

- Conceptually differentiate between a cognitively run movement and an automatic/feedforward motor program controlled by the CNS.

- Discuss the difference between new motor learning, as seen in a child, and relearning of movement patterns, as seen in a patient with CNS dysfunction.

INTRODUCTION

Motor learning, motor control, and *neuroplasticity* are three areas of interest to the PT and PTA when working with patients of various ages diagnosed with disease or trauma to the CNS. New advances in research in the areas of neurophysiology, theories of motor learning and control, and adaptation of the nervous system following injury (neuroplasticity) are directing evaluations and interventions employed by PTs and, thus, interventions delegated to the PTA. Although the specific rationale for each component of an intervention design is the responsibility of the PT, a general understanding of the theory within these three areas and their relationship to treatment practice enhances the PTA's knowledge and the rationale for why specific interventions for a particular patient may or may not be delegated. Similarly, explanations can be identified that explain why certain practice environments need to be the responsibility of a caregiver or family member. Table 3-1 identifies the differences among these three conceptual areas of CNS function as well as the time

Table 3-1

Differentiation Among Motor Control, Motor Learning, and Neuroplasticity

	Control Function	Neuromechanism
Motor Control	Using existing synaptic connections and existing programming.	*Neurotransmitters:* 10th to 100th of milliseconds to respond. *Neuropeptides:* hours or days for transmission to synapse; response can be hours, days, months, or lifetimes.
Motor Learning	Modification of existing motor programs and synaptic firing patterns.	Repetition of practice of new motor format takes months, days, or weeks and needs continual practice.
Neuroplasticity	Modification of surviving cellular structure to reform primary function, assume a different function, and regain control of sensory processing and motor programming.	Based on environmental demands placed upon the organism and potential for the organism for neuroplasticity. Repetition of practice takes weeks, months, or years and continual environmental demand.

parameters needed for the CNS to control, learn, and adapt to the motor requirements of the environment.

Theories within the areas of motor learning, motor control, and neuroplasticity will be introduced in this chapter. For theories of development and how they affect stages of learning, see Chapter 2. Before discussing how theories might guide intervention decisions, a clear definition of each topic and the specific role it plays in functional movement will be introduced. Once each topic has been discussed, the interaction of these theories will be presented through case examples as possible explanations for selected treatment sequences and required intervention changes. For specific intervention techniques appropriately delegated to the PTA, refer to Chapter 5. The goal of this chapter is discussion of theory and its application to the practice of physical therapy.

The roles of the PT and PTA are directly linked to functional movement limitations. Those limitations can be linked to disease, pathology, trauma, or pre-existing life experiences that affect a specific system and to interactions among the functions of the cardiopulmonary, integumentary, musculoskeletal, and neuromuscular systems. Regardless of the specific system involvement, the individual's ability to learn new movement options (motor learning), control that movement in functional activities (motor control), and regain motor function following direct or indirect CNS insult (neuroplasticity) is regulated by the existing potential of an individual and by the environment created for learning. Although this chapter will focus upon individuals who have identified CNS problems, PTs and PTAs need to remember that the theories presented within this chapter relate to motor output and functional limitations despite what the identified medical problems or diseases may be.

This chapter's organizational structure begins with a historical perspective and then proceeds to motor learning, motor control, and neuroplasticity. This order was selected to help the reader understand how treatment philosophies have evolved and to emphasize theory in the order consistent with CNS processing. Learning a behavioral sequence or motor program must occur before the individual's ability to control that motor pattern or behavior. Some motor learning occurs in utero and is often called reflexive or preexisting motor programs. In a 6-month gestational-aged infant born premature, the heart muscle and most autonomic smooth muscle control has already been established; however, the skeletal muscle tone characteristics observed will be flaccid with no muscle control evident. These types of observations help therapists understand that motor learning occurs very early in the development of a fetus. Motor learning will continue throughout life as long as the environment asks for change and the CNS has the pliability and desire to so.

HISTORICAL PERSPECTIVES

Regaining movement function through therapeutic exercise has been a central theme for the field of physical therapy since the profession's beginning. The decision of how best to regain or learn motor skill in various functional activities has always been based on the best science theory of the time. In the first half of the 20th century, exercises were based on theories of reinforcement, existing muscle physiology, and practice schedules related to maximal and submaximal strength of existing muscles. In the mid-20th century, treatment techniques in the area of neurorehabilitation began to be explained using theories of neurophysiology, neuroanatomy, and childhood development. The accepted neurophysiology was based on research done by the physiologist Sherrington.[1] His understanding of the nervous system was based on the responses of animals under anesthesia, the accepted research neuromechanisms protocol, and observed movement development of children. The theory was based on the assumption that functional movement was under a rigid hierarchical control within the nervous system. It was during this era that treatment approaches, such as proprioceptive neuromuscular facilitation[2] (PNF), Bobath,[3] Rood,[4] Ayers,[5] Johnstone,[6] and Brunnstrom,[7] were developed. The therapists that developed these various approaches had one thing in common. They all tried to use theories regarding how the nervous system was regulated. They were very keen observers of movement, normal and abnormal. Although the basic science knowledge of the time had errors and the theory needed to change, due to the evolution in understanding of motor control, motor learning, and neuroplasticity, the movements observed by therapists during that time are the same movements observed by therapists today. Theories will change as new research opens new avenues of science analysis, but keen visual observations of functional movements and limitations will always remain a critical skill for the PT and PTA. Many of the previously mentioned approaches are still used and retain similar treatment applications and interventions; however, the treatment rationale for each of the various approaches utilizes more current research and basic science to explain its validity. In the 1970s and 1980s, some therapists[8,9] were teaching integrated approaches based on a systems model and functional training versus a more traditional Sherringtonian/Hierarchichal sequential model. Once physiologists and neuroanatomists began to analyze movement while the animals were awake, they realized that the Sherrington model was not as accurate as Bernstein's model[10,11] presented decades before. Since the later part of the 20th century, therapists have known and/or taught a systems versus a hierarchical model for CNS control and learning. Only within the last 10 years has the concept of neuroplasticity evolved and begun to take part in decision-making regarding patient interventions following CNS injury.

MOTOR LEARNING

Motor learning is the study of how individuals acquire, modify, and retain motor memory patterns so that programs can be used, reused, and modified during functional activities. Examples of these functional motor memory patterns include rolling, head control in all planes of movement, coming to stand, toilet training, feeding, walking, running, skiing, mountain climbing, spelunking, playing group sports, or any other combination of simple to complex motor behaviors synthesized to allow for success at the motor task.

Principles of motor learning can be summarized as "(1) Learning is a process of acquiring the capability for skilled action; (2) learning results from experience or practice; (3) learning cannot be measured directly – instead, it is inferred based on behavior; and (4) learning produces relatively permanent changes in behavior, thus short-term alterations are not thought of as motor learning."[12] Motor learning is a complex process reflecting the nervous system's response to a task-specific activity that emerges from an interaction between the need to perform the task and the environment within which the task is being performed.[13,14,15] The difference between a short-term change in behavior and motor learning can be demonstrated when a PTA is working with a patient on rolling from supine to sidelying. At the beginning of the treatment session, the patient may need both verbal and physical assistance to complete the task, yet, by the end of the session, is able to roll independently. The next day, the patient may not roll independently from supine to sidelying even with verbal cueing but is more quickly able to roll without assistance. This is an example of a short-term alteration, where permanent motor learning has not occurred. When the patient is consistently capable of rolling independently over time (a relatively permanent change in behavior), motor learning has occurred.

A variety of components affect motor learning. Thus, how movement is expressed is a synopsis of the interaction of all the components. The context within which a motor program is practiced, the schedule of practice, the stage of motor learning of the behavior, how feedback is applied, and the type of feedback applied are the major components of motor learning. Each are discussed separately.

Practice Context

Practice context refers to the way a therapist chooses to teach the motor activity. There are four context categories: whole learning, pure-part learning, progressive/sequential-part learning, and whole to part to whole learning.

Whole Learning

Whole learning refers to practicing a behavior or task in its entirety. Simple and discrete motor tasks, such as rolling over in bed, sit to stand, or scratching one's head, generally require whole learning. Asking an individual to stand up from a chair is a whole program. Asking that same individual to scoot forward, place both feet 6 inches apart, shift weight over the feet, and then stand up requires four steps or components. Therefore, asking an individual to stand up requires one program that incorporates all the components but is practiced as a whole activity. When a specific impairment such as strength, range, or balance is identified, a PT may ask a PTA to treat the impairment or impairment train (ie, strengthening, ranging, balance training under specific environments, practicing specific synergist movement parts, etc), but then the activity must be practiced as a whole program for motor learning to occur. To assume that strengthening of a muscle will automatically lead an individual to be able to perform a function skill, such as standing up from a chair, can be neither substantiated in the literature nor observed in clients.

Pure-Part Learning

Pure-part learning is used for complex activities where the component parts are discrete motor programs in and of themselves. When learning a tennis serve, an individual needs to learn (1) how to throw the ball into the air vertically with a specific height expected and using the nondominant arm, and (2) how to traject the dominant arm while holding the racket in order for the face of the racket to hit the ball overhead with a specific angle and force of the racket. It does not matter whether the individual is taught first how to throw and second how to traject the racket. Ultimately, both need to be learned and then practiced together as a whole activity. Though it is not critical which part is taught first, they must come together in order for motor learning to occur. As a clinical example, a PT asks a PTA to teach an individual to stand up from and sit down onto a chair. The first part of the activity, to attain and stop at the vertical upright standing pattern, requires the strength, range, postural control, and balance needed to shift one's weight over one's feet; concentrical contact from sit to stand using posture, balance, and movement pattern; and knowledge of where vertical is in space. The second discrete part

of this motor program requires going from stand to sit. Eccentric control over the same patterns is required; thus, the two movements are unique in their programming. At times, a PTA may be asked to place a patient in standing and practice one-quarter of both parts of the pattern (ie, sit down a little and then rise to stand with control). The PT may instruct the PTA to have the patient practice one-quarter of both patterns (two unique programs) and then slowly increase the range of the activity. The ultimate goal is to have the patient practice the whole program once both parts are learned. This is an example of pure-part learning even though only one-quarter of both patterns are initially practiced. The decision to start in standing should be determined by the PT. There are many reasons a PT might have for beginning in standing. Nevertheless, if not stated specifically, the PTA should ask the PT before beginning intervention. Starting in sit or in standing will lead to independence of the patient in the sit to stand to sit program as a whole, but one way may be easier for the patient to learn and, thus, reduce intervention time.

Progressive/Sequential-Part Learning

Progressive/sequential-part learning is employed when teaching intermediate skills and serial tasks that require many steps that must be performed in a specific sequence in order to be considered successful. When practiced, the learning always begins with the same initial step and follows in sequence with additional steps. Line dancing is an example of a sequential part task. If the components of the dance are taught to individuals as unique parts, different groups of people will put those parts together in different sequences, thus creating chaos on the dance floor. In a therapeutic environment, a PTA may be asked to teach a patient how to stand up from a wheelchair (w/c). This task consists of three activities: lock the brake on the w/c, pick up the foot pedal, and then come to stand. Although these three activities are separate parts of the whole, teaching the patient to perform them in a specific sequence or order will help the patient to not only learn the activity but also the sequential series within which it should be performed. This is especially true when patients have specific types of perceptual impairment. Thus, if not instructed, again the PTA should ask the PT whether this type of motor learning is appropriate for a specific patient. Every PT and PTA has or will have a patient that stands up and then tries to either lock the brake or pick up the foot pedals. Often, the result is the practitioner writing up an incident report because the patient falls.

Whole to Part to Whole Learning

Whole to part to whole learning is the most frequently used in the clinical environment. An individual is first asked to perform the whole task; the clinician then breaks down the task into separate components and reconstitutes the entire program. The purpose is to have the patient execute the whole task so that the PT can complete a task analysis. In a task analysis, the PT needs to recognize what parts of the task are missing, what components of the movement are functioning, and what parts function intermittently and in limited ranges or positions in space. From this analysis, a PT should be able to direct the PTA regarding what components need to be practiced, when or in what sequence, and a given improvement indicating when the PTA should again begin practicing the whole task. This type of practice generally incorporates impairment training, which needs to then be incorporated into the program as a whole.

If a PTA is not sure whether the task should be taught through whole, pure-part, sequential-parts, or whole to part to whole learning, then asking the PT would be very appropriate prior to beginning the intervention. If the PT has not learned to incorporate this type of analysis into the clinical decision-making in his or her verbal explanation, then the PTA can help the PT with the verbal explanations given in this chapter. Many clinicians, whether they are PTs or PTAs, make decisions based on experience or gut-level feeling. *Efficacy of practice* has become an accepted term, and both clinicians need to be able to verbalize what they are doing using terminology that is considered standard of practice for that level of clinician.

Practice Schedule

This motor learning component refers to the frequency at which the patient practices the task. There are three categories of *practice schedule*: mass, variable, and random practice.

Mass Practice

Mass practice is used to learn or relearn a skill that is essential for ADLs. Regardless of how simple or complex the functional task, initially the individual needs to mass practice the whole task. Thus, if parts of the task need to be learned as discrete components, they can be taught using pure-part, sequential-part, or whole to part to whole learning. However, to achieve motor learning, the entire pattern/motor program must be practiced frequently enough for the CNS to learn the pattern as a whole. A PT may delegate any components of the whole task or the whole activity itself, but in order for the learner to initially retain the learning mass, practice is essential. In an inpatient rehabilitation level of care, a patient comes to the PT clinic once, twice, or three times a day to practice the functional skills within a mass-practice clinical environment. A PT will need to determine the skill level by which the patient is performing in order to determine if it is appropriate to delegate the intervention to a PTA. If the only way a patient can perform a task is with constant correction of error and constant manual contact, then delegation of the task to a PTA is inappropriate. If, on the other hand, the patient needs to either practice with guidance in order to stay within the motor program or needs to work on specific components or impairments, delegation to a PTA is very appropriate.

Mass practice, from a practical perspective, is the opportunity for the patient to repetitively practice a motor pattern or functional movement with few interruptions; this helps limit distractions that can hinder the CNS from remembering the program being taught. Normal motor development, as discussed in Chapter 2, is an excellent illustration of the role of mass practice in a child's development of functional movement. For example, a child may try to succeed at a movement task such as rolling over. Once the child experiences success, the child will practice this activity repeatedly. The parents may become very frustrated because the child may roll off a bed or will try to roll when being bathed or having a diaper changed. The child's CNS knows that, in order to learn that motor program, this type of practice is critical. Once the motor program is established within the CNS, the individual will no longer need to mass practice unless the external environment changes. For example, if an individual learns through mass practice to walk on a hard, flat surface, that person should be able to automatically use that program within that environment. If the person now wishes to walk on grass, or up or down a hill, the environment for walking has changed, and mass practice will again be necessary in order to learn the variations of walking as an automatic adaptation. As an individual begins to automatically run motor or movement programs during daily activities, the amount of practice needed is reduced. Similarly, the number of tasks the CNS might be asked to do, whether motor or cognitive, should increase between practicing the specific functional movements. Motor learning requires mass practice, but the PT must realize that if the individual stops performing a task, learning can deteriorate. Thus, following inpatient rehabilitation, a patient is often scheduled for outpatient rehabilitation, which may be daily, three times a week, etc. This second type of practice schedule is termed intermittent/scheduled practice.

Intermittent/Scheduled Practice

Intermittent/scheduled practice is used when the program is available to the patient's CNS, but impairment errors occur and practice is still needed to insure long-term motor memory. This type of practice is generally used in outpatient rehabilitation, private practice, and home health visitation. PTA's are often employed in all three environments, and thus, delegation to the PTA of specific impairment training and practice of specific functional tasks is very appropriate. The specific frequency of intervention and practice identified by the PT should correlate with the needs of the patient and proceed from more frequent to less frequent as the patient progresses with independence. Unfortunately, the number of visits a patient receives in this setting is often limited by insurance policies, the availability of clinics, and the availability of therapists. These limitations may not be to the advantage of the patient but are a reality of health care delivery today. Even when practicing a large number of activities, with too limited time to truly embed the learning of any motor program, the patient does not generally gain long-term independence. Greater independence for the patient is achieved by selecting and practicing programs critical to independence as well as programs or activities that the patient is highly motivated to practice. The decision about what to practice should be made by the PT; the practice itself certainly can be delegated to the PTA. There may be certain functional activities that the patient is mass practicing while others are on a distributed practice schedule.

Random Practice

Random practice refers to practice done independently without a scheduled frequency of practice. Random practice is, ultimately, the responsibility of the patient and/or caregiver. Once the patient can practice independently or with stand-by assistance, the activity must become part of one's daily-living life skill. Generally, neither the PT nor the PTA must be present during random practice; however, follow-up visits may be indicated to insure that practice has been incorporated into the patient's lifestyle. The arrangement of a daily-living random practice schedule or home program is the PT's responsibility, but the PTA may be given the responsibility of monitoring these. As an example, a patient may independently come out of the chair and walk to the bathroom or kitchen. Simultaneously, due to a medical condition, he must drink a glass of water hourly. If the patient is told that he needs to get up and go to the kitchen or bathroom for a glass of water every hour, he will automatically practice sit to stand, stand to sit, as well as walking a certain distance. The patient is empowered to the responsibility of drinking the water, but the whole activity incorporates functional movements that are practiced automatically as part of the daily routine.

Stages of Motor Learning

There are three *stages of motor learning*. Remember that a complex motor activity may consist of a variety of motor programs. Following injury to the brain, the memory of each program may need to be evaluated by the PT. It is the PT's decision to run certain aspects of an entire program. Delegation of that activity can be given to the PTA. For example, an individual who has suffered a traumatic brain injury (TBI) may need to relearn specific components of a task. The PT may ask the PTA to bring the patient to standing using the right LE. If both legs were used, then the left leg might go into a strong extensor pattern, such as hip extension and adduction, knee extension and ankle inversion, and plantar-flexion. Thus, the right leg is ready to stand, but the left is not. The PTA may be instructed to bring the patient to stand, then bend the left LE at the knee, and place the left knee on a stool. In this way, the right leg can practice all components of standing and the left leg can still practice postural control of the hip without going into a strong extensor pattern. While delegation to the PTA is appropriate, the PT should make the decision regarding the best treatment intervention.

Stage 1:
Cognitive Stage/Acquisition of a Motor Skill

Stage 1 is the phase when the patient is learning a new skill or relearning an old one as a whole activity. At this stage, an individual needs to practice often and needs a lot of external feedback from the practitioner in order to be successful. However, allowing the patient to practice and self-correct is important during this initial stage. For example, if a patient is coming to stand and shifts his or her weight to the lateral aspect of the foot, then there is a greater likelihood of falling; however, if he or she self-corrects, then the boundaries of the activity are being practiced and learned. Giving the patient time to self-correct before providing the external feedback is important. The patient, when instructed to stand up, needs to make those errors in order to move to the second stage of motor learning. Practicing a program with error means practicing within the instructed task. If a PT asks a patient (Mr. X) to stand, and as Mr. X executes the task, he starts to fall, then he is no longer in the coming to stand pattern. He is then practicing falling! In this example, Mr. X is not self-correcting the error and is not learning how to come to stand.

There are many ways to encourage an individual to stay within the pattern, and the PT should instruct the PTA in specifics, if necessary. Teaching the patient to respond to inherent/intrinsic feedback from within his or her body is a critical component of this stage of learning. When in the acquisition stage of motor learning, the environment used for practice should be consistent, and the type of practice is generally mass practice. Once a patient begins to automatically respond to the demands of the external environment by the use of an appropriate motor program (eg, automatically stepping when the weight of the body is forward enough on the foot to trigger a stepping reaction), the program itself often runs as a feed-forward pattern. This feed-forward pattern means that the individual no longer needs feedback for the CNS to know that walking is the appropriate response. As an example, the feed-forward mechanism is similar to that of a DVD player. Once the equipment is told to run the movie, the player will continue running the movie until it is told to stop. Likewise, the motor system, due either to the external environment or internal environment of the individual (motivation, cognitive decision, etc), is told to walk. That motor system will continue to walk the musculoskeletal system until some aspect of the CNS changes that decision. Feedback to the CNS is often the critical component of the CNS's decision to change a program. Thus, as a PTA begins to understand the stages of motor learning, consideration of feedback variables will need to be incorporated into these appropriate stages.

Stage 2:
Associative Stage/Refinement

Stage 2 is the stage when a patient can run the program within specific environmental constraints, will have a decrease in error during the activity, and will apply less effort during performance. Generally, the environment used during performance is consistent, although variance in the specific components is present. For example, if Mrs. Y is able to sit on a hard surface as long as she does not reach and perturb herself more than 20 degrees, then she has learned the program but is limited in range, power, and/or balance when perturbed beyond her range. She is in the refinement phase. A PT may delegate an activity of reaching for objects in space slightly beyond the 20-degree mark. The PTA should be instructed in retaining the same environment (eg, a hard surface) while allowing the patient to refine the movement and self-correct. At this stage, a patient is enlarging control within a specific environment.

Stage 3:
Autonomous Stage/Retention

Stage 3 is the stage when the patient moves to a variety of different environments and retains control of the whole program. The PT should instruct the PTA regarding changes in programming. Continuing the previous example, once the PT determines that the patient has learned the sitting program on a hard surface, the PTA may be asked to move to a compliant surface, such as a ball. The true hallmark of learning is the ability to retain the skill and transfer the skill into different settings. At this time, practice is usually random and part of everyday life.

Feedback

There are two types of feedback: intrinsic and extrinsic. Feedback is dependent upon sensory input. When patients have sensory loss, often feedback mechanisms are lost or inconsistent, and compensation through alternative sensory systems is indicated.[16-18]

Intrinsic Feedback

Intrinsic feedback is based upon sensory responses inherent to the patient's body as part of the desired movement itself. For example, the muscles and joints tell the CNS where the trunk and limbs are in space and which limbs are in an open or closed chain. The vestibular system within the inner ear tells the CNS where the head is in space. Both sensory mechanisms are inherent and the primary input for refinement and retention of postural and movement programs. The PT should determine whether there is conflict or loss in inherent feedback. If deficits exist, the PT should delegate the specific activities that either allow the patient to regain accurate sensory awareness during the activity or substitute another sensory system. Lack of appropriate intrinsic feedback or compensatory input systems will lead to error that is not corrected and, thus, failure in obtaining functional independence. Fortunately, motor learning can often be obtained through neuroplasticity, even with severe sensory deficits. This topic will be discussed later.

Extrinsic Feedback

Extrinsic feedback is based upon an outside source providing feedback. Biofeedback, the auditory feedback from a therapist's voice, use of a mirror, and proprioceptive input feedback that the therapist uses during handling techniques are a few of the many extrinsic feedback mechanisms used by PTs and PTAs. This type of feedback can lead to better performance during a motor activity, but until the patient self-corrects using inherent feedback, independence is not obtained. There are two types of extrinsic feedback.[19] Knowledge of performance (KP) feedback uses a sensory system (eg, the therapist's voice) to inform the patient as to whether the quality or efficiency of the movement pattern is achieved. A PTA may say, "You are doing fine Mr. B, but you need to keep your balance over your feet," "you need to push down on your walker," or "put your foot farther forward." Knowledge of results (KR) feedback informs the patient as to whether the task is accomplished or how close the movement comes to accomplishing the task. The PTA may say, "Mrs. J, you came to standing without my help" or "you should not sit down without looking because you just sat on Mr. M." Both types of feedback give the learner information regarding error. Constant feedback leads to immediate behavioral performance, but the patient will learn to rely on external feedback and will not develop a need to process inherent information necessary to learn the task independently. As an example, a PTA verbally corrects many aspects of walking, and the patient does very well by the end of the morning session. In the afternoon, when the patient is asked to walk again, his performance is the same as the beginning of the morning and does not show the changes made by the end of the morning session. Obviously, the patient here is depending upon external feedback from the PTA and not learning to perform the task independently.

Three schedules of external feedback can be used: (1) summed feedback, which provides feedback after a set number of trials of the task (eg, after every other or every third trial); (2) faded feedback, which initially provides feedback after every trial, then decreasing to every other trial, every third, every fourth, etc; and (3) bandwidth feedback, which provides feedback only when the performance of the task is beyond a given range for error. Another way to vary external feedback is by providing delayed feedback, in which the PTA withholds the feedback for a short time (eg, a 5-second delay).[20] The most effective feedback schedule for motor learning is a faded schedule, where external feedback becomes increasingly intermittent throughout patient trials (practice). Delayed feedback also allows for improved motor learning by providing the patient time to self-assess performance. However, the specific feedback schedule depends on the patient and the task to be learned and practiced. When the PTA has doubt regarding performance, asking the PT for additional direction is very appropriate.

MOTOR CONTROL

Motor control is the study of how an individual controls movement already acquired.[21-23] The sciences leading to an understanding of motor control are neurophysiology, neuroanatomy, kinesiology, movement science, exercise physiology and bodily systems interacting with the motor system during an activity (eg, the heart, circulation, digestion, and breathing). It is not the PTA's responsibility to know what movement dysfunctions correlate with what types of lesions, the location of lesions, or status of a lesion, but it is the responsibility of the PTA to recognize a change in the control of a pattern or functional skill and inform the PT. This can be a critical health issue when the change seems to be toward dysfunction versus function. One of the challenges in understanding motor control is realizing that the PT's or the PTA's motor control over his or her body affects feedback to the patient. The patient's ability to perform a task is dependent upon his or her own inherent mechanisms, which may vary

from those of the therapist's regardless of a CNS lesion. The most obvious difference is probably anthropometric. The clinician's height, weight, flexibility, strength, endurance, etc affect the motions that can be reinforced through feedback to the patient. In addition, these same body parameters affect how a patient can perform movement. The easiest example to articulate is observing how a short versus a tall person comes out of a chair. Look at your fellow classmates and you will be surprised at the difference. Motor control means the control an individual has given the unique characteristics of that individual. Differences occur before injury or disease as well as following. It is up to the PT to guide the PTA's interventions in order to optimize the functional recovery of the patient.

When analyzing motor control of a specific movement, such as walking, the therapist will look at many motor programs that are running simultaneously. These programs include the following: automatic walking, postural control of the head, axial muscles and trunk in open and closed chain environments, balance programs from heel strike to heel strike of both legs, arm swing and how it perturbs the patient, and the environment within which the patient is walking (eg, wood floor, shag rugs, cement walkway, grass on level ground versus up and down inclines). Each one of these programs is a movement sequence being controlled by the CNS. The CNS must control and modify all of these programs simultaneously in order for the therapist to observe normal walking within the environment specified. Some patients may lose one of the multitudes of programs, and thus, a PTA may be instructed to run a complex program, such as walking, under controlled environments, such as with a body-weight bearing overhead suspension system. The suspension system and a treadmill reduce the individual's need to run adequate postural programs and reduce the variable power production used throughout the gait cycle. The frequency of stepping can be controlled externally, and foot placement can be assisted by a clinician. As the patient gains control of posture, walking, balance power, stepping frequency, and symmetrical stride length, the amount of suspension can be reduced, which demands more motor control by the patient.

NEUROPLASTICITY

Neuroplasticity is defined as the brain's ability to adapt and use cellular adaptations to learn or relearn functions previously lost due to cellular death by trauma or disease at any age. The changes occur in response to a variety of external and internal demands placed upon the individual's CNS. Within an optimal treatment environment, the resultant behavior leads to functional recovery and allows the individual to regain or attain a higher quality of life. In reality, neuroplasticity occurs throughout life. Internal adaptations of the CNS to height, weight, endurance, normal and chronic disease, and cellular death over a lifetime allow all of us to maintain function as our bodies change. Similarly, external environments vary over a lifetime, such as climate, exercise level, dietary demands, and changes in habitat. The CNS needs to modify and change previously effective motor programs and their parameters in order for each of us to be flexible, adaptable, and disease free. When trauma or disease causes dramatic observable changes in behavior, then everyone around becomes aware of those variances. Theory from the early- to mid-20th century lead therapists to believe that once cellular death had occurred, there was nothing that could be done except compensation. It was believed that plasticity within the CNS is not possible. Therapists working with patients with CNS disease or trauma could not reconcile the discrepancy between theory and patient recovery following disease or trauma. Therapists have always dealt with function and physicians with pathology. Often, the pathology, according to the physician or basic scientist, would indicate that function was impossible, yet therapists dealing with behavior found that patients often got better and regained lost motor function. In the last two decades, with the advent of better measurement tools and research on live animal models, scientists and researchers have discovered that the brain is much more plastic than previously thought. It has been found that, given an appropriate environment to learn in, the *brain can learn or relearn* despite cellular damage.[14,15,24-28]

Neuroplasticity gives the basic science efficacy for behavior that therapists have observed since the beginning of the profession. Previously, clinicians, especially master clinicians, had difficulty or could not explain how patients regained function; however, they could observe and measure those behaviors. As a clinician and therapist, this author always believed that "If a motor behavior looked right to me or other people, was easy and enjoyable for the patient, then somehow the intervention was creating change in the direction of normality and functional recovery no matter the theory." Neuroplasticity helps to explain why patients were regaining function even though the medical system of the time said they could not. This theory has helped guide therapists with intervention delineation. The CNS will always try to succeed at a task presented as long as the individual is motivated to succeed. If the environment used to teach a task is too difficult, then a patient will substitute other programs to try to succeed at the task. For example, if a patient cannot flex the hip at push-off, he or she will circumduct the hip or use some alternative movement pattern to succeed

at bringing the limb forward. These alternatives are easily identified and, if practiced, will become a new program for the patient; it will, however, require more energy because it is less efficient. It will affect synergy patterns, postural control, balance, and needed power throughout the range. Therefore, it would be better to try to trigger the patient's normal walking patterns before choosing some compensatory solution. The complex theory and its relationship to function are not the responsibility of the PTA, but that does not mean that sensory input to the eyes and ears and kinesthetic feelings may not lead to solutions to patients' functional recovery. Thus, it is the PTA's job to become a keen observer of functional movement and report changes in those behaviors to the PT. A patient's movement or postural problems are usually answered by the patient's motor responses.

CONCLUSION

If a patient has never learned normal motor programs (eg, in the case of trauma at birth), the movement pattern must be mass practiced in an environment where success is possible, reinforcement accurate, and potential actualized. If the individual has already learned a movement strategy (eg, walking) and suffers a trauma (eg, drowning), traumatic head injury, or stroke, the potential exists to regain a previously learned pattern or to learn a new one in the intervention environment of the therapist. An individual must first learn a pattern or task-specific program, and then practice enough for the control over that program to become automatic, as in the feed-forward motor program. A learned program is similar to a videotape placed in a recorder. The CNS determines the pattern and will run the program (or videotape) until the CNS is told to change it. As an example, the therapist places the client in an environment where the patient's CNS determines that walking is the appropriate program to run. The type of walking observed tells the therapist what programs are interacting and being controlled by the patient. That person runs the motor control of walking until either the CNS tells it to do something else, or the motor control of that individual cannot self-correct the error, and thus, the environment forces a new program. The person falling because of a surface change for which the person cannot compensate is an example of external environmental change that forces a change in programming and loss of motor control over walking. Understanding motor learning and what patterns the CNS can use to control the motor system's response to a required movement can give tremendous insight into the prognosis of a patient with movement dysfunction following insult to the CNS. How the map fits together will be influenced by the PT, the PTA, the patient, and the environments within which the patient can learn. The following case examples should help the PTA understand the theoretical principles presented within this chapter.

CASE STUDIES

The specific case examples following are patient examples similar to those discussed in later chapters. The PTA is not expected to be able to answer these clinical questions after reading this chapter. Instead, the PTA can use these cases to help integrate the information presented in this chapter with information presented in all the clinical problems chapters. It is recommended that the learner read this chapter, the case examples, and questions in order to identify appropriate questions regarding motor learning, motor control, and neuroplasticity as they relate to patient care. After reading and analyzing any clinical problem chapter, the PTA can return to this chapter, find an appropriate case, and then progress through the questions and answers in order to better integrate this material into clinical intervention decisions.

Case #1

The patient is a 6-month-old child diagnosed with spastic diplegia. She was born 8 weeks premature and was extremely flaccid at that time. The child's gestational age would be placed at 4 months, giving the child the 8 weeks she should have remained in utero. However, the tonal characteristics of the child are extensor dominant in the trunk and LEs. The child has more control over the arms than legs but loses function of the arms when placed in positions that require a lot of trunk stability, such as sitting or pressure on the feet in standing. The child does not have adequate head control and is unable to roll over, come to sitting, or sit independently. The PT has asked the PTA to first do a handling technique with rotation of the trunk in sidelying. The PTA should rotate the lower trunk on the upper trunk to facilitate rolling and, initially, have one of the patient's LEs lead with hip and knee flexion (without holding the ball of the foot). Second, the child should be placed on the PTA's bent knees with the head in vertical and, with small degree changes of the trunk, the PTA should facilitate small movements of the head and, thus, assist the child in gaining head control.

Questions

1. Why has the PT asked the PTA to do these activities?

2. Is the request within the domain of the PTA?

3. At what stage of motor learning is the child?

4. What type of practice context would you choose? The response needs to relate to whole, pure-part, sequential-part, and whole to part to whole learning.

5. What type of practice schedule would you expect the PTA to use? When considering the practice schedule, what type of feedback would be used initially, and how would that feedback be changed as the patient improves?

6. Why would you expect change, and what might it look like? When or why would you ask the PT to change the interventions delegated?

Case #2

The patient is a 5-year-old male who suffered an anoxic event due to drowning. Before the injury, he was an active, healthy child in kindergarten and doing very well. The child was in a coma for 1 week and in a vegetative state for 3 weeks. He is now stable and has been sent to neurorehab for physical therapy. The patient can roll and come to sitting although his trunk tone is reduced. He can sit independently as long as he does not have to move but cannot stand up from sitting. The PT has asked the PTA to first place the patient in sitting, the PTAs using his or her own leg to support the patient's trunk from behind, bringing the boy into a vertical postural pattern. The PTA is then to ask the child to reach for toys and hand them to his mother. Next, using a large ball, the PTA should roll the child into a vertical posture on his knees and then, using toys and manipulating the ball, the PTA should demand that the child maintain and/or regain upright posture during play.

Questions

1. Why has the PT asked the PTA to do these activities?

2. Is the request within the domain of the PTA?

3. At what stage of learning is the child?

4. What type of environmental context would you chose?

5. What type of reinforcement schedule would you expect the PTA to use?

6. Why would you expect change, and what might it look like? When or why would you ask the PT to change the interventions delegated?

Case #3

The patient is a 27-year-old male who suffered a TBI following a head-on collision while driving his car without a seat belt. He has been in the ICU for 4 days and has been transferred to the rehab unit today. The PT has evaluated the patient. At this time, he is conscious but has extremely low tone. He is unable to come to sitting or standing independently, and he does not have enough tone to sit independently. The PT has asked the PTA to sit the patient on the side of the bed with the feet supported, first by raising the head of the bed, then guiding the patient into sitting. The PTA can either kneel behind the patient on the bed with a ball in the patient's lap and the patient's arms over the ball, or the PTA can sit in front of him and make sure his weight is forward over his pelvis with his arms on the PTA's shoulder. The goal is to increase the length of time the patient is able to sit semi-independently. As the patient gains control and strength, have him begin to reach for real targets, such as a cup or ball, while maintaining trunk and pelvic control. The goal is to increase the length of semi- or independent sitting. This is accomplished through the patient being challenged by perturbation of his weight over his hips during reaching.

Questions

1. Why has the PT asked the PTA to do these activities?

2. Is the request within the domain of the PTA?

3. At what stage of learning is the patient concerning sitting?

4. Is the PTA working on new learning or relearning an old program?

5. What type of environmental context would you choose (quiet or noisy, hard or soft surface)?

6. What type of reinforcement schedule would you expect the PTA to use?

7. Why would you expect change, and what might it look like? When or why would you ask the PT to change the interventions delegated?

Case #4

The patient is a 59-year-old male with the medical diagnosis of Parkinson's disease. He is able to do all functional activities at a certain rate, but he has great difficulty regaining his balance if he trips and difficulty initiating changes such as sit to stand and stand to walk. He especially complains of problems turning (eg, turning into the bathroom or turning and walking back to the dining room with his food). First, the PT asks the PTA to teach the patient to use a partial rotation pattern when coming to sit versus the adult sitting pattern he is using. The PT also asks the PTA to have the patient practice going from sit to stand to sit on a variety of surfaces, with the chair or stool at a variety of levels. The PT delegates placing this patient on the treadmill, first at his normal gait pattern and then changing the settings to encourage fluctuation in walking speed and height of incline. The fourth task for the PTA is to create a maze for the patient to walk through that requires him to turn at each corner. Initially, he should be instructed to just walk, and then he should progress to walking through the maze facing a specific direction. Once he can do this independently, the activities will become his home exercise program, which he must practice in order to maintain function for as long as possible. Additionally, there are other activities the PT may delegate to the patient's significant other or caregiver because the patient still needs to continue practicing but does not need a PT or a PTA to help with these functions at this time.

Questions

1. Why has the PT asked the PTA to do these activities?

2. Is the request within the domain of the PTA?

3. At what stage of learning is the adult concerning walking?

4. Is the PTA working on new learning or relearning an old program?

5. Why did the PT select the specific environmental context, and why should it work?

6. What type of reinforcement schedule would the PTA expect to use?

7. Why would you expect change, and what might it look like? When or why would you ask the PT to change the interventions delegated?

Case #5

The patient is a 71-year-old male with the medical diagnosis of a mild right cardiovascular accident (CVA) with resulting left hemiplegia. He can sit independently but does not have equal weight bearing on the left hip. With assistance, he can come to standing with the majority of weight on his right leg. The PT has delegated to the PTA the activity of weight shifting in sitting. Specifically, the PTA is to have the patient reach with his right arm over to the left side as far as possible and increase that range as the patient improves. If he can use the left arm to do the same, then the PTA is to also include that extremity. Second, the PTA is to assist the PT in placing the patient in a harness in order to do supported weight bearing on the treadmill. Once the patient is in the position and the PT determines the pace and degree of body weight support, the PTA will be assisting the patient with his left leg in order to practice walking.

Questions

1. Why has the PT asked the PTA to do these activities?

2. Is the request within the domain of the PTA?

3. At what stage of learning is the adult concerning walking?

4. Is the PTA working on new learning or relearning an old program?

5. Why did the PT select the specific environmental context?

6. What type of reinforcement schedule would you expect the PTA to use?

7. Why would you expect change, and what might it look like? When or why would you ask the PT to change the interventions delegated?

Suggested author answers are available at www.slackbooks.com/neuroquestions.

REFERENCES

1. Liddell EG. Cajal and Sherrington. *Lect Sci Basis Med.* 1956-1958;6:100-115.

2. Knott M, Voss DE. *Proprioceptive Neuromuscular Facilitation.* New York, NY: Harper and Row; 1968.

3. Bobath B. *Abnormal Postural Reflex Activity Caused by Brain Lesions.* 3rd ed. Frederick, Md: Aspen Publications; 1985.

4. Rood M. The use of sensory receptors to activate, facilitate, and inhibit motor response, autonomic and somatic, in developmental sequence. In: Scattely C, ed. *Approaches to Treatment of Patients with Neuromuscular Dysfunction.* Third International Congress, World Federation of Occupational Therapists. Dubuque, Iowa: William Brown Group; 1962.

5. Ayers AJ. *The Development of Sensory Integration Theory and Practice.* Dubuque, Iowa: Kendall/Hunt Publishing; 1974.

6. Johnstone M. *Restoration of Normal Movement after Stroke.* New York, NY: Churchill Livingstone; 1995.

7. Brunnstrom S. *Movement Therapy in Hemiplegia.* 2nd ed. Philadelphia, Pa: JB Lippincott; 1992.

8. Carr JH, Sheperd RB. *Movement Science: Foundations for Physical Therapy in Rehabilitation.* Frederick, Md: Aspen Publishers; 1987.

9. Umphred, DA. *Neurological Rehabilitation.* 1st ed. St Louis, Mo: CV Mosby; 1985.

10. Bernstein N. *Coordination and Regulation of Movement.* New York, NY: Pergamon Press; 1967.

11. Tuller B, Turvey MT, Fitch HI. The Bernstein perspective II: the concept of muscle linkage or coordinative structure. In: Kelso JAS, ed. *Human Motor Behavior. An Introduction.* Hillsday, NJ: Erlbaum; 1982.

12. Shumway-Cook A, Wollacott M. *Motor Control: Theory and Practical Applications.* Philadelphia, Pa: Lippincott, Williams, and Wilkins; 1995:24.

13. Candia V, Weinbruch C, Elbert T, Rockstroh B, Ray W. Effective behavioral treatment of focal hand dystonia in musicians alters somatosensory cortical organization. *Proc Natl Aca Sci USA.* 2003;100(13):7425-7427.

14. Nudo RJ. Functional and structural plasticity in motor cortex: implications for stroke recovery. *Phys Med Rehabil Clin N Am.* 2003;14:S57-76.

15. Ward NS, Brown MM, Thompson AJ, Frackowiak RS. Neural correlates of motor recovery after stroke: a longitudinal fMRI study. *Brain.* 2003;126:2476-2496.

16. Kuo AD. The relative roles of feedforward and feedback in the control of rhythmic movements. *Motor Control.* 2002;6(2):129-145.

17. Sullivan KJ, Knowlton BJ, Dobkin BH. Step training with body weight support: effect of treadmill speed and practice paradigms on poststroke locomotor recovery. *Arch Phys Med Rehabil.* 2002;83(5):683-691.

18. Winstein CJ. Knowledge of results and motor learning: implications for physical therapy. *Phys Ther.* 1991;71:140-149.

19. Schmidt RA, Lee TD. *Motor Control and Motor Learning: A Behavioral Emphasis.* 3rd ed. Champaign, Ill: Human Kinetics; 1999.

20. O'Sullivan SB. *Physical Rehabilitation: Assessment and Treatment.* 4th ed. Philadelphia, PA: FA Davis; 2001.

21. Horak FB, Henry SM, Shumway-Cook A. Postural perturbations: new insights for treatment of balance disorders. *Phys Ther.* 1997;77(5):517-533.

22. Shumway-Cook A, Patla A, Stewart A, Ferrucci L, Ciol MA, Guralnik JM. Environmental components of mobility disability in community-living older persons. *J Am Geriatr Soc.* 2003;51(3):393-398.

23. Woollacott M, Shumway-Cook A. Attention and the control of posture and gait: a review of an emerging area of research. *Gait Posture.* 2002;16(1):1-14.

24. Das A, Franca JG, Gattass R, Kaas JH, Nicolelis MA, Timo-Laria C, Vargas CD, Weinberger NM, Volchan E. The brain decade in debate VI. Sensory and motor maps: dynamics and plasticity. *Braz J Med Biol Res.* 2001;34(12):1497-1508.

25. Hashino O. Neuronal bases of perceptual learning revealed by a synaptic balance scheme. *Neural Comput.* 2004;16(3):563-594.

26. Jackson PL, Lafleur MF, Malouin F, Richards C, Doyon J. Potential role of mental practice using motor imagery in neurological rehabilitation. *Arch Phys Med Rehabil.* 2001;82(8):1133-1141.

27. Kandel ER, Schwartz JH, Jessel TM. *Principles of Neural Science.* 4th ed. New York, NY: McGraw-Hill; 2000.

28. Sapolsky RM. Stress and plasticity in the limbic system. *Neurochem Res.* 2003;28(11):1735-1742.

Chapter

4

EXAMINATION PROCEDURES

Rolando T. Lazaro, PT, MS, DPT, GCS

KEY WORDS

balance examination
neuromuscular examination
sensory testing

CHAPTER OBJECTIVES

- Discuss the purposes of a neuromuscular examination.

- Identify the reasons for performing the particular neuromuscular examination procedures.

- Discuss the role of the PTA in the examination of patients and clients referred to physical therapy.

- Identify and discuss when and which neuromuscular examination procedures may be performed by the PTA.

INTRODUCTION

Integral to the effective physical therapy management of any patient or client is the foundation of a sound examination and evaluation. A complete examination allows the identification of problems that can be appropriately managed through physical therapy intervention. In addition, the examination enhances the patient's achievement of optimal health and well-being by identifying the interactions of various body systems as they relate to the patient's signs, symptoms, and progress with rehabilitation. This examination process also protects the patient by identifying potential life-threatening or emergency conditions and/or the need to refer to other individuals who will be able to better manage aspects of the patient's care.

Examination is defined by the *Guide to Physical Therapist Practice*[1] (the *Guide*) as "a comprehensive screening and specific testing process leading to diagnostic classification or, as appropriate, to a referral to another practitioner."[1] Evaluation is defined as "a dynamic process in which the PT makes clinical judgments based on data gathered during the examination."[1] PTAs are well qualified to perform portions of an examination under the direction of the PT.

Knowledge of the results of the examination and evaluation allows the PTA a better understanding of the impairments, functional limitations, and clinical decisions involving intervention by either the PT or the PTA. It is important to remember, however, that it is the PT's responsibility to analyze the results of the examination, classify them into syndromes or clusters (termed physical therapy evaluation[1]), and make any other pertinent clinical decisions regarding the establishment of the prognosis, which includes the goals, plan of care, and specific interventions to be used. A PTA will certainly learn through experience the interactions among examination, prognosis, and intervention design, but the responsibility for each is the PT's. In this respect, it is important for the PTA to effectively communicate to the PT the results of tests and measures used for reexaminations and any other important information; this allows the PT to make the best decisions regarding the patient's care.

There are typically three types of "formal" examinations and evaluations used when a patient receives physical therapy: (1) an initial examination and evaluation, (2) an interim examination and evaluation, and (3) a discharge examination and evaluation. Not all components of an examination are repeated for the second two types of examinations. This chapter will focus on the initial examination and evaluation process and include discussion of the role of the PTA in the interim and discharge examinations. Following the *Guide*, this *neuromuscular examination* should consist of the patient or client history, a review of systems, and tests and measures appropriate to the medical diagnosis and movement dysfunctions identified by the therapist.[1]

Many textbooks[2,3] offer a comprehensive discussion of the musculoskeletal examination, and the PTA is encouraged to be familiar with the components of these examinations, especially those tests and measures frequently delegated to the PTA. The neuromuscular examination includes tests and measures typically used during a musculoskeletal examination but obviously delves more thoroughly into the assessment of the neuromuscular system. Examples of common musculoskeletal tests and measures used with neuromuscular patients include anthropometric measurements (eg, circumferential and length measurements), ROM and flexibility measurements, joint integrity and mobility measurements, pain assessment, postural assessment, and assessment of muscle performance (eg, strength, power, and endurance). This chapter will not discuss these tests and measures but will emphasize those that focus on the neuromuscular system.

THE PATIENT HISTORY

A thorough investigation of the patient's history assists in the understanding of the chronology of the complaints and provides important information that may be pertinent to the patient's future care. This information may be partially obtained from the patient's medical chart, intake form, or other supporting medical documentation. A PTA may be asked to instruct the patient or family in reporting the patient's history before the PT observes the patient. This information is documented on an intake form that is generally standardized to the clinic and/or specific to the patient's medical history. Although a PTA may be asked to assist in obtaining history, interpretation of that history is the responsibility of the PT.

Another important aspect of the patient history is to identify the specific patient goals. This component of the history helps the therapist investigate the patient's understanding of the cause of the illness or disease and the patient's expectations regarding therapy. For example, a PT or PTA may think that ambulation with an assistive device on a hard surface is a realistic expectation while the patient expects to be playing golf when he returns home. Finding avenues to allow the patient to achieve ambulation without taking away the hope of golf is part of the empowerment model. Knowledge of the goals of the patient, family, physicians, and therapists becomes especially important when considering the effect of the patient's culture and belief systems because they apply to the entire disease-illness-wellness continuum.

The interview portion of the patient history must be conducted in a private area to allow the patient to honestly answer the therapist's questions and feel safe that no one else can hear the answers. It is imperative that the PT or PTA assures patient confidentiality within the environment where the examination takes place. Ensuring privacy allows trust to develop between the patient and the therapist, which is paramount to optimal care.

SYSTEMS REVIEW

The next portion of the patient examination is the review of systems. This is the process where the clinician "clears" several systems that are potentially involved or implicated in the patient's performance or progress.[1] Another reason for performing a review of systems is to identify potential system abnormalities that may necessitate a medical referral. It is important to remember that the PT must perform the systems review on a *systems* level. It is not the PT's responsibility to diagnose a medical disease or pathology. However, it is important for him or her to determine whether a particular body system (GI, urinary, cardiopulmonary, etc) is problematic and, therefore, needs assessment by a health care practitioner who is able to diagnose the condition.

Another important aspect to remember about the review of systems (and during treatment) is that the PT and PTA must be able to recognize signs and symptoms of medical emergencies, wherein the patient must be referred to other health care practitioners to receive the necessary attention. As more patients with increasingly complicated medical histories or more active secondary pathologies access physical therapy, cognizance of potential medical emergencies is imperative. The review of systems is outside the scope of the PTA; therefore, delegation to the PTA is not appropriate for interim or discharge reexaminations.

TESTS AND MEASURES

The third portion of the patient examination involves the selection of appropriate tests and measures that will provide the PT with the most accurate reflection of the patient's movement dysfunction. The selection of the appropriate tests and measures is within the purview of the PT. To assist the PT with completion of interim and discharge examinations, the PTA performs tests and measures as delegated by the PT. Communication is important between the PT and PTA for appropriate selection of tests and measures, as this leads to better care for the patient. For example, if the PTA identifies additional clinical signs and symptoms when performing the delegated tests and measures, she or he should communicate this to the PT so that the PT can determine additional tests to be performed and who should perform them.

As a reference, the *Guide* provides a list of the more common tests and measures performed on a patient based on a particular practice pattern presentation. It should be noted, however, that the *Guide* is a *guide:* it reflects the most common practice guidelines available to PTs and PTAs at this time. The reader is referred to the *Guide* for details on the categories of and types of tests and measures that may be used for each neuromuscular practice pattern. It is important to note that not all of the categories of tests and measures are appropriate for all patients or clients with neuromuscular disorders. It is beyond the scope of this text to address all of the tests and measures that may be used for each patient with a neuromuscular disorder. The following are the most commonly used tests and measures appropriate for patients with neuromuscular disorders and those frequently delegated to the PTA for data collection as a component of reexamination and reevaluation.

Vital Signs

This text will not cover the procedures to assess vital signs but will address the importance of their assessment for patients with neurologic disorders.

Assessment of vital signs is a very important aspect of the patient's examination. The assessment establishes the integrity of the patient's baseline cardiopulmonary functions and screens any potential emergencies that may occur during the physical therapy session. BP, pulse, and respirations must be assessed and documented, especially for older patients or patients with multiple medical issues. As appropriate, pulse oximetry may be assessed for documentation of the patient's oxygenation level. Vital signs are also frequently taken at each treatment session.

Observation

Observation involves the identification of potential abnormalities during visual inspection. During the initial examination, observation is the responsibility of the PT. The PTA must be able to communicate to the PT clinically relevant observations made during treatment and reexamination that may affect the patient's progress. PTAs may be directly involved in performing observations and documenting these as components of daily treatment and reexaminations. Under this heading, the PTA might make note of the patient's general movement patterns, the ease by which the patient moves, as well as the patient's general affect and ability to communicate. The PTA might also document areas of swelling/edema, atrophy, skin integrity, contractures, and other skeletal or joint abnormalities. Once these aspects are noted, more in-depth examination procedures (eg, circumferential measurements, wound assessment, or goniometry) may be performed.

Arousal, Attention, and Cognition

The accurate assessment of the patient's arousal (level of consciousness), attention, and cognition will provide the clinician with important information. This information includes the ability of the patient to voluntarily participate in therapy as well as other factors (eg, memory or ability to follow directions) that may affect the patient's progress.

Arousal is the physiological readiness of the individual for activity and is characterized by responsiveness to stimulation.[4] In terms of levels of consciousness, common descriptors include alert (awake and attentive), lethargic (appears drowsy or falls asleep), obtunded (hard to arouse from sleep and confused when awake), stuporous (responsive only to strong, noxious stimuli), comatose (nonresponsive to any type of stimulation), and persistent vegetative state (state of unconsciousness with irregular sleep/wake cycles and inconsistent response to stimulation).[4,5]

Attention is awareness of the environment and ability to focus on a specific stimulus without distraction.[4,5] In terms of orientation, the individual is assessed according to orientation to person, place, time, and situation. Documentation of orientation is often abbreviated as "oriented x 4," referring to the four domains. When a patient is not oriented to one or more domains, it is documented with the domains of disorientation listed within parentheses, for example, "oriented x 2 (place, situation)."[4]

Both short- and long-term memory are also assessed, though impairments of short-term memory will have the greater impact upon the successful outcome of physical therapy management. Short-term memory can be assessed by verbally providing a list of numbers (7 digits) or words (5 to 7 or a short sentence) to the patient, asking the patient to immediately repeat the list, then asking him or her to recall the list again after 5 minutes (min), then 30 min. Normal memory allows an individual to recall the entire list after 5 min and at least two of the items after 30 min. Long-term memory can be assessed by asking the patient questions such as date and location of birth, date of marriage, and historical facts.[4]

The therapist may also examine the patient's ability to follow directions (one-step or multi-step commands). Some of these specific cognitive tests and measures are performed by the PT and should not be delegated. However, PTAs should to be able to recognize changes in a patient's state or level of consciousness, recognize the level of recall, recognize a patient's orientation level, and determine a patient's ability to process and respond to commands. In addition, it is important for a PTA to understand the ramifications of the results of all of the tests and measures and how they affect the success of interventions. For example, if a PT determines that a patient cannot understand more than a two-step command, then asking a patient to lock the w/c, scoot forward in the chair, lean forward, and stand up involves two more steps than that patient can comprehend. A change in the level of consciousness must always be communicated to the PT or appropriate medical professionals.

Sensation

Assessment of the patient's sensory integrity allows the therapist to identify the extent of impairment of the sensory system brought about by the particular pathology or injury. By looking at the specific patterns and location of sensory loss or abnormality, the PT may hypothesize which of the specific components of the nervous system have been damaged and which are processing accurately. The therapist may also look at the implication of sensory loss in the loss of function and the potential secondary risks due to sensory impairment. Lastly, knowledge of sensory impairment assists the PT in establishing an appropriate prognosis, goals, and a treatment plan. A PTA may be asked to perform any or all of these sensory tests on a patient for a reexamination; however, interpretation of this information must be part of the PT evaluation process.

Sensations that may be tested include the following:

- **Exteroceptive and proprioceptive senses:** Light touch, superficial pain, temperature, pressure, vibration, joint position (proprioception), and movement sense (kinesthesia).

- **Combined sensations (cortical sensations):** Examples include two-point discrimination, tactile localization, texture recognition, stereognosis, graphesthesia, and barognosis.

To begin sensory assessment, the clinician asks the patient to describe what she or he is sensing (or not sensing) and to outline the area of sensory abnormality on him- or herself. The clinician then performs a "quick scan" of sensation by running his or her relaxed fingers over the skin to be tested and a corresponding area of normal sensation, as appropriate. This step allows the clinician to identify areas of sensory abnormality that the patient may not have identified and to examine the color, texture, and plasticity of the skin itself. The clinician then performs a more detailed test of the area or areas in question. For all tests, the patient has eyes closed, vision blocked by a blindfold, or a clipboard placed below the patient's chin to impede looking down. The patient is encouraged to respond as quickly as possible to each stimulus.

Sensory Testing Protocols: Exteroceptive and Proprioceptive

- **Light touch:** Use a piece of cotton or the end of a cotton swab to lightly stroke the skin. Request from the patient, "Tell me when you feel me touching you"[4] (Figure 4-1).

- **Superficial pain:** Cut a tongue depressor in half so that there is a blunt and a sharp end, or pull apart a paperclip. Apply uniform pressure with each application of the stimuli. Alternate the sharp and dull stimuli randomly. Request from the patient, "Tell me whether this feels sharp or dull."[4]

- **Temperature:** Fill one test tube with hot water, the other with cold water. Touch the skin with the test tube and request from the patient, "Tell me whether this feels warm, cold, or you are unable to tell."[4]

- **Deep pressure:** This is usually used for patients with altered mental status. Apply a knuckle to the sternum (sternal rub), or squeeze the Achilles tendon or the web space between the thumb and the index finger. Observe the response to painful stimulus.

- **Pressure:** Using your thumb or fingertip, apply pressure firm enough to indent the skin, and request from the patient, "Tell me when you feel the stimulus by saying 'now.'"[4]

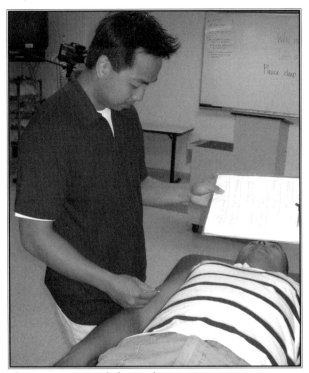

Figure 4-1. Testing light touch sensation.

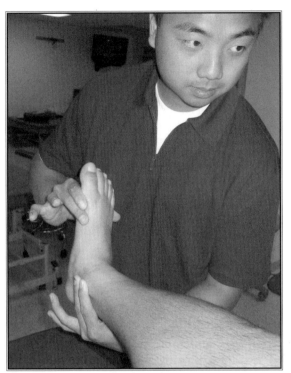

Figure 4-2. Testing proprioception.

- **Vibration:** Strike a tuning fork that vibrates at 128Hz and hold it against boney prominences such as the sternum, elbow, or ankle. Request from the patient: "Tell me when you feel the vibration, and tell me when it goes away."[4]

- **Proprioception:** Use a fingertip grip over the boney prominences of the lateral joint surfaces. Tell the patient which words to use to identify the ROM positions (eg, initial, mid-, or terminal range). Move the joint(s) through a ROM and then hold it (them) in a static position. Ask the patient to verbally describe the position or to duplicate the position of the joint(s) on the opposite limb[4] (Figure 4-2).

- **Kinesthesia:** Use a fingertip grip over the boney prominences of the lateral joint surfaces. Move the joint passively in small increments up and down or medially and laterally, and ask the patient to indicate the direction of movement: "Is this up or down?" or "Is this in or out?" An alternative is to use the same grip, passively move the extremity, and ask the patient to move his other extremity to match your movements (called a mirroring test).[4]

Grading Sensation (Exteroception)

A PT may ask the PTA to place sensory information on a body-chart examination sheet so that future tests can reflect progress or changes in sensory awareness and discrimination. When a patient has only one side involved (eg, following a stroke) or minimal involvement that varies from limb to limb, sensation is graded NORMAL when the person perceives the sensation with the strength similar to the sensation felt on the normal side of the body. Sensation is graded IMPAIRED when the person perceives the sensation with more than 50% but less than 100% accuracy or when the person takes an abnormally long time to respond. Sensation is graded ABSENT when the person demonstrates less than 50% accuracy.

Sensory Testing Protocols: Combined (Cortical) Sensations

- **Two-point discrimination:** Several instruments are available for assessing two-point discrimination. A common one looks like a caliper and allows the therapist to move the two points closer together or farther apart. The therapist applies the caliper with the two tips apart and touching the patient's skin. In successive applications, the therapist then places the tips closer together and asks the patient to say when the two points are perceived as one. Several tables indicating normative values for two-point discrimination for different parts of the body are found in the O'Sullivan and Schmitz text *Physical Rehabilitation: Assessment and Treatment*.[4]

Table 4-1
Modified Ashworth Scale

0	No increase in muscle tone.
1	Slight increase in muscle tone, manifested by a catch and release or minimal resistance at the end of the ROM when the affected part is moved in flexion or extension.
1+	Slight increase in muscle tone, manifested by a catch followed by minimal resistance throughout the remainder (less than half) of the ROM.
2	More marked increase in muscle tone through most of the ROM but affected part easily moved.
3	Considerable increase in muscle tone; passive movement difficult.
4	Affected parts rigid in flexion and extension.

Adapted from Bohannon RW, Smith MB (1997). Interrater reliability of a modified Ashworth scale of muscle spasticity. Phys Ther. 1987;67(2):206-7.

- **Tactile localization**: The therapist touches the patient on different areas of his or her body then asks the patient to point to where she or he was touched.[4]

- **Texture recognition**: The therapist gives the patient cutouts of fabrics with different textures then asks the patient to describe the texture perceived (soft, rough, thick, thin, etc).[4]

- **Stereognosis**: Common items (eg, paperclips, keys, dice, coins) are placed in the patient's hand, and the patient is asked to identify the object by touching and feeling it.[4]

- **Graphesthesia**: The therapist "writes" letters or shapes on the patient's skin and the patient is asked to identify each letter or shape drawn.[4]

- **Barognosis**: The therapist gives the patient objects of different weights and asks the patient to identify which item is heaviest.[4]

Scoring for tactile localization, texture recognition, stereognosis, graphesthesia, and barognosis is the same as for the exteroceptive and proprioceptive senses.

Motor Examination

There are several areas to assess that will allow the therapist to make determinations as to the integrity of the motor system in a neurologically involved individual, and some of these tests are mentioned below.

Assessment of Muscular Tone

Muscle tone has been defined in a variety of ways[6-9] but, for the purposes of this text, is defined as the ability or the readiness of the muscle to contract, which is dependent upon the excitation of the motor pool in the spinal cord. There should be an appropriate amount of tone present to allow the individual to perform a movement that is synergistic, appropriate in strength and intensity, efficient, and purposeful. In neurologically involved patients, a range of tone can be found. Flaccidity is a term denoting the absence of tone, while hypotonicity is a state of decreased tone. On the other side of the spectrum, hypertonicity is a state of increased tone, while rigidity is a state of severe hypertonicity that results in an inability to move the extremity, passively or actively, and with limitation in all directions. Spasticity is an abnormal velocity-dependent muscle tone; the faster the limb is moved and the muscle is lengthened, the more resistance is felt in the muscle. With spasticity, the amount of resistance felt increases with increasing amplitude and velocity of the lengthening of the muscle.[9] To assess tone, the therapist moves the limb slowly and passively, feeling for resistance or lack of resistance to movement. To assess spasticity, the extremity is moved at varying speeds and resistance to movement is again assessed. The Modified Ashworth Scale[10] can be used as a more objective assessment of tone and is presented in Table 4-1.

Assessment of Strength

Manual muscle testing is performed to identify possible decreases in strength due to impingement in the nervous system or damage to the motor cortex or tract systems conveying motor information. Appropriate manual muscle testing protocols can be found in the texts written by Hislop and Montgomery[11] and Kendall and McCreary.[12] The PTA needs to understand the difference between weakness in a muscle due to a musculoskeletal and peripheral nerve injury versus weakness due to a CNS injury. Weakness in the peripheral system means a problem along the nerve, at the muscle/nerve junction, or within the muscle tissue itself. Weakness due to CNS damage is caused by a problem with the spinal cord or brain and comes from inside the spinal or cranial skeletal system. Weakness can also be due to disuse, which is not a pathology but an impairment caused by inactivity.

Table 4-2
Synergy Patterns of the Extremities

Limbs	Flexion Synergy Components	Extension Synergy Components
Upper	Scapular retraction, elevation, or hyperextension. Shoulder abduction, external rotation. Elbow flexion.* Forearm supination. Wrist and finger flexion.	Scapular protraction. Shoulder adduction*, internal rotation. Elbow extension. Forearm pronation.* Wrist and finger flexion.
Lower	Hip flexion,* abduction, external rotation. Knee flexion. Ankle dorsiflexion, inversion. Toe dorsiflexion.	Hip extension, adduction*, internal rotation. Knee extension.* Ankle plantarflexion*, inversion. Toe plantarflexion.

Adapted with permission from O'Sullivan SO. Assessment of motor function. In: O'Sullivan SB, Schmitz TJ, eds. Physical Rehabilitation: Assessment and Treatment. *4th ed. Philadelphia, PA: FA Davis; 2001.*

Assessment of Muscle Stretch Reflexes (or Deep Tendon Reflexes)

Muscle stretch reflexes (MSRs) assess the integrity of the reflex arc. This test is performed by using a reflex hammer to tap several muscle tendons with the purpose of eliciting a reflex response. A very strong response to the stimulus may indicate hyperactive MSRs (hyperreflexia) and typically suggests an upper motor neuron lesion. Decreased response to the stimulus may indicate hypoactive MSRs (hyporeflexia) and is typically suggestive of a lower motor neuron lesion. Although this test is administered by the PT, knowing the results from this procedure allows the PTA a better understanding of how the patient will present and of the patient's rehabilitation process.

Assessment of Synergy

Synergies are stereotypical movements that may be present and elicited in individuals with neurologic insults. Typical presentations of individuals with flexor or extensor synergy patterns are presented in Table 4-2.[13] The components marked with an asterisk (*) are generally the strongest or most prominent.

It is important for PTAs to identify these abnormal patterns and understand their implications in terms of facilitating normal movement. For example, the presence of a flexion synergy in the LE may inhibit the patient's ability to weight bear, thereby making functions like transfers and ambulation very difficult.

Assessment of Developmental Reflexes and Reactions

Developmental reflexes and reactions are assessed in pediatric patients to determine the child's level of development and if there are any delays. In adults, these reflexes are typically not present but may appear under conditions of fatigue or effort or following damage to the CNS.[9] The exceptions to this are higher level reactions such as the righting, protective, and equilibrium reactions, which persist throughout life in normal individuals. Patients with a brain injury (from a stroke or traumatic injury) may demonstrate the presence of the following reflexes: flexor withdrawal, extensor thrust, crossed extension, palmar grasp, symmetrical tonic neck (STNR), asymmetrical tonic neck (ATNR), symmetrical tonic labyrinthine (TLR or STLR), positive supporting, and associated reactions. The presence of these reflexes is considered abnormal when present beyond the age they are expected to be integrated.

The PT will perform the initial assessment for the presence or absence of developmental reflexes and reactions as part of the initial examination, when appropriate. The PTA may be delegated the assessment of selected reflexes and reactions as part of interim examinations, especially for pediatric patients. The importance of recognizing the presence or absence of developmental reflexes and reactions in pediatric patients is discussed in Chapters 7 and 8. The re-emergence of one or more of these reflexes or the absence of the higher level reactions in older children or adults can have a significant impact on muscle tone, the ability to isolate movements, balance, and functional skills such as feeding and ambulation.

There are several factors the PT and PTA must be mindful of to ensure an accurate assessment of these reflexes and reactions. These factors include the following:

1. Appropriately positioning the patient to allow for the expected movement response.

2. Adequate magnitude and duration of the test stimulus.

3. Sharp observation skills, in order to detect subtle movement changes and abnormal responses.

4. Palpation skills used to assist in identifying changes in muscle tone that are not easily observed.[9] A suggested reflex scoring scale from the O'Sullivan and Schmitz[9] text is presented below:

0+ Absent

1+ Tone changes: slight, transient with no movement of extremities

2+ Visible movement of extremities

3+ Exaggerated, full movement of extremities

4+ Obligatory and sustained movement, lasting for more than 30 seconds

Reflex testing procedures have been effectively presented by multiple authors, and detailed explanations can be found in the texts by Barnes[14] and Fiorentino.[15] Table 4-3 presents an overview of the assessment of developmental reflexes.

Coordination

Coordination is the ability to perform smooth, accurate, controlled motor responses that are characterized by appropriate speed, distance, direction, timing, and muscle tension.[16] Assessment of coordination allows the clinician to assess the ability of synergistic muscle groups to produce a smooth, coordinated, purposeful movement. Coordination tests are performed in the nonweight-bearing positions and weight-bearing postures. Inability to perform the tests when there is ample ROM and strength indicates a problem with coordination.

Examples of nonweight-bearing coordination tests include the following:

- **Nose-finger-nose**: The therapist asks the patient to touch his nose using his index finger, then to touch the therapist's finger, then again to touch the patient's nose. Inability to perform this test with a smooth coordinated movement is termed dysmetria (past pointing) (Figure 4-3).

- **Rapid alternating movement**: The therapist asks the patient to hold his elbows flexed at 90 degrees and close to the body and then perform alternate pronation and supination of the forearm. Inability to perform rapid alternating movements is termed dysdiadochokinesia.

- **Heel to shin**: The patient is positioned in supine. The patient is then asked to lift one leg up, use the heel of that leg to touch the kneecap of the contralateral leg, and then slide the heel down the shin.

Examples of coordination tests that can be performed with the patient in a weight-bearing posture include the following:

1. Have the patient stand with a narrow BOS (feet together).

2. Have the patient stand with one foot directly in front of the other with the toe of one foot touching the heel of the other.

3. Have the patient in standing and have him or her take steps following footprints placed on the floor by the therapist.

4. Have the patient walk along a straight line drawn or taped to the floor.

5. Have the patient walk sideways, backward, or using cross steps.

The reader is referred to the O'Sullivan and Schmitz text[16] for a more thorough listing and description of tests for assessing coordination. In terms of documenting the results of the coordination test, several scales may be used to provide an objective assessment of coordination; however, the validity or reliability of these scales has not been proven. The following presents a "basic" way of grading coordination:

- A NORMAL rating is characterized by the performance of the test in a smooth, accurate, and controlled motion;

- An IMPAIRED rating is when the movement is slow or jerky.

- An ABSENT rating is used if the patient is unable to perform the test.

The PT administers the appropriate tests to a patient during the first examination in order to obtain baseline measurements. If the patient is unable to complete the tests at the initial examination, the PT will administer them at a reexamination. It is important for PTAs to be familiar with the different types of tests so they can integrate the concept behind each test into an intervention during a treatment session. To determine if there have been any changes in the patient's coordination, a PTA can administer any of these coordination tests after the initial assessment by the PT. The PT may also ask the PTA to monitor coordination activities and alert the PT if changes occur before an interim examination.

Cranial Nerve Assessment

Another important component of a neurologic examination is the assessment of the integrity of the cranial nerves. These nerves originate in the brainstem and innervate the head, neck, and face. This assessment allows the clinician to determine how the specific

Table 4-3
Developmental Reflexes and Reactions Assessment

Reflex	Testing Position and Stimulus	Response
Flexor withdrawal	Supine or sitting position. Noxious stimulus (pin prick) to sole of foot.	Toes extend, foot dorsiflexes, entire leg flexes uncontrollably.
Crossed extension	Supine position. One leg fixed in extension. Noxious stimulus to ball of foot of the leg fixed in extension.	Opposite leg flexes, then adducts and extends.
Traction	Start in supine position. Grasp forearm, and pull up from supine into sitting position.	Flexion of the shoulders, elbows, wrists, and fingers.
Moro	Sitting position. Sudden change in position of head in relation to trunk; drop patient backward from sitting position.	Extension, abduction of arms, hand opening, and crying followed by flexion, adduction of arms across chest.
Startle	Any position. Sudden loud or harsh noise.	Sudden extension or abduction of arms; crying.
Palmar grasp	Any position. Maintained pressure to palm of hand.	Maintained flexion of fingers.
Plantar grasp	Supine or sitting position. Maintained pressure to ball of foot under toes.	Maintained flexion of toes.
Asymmetrical tonic neck (ATNR)	Any position (commonly tested in supine). Rotation of the head to one side.	Flexion of arms and legs on skull side, extension of arms and legs on chin side. ("bow and arrow" or "fencing posture"). Response may be stronger in the arms than legs.
Symmetrical tonic neck (STNR)	Any position (commonly tested in supine). Flexion or extension of the head.	With head flexion: flexion of arms, extension of legs. With head extension: extension of arms, flexion of legs.
Symmetrical tonic labyrinthine (STLR or TLR)	Prone or supine position.	With prone position: increased flexor tone or flexion of all limbs. With supine position: increased tone or extension of all limbs.
Positive supporting	Upright standing position. Contact to the ball of the foot.	Rigid extension (co-contraction) of the legs.
Associated movements or reactions	Any position. Resisted voluntary movement in any part of the body.	Involuntary movement in a resting extremity or increase in tonic muscle tension.
Neck righting acting on the body (NOB)	Supine position. Passively turn head to one side.	Body rotates as a whole (logrolls) to align the body with the head.
Body righting acting on the body (BOB)	Supine position. Passively rotate upper or lower trunk segment.	Body segment not rotated follows to align the body segments.
Labyrinthine head righting	Upright position (standing or sitting). Blindfold eyes; alter body position by tipping body in all directions.	Head orients to vertical position with mouth horizontal.
Optical righting	Upright position (standing or sitting). Alter body position by tipping body in all directions.	Head orients to vertical position with mouth horizontal.

Table 4-3 (continued)
Developmental Reflexes and Reactions Assessment

Reflex	Testing Position and Stimulus	Response
Upper extremities Protective extension (PE) forward, sideward, and backward	Sitting, kneeling, or standing position. Displace the COG outside of the BOS.	*Forward:* fingers and elbows extend, shoulders flex to support and to protect the body from falling. *Sideward:* fingers and elbows extend, shoulders abduct. *Backward:* fingers and elbows and shoulders extend.
Lower extremities Protective staggering forward, backward and sideward	Standing. Displace the COG outside of the BOS.	*Forward:* subject steps forward when balance displaced forward. *Backward:* subject steps backward when balance displaced backwards. *Sideward:* subject steps to side or crosses one foot over the other when balance displaced sideward.
Equilibrium reactions (ER): tilting	Supine, sitting, or standing position on a moveable object such as a balance board or ball. Displace the COG by tilting or moving the support surface.	Curvature of the trunk toward the upward side along with extension and abduction of the extremities on that side; protective extension on the downward side.
Equilibrium reactions: postural fixation	Sitting or standing position. Displace the COG in relation to the BOS but not outside of BOS. Can also be observed during voluntary activity.	*Sideward force:* curvature of the trunk toward the external force with extension and abduction of the extremities on the side to which the force was applied. *Backward force:* trunk flexion, extension of elbows with flexion of shoulders, and in standing plantarflexion of ankles. *Forward force:* trunk extension, extension of arms, and in standing. Dorsiflexion of ankles.

Adapted from Barnes MR, et al. The Neurophysiological Basis of Patient Treatment, Vol II: Reflexes in Motor Development. *Atlanta, Ga: Stokesville Publishing; 1978.*

---

neuromuscular disease or pathology has affected the patient's function as well as to differentially diagnose whether a particular movement disorder is caused by a central or peripheral nervous system abnormality. Cranial nerve testing is performed during the initial examination by the PT and is not commonly repeated in a reexamination. PTAs should be familiar with the purposes and the results of these tests to have a basic idea of some impairment that may affect a patient's ability to participate in physical therapy. The PTA can also notify the PT if changes in the function of any of the cranial nerves are noticed. Following are examples of cranial nerve tests.[17,18]

- **Cranial Nerve I: Olfactory Nerve** – Ask the patient to close his eyes. Hold one nostril closed, and introduce a cotton swab dipped in a substance with a non-noxious odor (eg, coffee, lemon, vanilla) up the other nostril; then ask the patient to identify the odor.

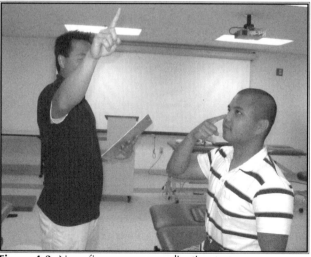

Figure 4-3. Nose-finger-nose coordination test.

- **Cranial Nerve II: Optic Nerve** – To test visual acuity, have the patient cover one eye. Hold a magazine about 2 to 4 feet away, and ask the patient to read a specific line. To test the visual field, sit in front of the patient. Ask the patient to cover one eye and look straight ahead with the other. The examiner places a finger out of the field and gradually brings it into view and asks the patient when she or he first sees the object.

- **Cranial Nerves III, IV, and VI: Oculomotor, Trochlear, and Abducens Nerves** – The examiner holds up a pen approximately 12 inches from the patient's face and asks the patient to keep his or her eyes on the pen. Examiner then moves the pen up and down (CNIII), down and in (CNIV), toward the nose to see if the two eyes converge (CNIII), and to both sides (CNVI). The ability of the eyes to track equally and appropriately is also observed during this test.

- **Cranial Nerve V: Trigeminal Nerve** – The examiner tests light touch and sharp/dull sensation of the face or tests the strength of muscles of mastication.

- **Cranial Nerve VII: Facial Nerve** – The examiner performs a manual muscle test of the muscles of facial expression.

- **Cranial Nerve VIII: Vestibulocochlear Nerve** – To test hearing, the examiner rubs his or her fingers close to the patient's ears and checks if the patient can hear it. To test the vestibular component, the examiner asks the patient to stand on a foam surface with eyes closed and observes excessive sway.

- **Cranial Nerve IX: Glossopharyngeal Nerve** – The examiner can assess the gag reflex by moving the tongue depressor around and in the back of the mouth, checking for a gag.

- **Cranial Nerve XII: Hypoglossal Nerve** – The examiner asks the client to protrude his tongue to check for fasciculations, which are odd, nonvolitional movements on the surface of the tongue. Another test is to have the patient protrude his tongue and then observe if she or he can move it rapidly from side to side.

Balance

Assessment of balance is an important component of the neuromuscular examination. Balance is essential for an individual to maintain postural stability or equilibrium in which the center of mass (COM) is maintained within the boundaries of the BOS.[13] The *limits of stability (LOS)* is defined as "the maximum angle from vertical that can be tolerated without loss of balance."[19]

In sitting, the motor or balance strategies used when the COM moves beyond the LOS include movements of the trunk over the hips. When the disturbance comes from the rear, the extensor muscles of the hip, trunk, and neck will activate to prevent the individual from falling forward. The hip flexors, quadriceps, abdominal muscles, and neck flexors activate when the disturbance (perturbation) comes from the front. If the perturbation is directed from the side, the lateral flexors of the trunk and neck will activate.[13] If the perturbing force is strong enough, protective extension of the UE on the opposite side of the force may be seen.

In standing, there are three balance strategies that have been identified when the LOS are reached while there is a disturbance of the COM. These are the ankle, hip, and stepping strategies. In the first two strategies, the BOS is fixed, while the COM is disturbed. In the *ankle* strategy, the COM shifts forward or backward over the ankle joints like a pendulum and is used when the balance disturbances are small.[13] When the *hip* strategy is used, the disturbances of the COM are typically larger and faster, and the COM shifts forward, backward, or laterally over the hip joints, depending on the direction of the disturbing force.[13] The third strategy, the stepping strategy, is used when there are large, fast balance disturbances and brings about a realignment of the BOS under the COM. The individual will demonstrate rapid steps or hops in the direction opposite of the disturbance. If the disturbing force comes from the rear, the individual may step or hop forward; when the force comes from the front, the steps will be backward; when the force comes from the side, the individual may take a step sideways or take a cross step.[13] The O'Sullivan and Schmitz[13] text offers a more detailed description of postural control, balance, and balance strategies.

It is important to determine the integrity of the balance system and its implications on other functional tasks (eg, sitting, standing, transfers, or gait). Because maintenance of balance involves multisystem interaction, a complete assessment of this system must be linked to other systems (eg, musculoskeletal or cardiopulmonary) and, thus, will be initially examined by the PT. Delegation of tests and measures for components of balance (eg, balance strategies, muscle power necessary for balance, reaction time to perturbations, range necessary for balance responses) may be given to the PTA for frequent examination of changes in the patient's response to volitional and of unexpected perturbation in sitting, standing, and during ambulation.

The clinician may want to determine a patient's functional balance grade. In the clinical setting,

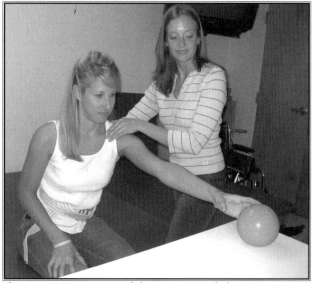

Figure 4-4. Assessment of dynamic sitting balance.

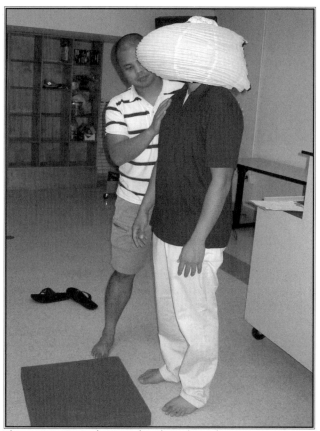

Figure 4-5. Typical set-up for clinical test for sensory interaction on balance (CTSIB).

important information can be obtained from assessing *static* and *dynamic* balance. Static balance is the patient's ability to maintain an upright position in a steady, nonmoving state, while dynamic balance is the patient's ability to maintain an upright posture while performing activities that move the COG within or outside of the BOS (Figure 4-4). Several textbooks[13,20] indicate the protocols for assigning functional grades for balance; however, the reliability and validity of these tests have not been assessed. Such functional grades are used routinely in the clinic environment despite the lack of evidence-based research to support them at this time.

To test static balance, the patient is asked to sit up (sitting balance) or stand (standing balance). Appropriate guarding is necessary to ensure that the patient is safe when performing these activities. To test dynamic balance, the patient is asked to sit or stand and perform activities that move his or her COG outside the BOS (eg, reaching forward or sideways). A sample balance grade scale is presented below:

- **Normal** – The patient is able to maintain steady balance without support (static) and is able to maintain steady position after being maximally challenged (dynamic) (challenge could be in the form of perturbations [push] or asking the patient to perform activities that will make the COG fall outside the BOS).

- **Good** – The patient is able to maintain balance without support (static) and is able to maintain position after being moderately challenged (dynamic).

- **Fair** – The patient is able to maintain position with handhold (static) and is able to accept minimal challenge (dynamic).

- **Poor** – The patient requires assistance of handhold and clinician support to maintain position (static) and is unable to accept any challenge (dynamic).

- **Unable** – The patient needs maximal assistance to maintain position.

Other tests of balance can be employed as a measure of the patient's stability in the sitting or standing position. In the Romberg test,[21] the patient is asked to stand with feet together with eyes open, then with eyes closed. A positive Romberg sign is noted if the patient is able to maintain an upright position with eyes open but demonstrates excessive sway or loses balance with eyes closed. The Sharpened Romberg test is done in the same position except that the feet are placed in a tandem position.[21] These two tests are used to determine increased sway, which may be due to problems within the somatosensory, visual, or vestibular systems or may demonstrate signs of cerebellar involvement. The Clinical Test for Sensory Interaction on Balance (CTSIB) is another test that assesses the integrity of the various systems responsible for balance (Figure 4-5). This test involves six sensory conditions in which trials of each condition are performed. The testing equipment includes a thick foam pad and a

Table 4-4
Terminology and Definitions of Assistance Levels

Term	Definition
Independent	Patient consistently performs the skill safely with no one present and in a timely manner. If an assistive device is needed, include the name of the device.
Supervision or Setup	Patient performs 100% of the task but requires verbal cueing, someone standing by, or someone must set up needed items.
Contact guarding	Patient performs 100% of the task but person assisting gives full attention to patient and has hands on patient for possible assistance or possible loss of balance.
Minimal assistance	Patient expends 75% or more of the effort for the task.
Moderate assistance	Patient expends 50% to 75% of the effort for the task.
Maximum assistance	Patient expends 25% to 50% of the effort for the task.
Dependent	Patient expends less than 25% of the effort for the task.

Adapted from Guide for the Uniform Data Set for Medical Rehabilitation (Adult FIM). *Version 4.0. Buffalo, NY: State University of New York at Buffalo; 1993..*

modified Japanese lantern. The CTSIB is described fully in the text *Neurological Rehabilitation*, edited by Umphred.[22] Other tests of balance have been developed and can be classified under Standardized Functional Tests (see page 52 for examples).

Functional Ability

As with all patients, it is important to examine the functional abilities of patients with neurologic pathologies. The most common functional mobility skills assessed include the following: rolling from side to side, transitioning from supine to sitting and sitting to supine, maintaining a sitting position, transfers, transitioning from sitting to standing and standing to sitting, maintaining a standing position, and locomotion in the form of walking or propelling a w/c. When working with pediatric patients, other postures and mobility skills may also be assessed, such as rolling prone to and from supine; transitioning into and out of different postures or positions (eg, prone on elbows, quadruped, kneeling, or half-kneeling), and coming to standing from the floor. PTs and PTAs must be aware that multiple patterns can be used to accomplish a mobility skill, and all of these patterns can be considered "normal." For example, when rolling from supine to the right side, a person could initiate the roll in several ways: using the left shoulder, reaching across with the left arm, using the pelvis, bending the left hip and knee and reaching across with the knee, or using the head. All of these patterns can be considered normal patterns for rolling.

When assessing functional ability, it is important to perform a qualitative assessment of the mobility skill or task and to document the findings by (1) describing the motion as normal or abnormal (if abnormal, including a description of what is observed), (2) describing how much, if any, assistance is necessary for the skill to be completed, and at times, (3) listing the amount of time it takes the patient to complete the task. Unfortunately, there is no universally accepted terminology for describing assistance levels. A sample terminology for describing assistance levels is derived from the Functional Independence Measure (FIM [Uniform Data System for Medical Rehabilitation, Amherst, NY])[23] and is listed in Table 4-4. When selecting the appropriate term, it is imperative that the PTA focuses on the amount of effort put forth by the patient for the task, not the effort of the PTA. A common mistake that health care students make is to describe how much effort they are putting forth for a task, not the amount of effort the patient is putting forth.

Use of Standardized Impairment and Functional Tests

Standardized tests have been developed as tools that aim to provide an objective assessment of a patient's impairments or functional performance. There are many tests available to the physical therapy community, and it is important to identify those tests that are truly important, valid, and reliable in assessing the patient's performance. While some tests have been developed for the elderly population, they are used for adult clients with neurologic pathologies. Examples of these tests are included as follows.

Berg Balance Scale

The Berg balance scale[24] involves the assessment of a patient's balance via the performance of several everyday tasks. It has been developed to test elderly patients' level of balance. This test involves 14 balance items, and the patient is rated in their ability to perform these tasks and given a score of 0, 1, 2, 3, or 4. This test takes 15 to 20 min to complete. Examples of tasks include sitting to standing, standing unsupported, reaching forward with outstretched arm while standing, retrieving an object from the floor, and turning 360 degrees. The higher the total score on the measure, the more independent the patient is.

Functional Reach Test

The functional reach test[25] has been developed by Duncan for use with an elderly population and involves the measurement of the patient's ability to reach forward while in standing, without falling (eg, how many centimeters the person can reach forward). Normative values have been determined and fall risk indicated for those individuals who test below specified levels. This test takes 5 min to complete.

Performance Oriented Mobility Assessment

The performance oriented mobility assessment test[26] (also known as the Tinetti Assessment Tool) has been developed for use with an elderly population and has balance and gait components. The test involves 16 items, some scored as 0 or 1 and others scored as a 0, 1, or 2. This test takes 10 to 15 min to complete. The patient is given a score corresponding to his or her performance on certain maneuvers (ie, coming to standing, initial standing balance, turning, initiating gait, step symmetry, and sway of trunk during gait). Cutoff scores have been determined to indicate fall risk.

Timed Up and Go

The timed up and go (TUG)[27] involves using a timer (stopwatch) to measure the time it takes for an individual seated in a firm chair with arms and a back rest to get up, walk 3 meters, turn around, walk back 3 meters, and then sit down. Normative values indicating an increased fall risk have been determined. Time to completion is dependent upon the patient but typically takes 5 min or less.

Fugl-Meyer Assessment of Physical Performance

The Fugl-Meyer assessment of physical performance[28,29] test has been developed for use with adult patients who have suffered a stroke and assesses motor impairment by looking at motor recovery, balance, sensation, and motion. This is a long test, taking 30 to 40 min to complete. Items are given a score of 0, 1, or 2 and include sensation in the UEs and LEs, movement in and out of synergy patterns, and sitting and standing balance.

Motor Assessment Scale

The motor assessment scale (MAS)[30] was developed by Carr and Shepherd for use with adult patients who have suffered a stroke, and it includes nine items, incorporating functional movements and tone. It takes 15 to 30 min to complete, depending upon the patient. Items include moving from supine to sidelying, supine to sitting on the side of the bed, walking, UE function, and general tone. Each item is given a score of 0, 1, 2, 3, 4, 5, or 6.

The Barthel Index[31]

The Barthel Index was developed by a PT over 40 years ago and measures the amount of assistance required by an individual on 10 items of mobility and self-care ADLs. It has been developed for use with adults with any diagnosis. The tool takes 5 to 20 min to complete, and each item is given a score of 0, 5, 10, or 15. Items include feeding, dressing, bathing, toilet transfers, transfers from w/c to bed, walking, and stair climbing.

Functional Independence Measure

The functional independence measure (FIM)[23] has been designed to assess the degree of assistance required by a patient at the beginning and end of rehabilitation. It is part of the Uniform Data System for Medical Rehabilitation (UDSMR), which collects data from participating rehabilitation facilities and issues summary reports of the data gathered. It consists of 18 items measuring physical, psychological, and social function. These are scored 1, 2, 3, 4, 5, 6, or 7. The physical items include self-care activities; bed, toilet, and tub transfers; ambulation; and w/c mobility.

CONCLUSION

This chapter provides the clinician an overview of the examination process, including the protocols for administration of more common tests that can be delegated to the PTA. Although the process of evaluation is the responsibility of the PT, the PTA can obtain additional information following the initial examination and evaluation regarding the patient's presenting movement dysfunction. This information flow further enhances the decision-making process and allows for the optimum level of care, leading to improved outcomes.

CHAPTER QUESTIONS

1. What is the purpose of a neuromuscular examination?

2. When is it appropriate for a PTA to be involved in the examination of patients with neurologic pathologies?

3. Which neuromuscular examination procedures may the PTA perform?

4. Describe the procedure for testing each of the following:

    a. Attention

    b. Short-term memory

    c. Light touch

    d. Superficial pain

    e. Proprioception

    f. Stereognosis

    g. Muscle tone

    h. Romberg test

5. What are three tests that can be used to assess balance?

6. When documenting the amount of assistance a patient needs for a transfer, what does the term moderate assistance mean?

Suggested author answers are available at www.slackbooks.com/neuroquestions.

REFERENCES

1. *Guide to Physical Therapist Practice.* 2nd ed. Alexandria, Va: American Physical Therapy Association; 2001:679.

2. Magee DJ. *Orthopedic Physical Assessment.* 4th ed. Philadelphia, Pa: WB Saunders; 2002.

3. Richardson JK, Iglarsh ZA. *Orthopedic Physical Therapy.* Philadelphia, Pa: WB Saunders; 1994.

4. Schmitz TJ. Sensory assessment. In: O'Sullivan SB, Schmitz TJ, eds. *Physical Rehabilitation: Assessment and Treatment.* 4th ed. Philadelphia, Pa: FA Davis; 2001.

5. Bottomley JM. *Quick Reference Dictionary for Physical Therapy.* 2nd ed. Thorofare, NJ: SLACK Incorporated; 2003.

6. Allen DD, Widner GL. Tone abnormalities. In: Cameron MH, ed. *Physical Agents in Rehabilitation: From Research to Practice.* 2nd ed. St Louis, Mo: Saunders; 2003.

7. Giuliani V. Spasticity and motor control. In: Montgomery PC, Connolly BH, eds. *Clinical Applications for Motor Control.* Thorofare, NJ: SLACK Incorporated; 2003.

8. Shumway-Cook A, Woollacott MH. *Motor Control: Theory and Practical Applications.* 2nd ed. Philadelphia, Pa: Lippincott, Williams, and Wilkins; 2001.

9. O'Sullivan SO. Stroke. In: O'Sullivan SB, Schmitz TJ, eds. *Physical Rehabilitation: Assessment and Treatment.* 4th ed. Philadelphia, Pa: FA Davis; 2001:532.

10. Bohannon RW, Smith MB. Interrater reliability of a modified Ashworth scale of muscle spasticity. *Phys Ther.* 1987;67(2):206-207.

11. Hislop HJ, Montgomery J. *Daniels and Worthingham's Muscle Testing: Techniques of Manual Examination.* 7th ed. Philadelphia, Pa: WB Saunders; 2002.

12. Kendall F, McCreary EK. *Muscles: Testing and Function.* 4th ed. Philadelphia, Pa: Lippincott, Williams, and Wilkins; 1993.

13. O'Sullivan SO. Assessment of motor function. In: O'Sullivan SB, Schmitz TJ, eds. *Physical Rehabilitation: Assessment and Treatment.* 4th ed. Philadelphia, PA: FA Davis; 2001.

14. Barnes MR, Crutchfield CA, Heriza CB. *The Neurophysiological Basis of Patient Treatment, Vol II: Reflexes in Motor Development.* Atlanta, Ga: Stokesville Publishing; 1978.

15. Fiorentino M. *Reflex Testing Methods for Evaluating CNS Development.* 2nd ed. Springfield, Ill: Charles C Thomas; 1981.

16. Schmitz TJ. Coordination assessment. In: O'Sullivan SB, Schmitz TJ eds. *Physical Rehabilitation: Assessment and Treatment.* 4th ed. Philadelphia, Pa: FA Davis; 2001.

17. Tan JC. *Practical Manual of Physical Medicine and Rehabilitation.* St Louis, Mo: Mosby; 1998.

18. DeMyer W. *Technique of the Neurologic Examination.* 4th ed. New York, NY: McGraw Hill; 1994.

19. Nahser L. Sensory neuromuscular, and biomechanical contributions to human balance. In: Duncan P, ed. *Balance.* Alexandria, Va: American Physical Therapy Association; 1990:5.

20. Mahoney F, Barthel D. Functional evaluation: the Barthel index. *Md State Med J.* 1965;14:61-65.

21. Lanska DJ, Goetz DG. Romberg's sign: development, adaptation, and adoption in the 19th century. *Neurology.* 2000;55:1201-1206.

22. Allison L, Fuller K. Balance and vestibular disorders. In: Umphred DA, ed. *Neurological Rehabilitation.* 4th ed. St Louis, Mo: Mosby; 2001.

23. *Guide for the Uniform Data Set for Medical Rehabilitation (Adult FIM).* Version 4.0. Buffalo, NY: State University of New York at Buffalo; 1993.

24. Berg K. Measuring balance in the elderly: validation of an instrument. *Physiother Canada.* 1989;41:304.

25. Duncan PW, et al. Functional reach: a new clinical measure of balance. *J Gerontol.* 1990;45:M192.

26. Tinetti ME. Performance-oriented assessment of mobility problems in the elderly. *J Am Geriatr Soc.* 1986;34:119-126.

27. Podsiadlo D, Richardson S. The timed "up and go": a test of basic functional mobility for frail elderly persons. *J Am Geriatr Soc.* 1991;39:142.

28. Fugl-Meyer A, Jaasko L, Leyman I, et al. The post-stroke hemiplegic patient: a method for evaluation of physical performance. *Scand J Rehab Med.* 1976;7:13.

29. Duncan PW, Propst M, Nelson SG. Reliability of the Fugl-Meyer assessment of sensorimotor recovery following cerebrovascular accident. *Physical Ther.* 1983;63(10):1606-1610.

30. Carr JH, Shepherd RB. Investigation of a new motor assessment scale for stroke patients. *Physical Ther.* 1985;65(2):175-180.

31. Montgomery PC, Connolly BH. *Clinical Applications for Motor Control.* Thorofare, NJ: SLACK Incorporated; 2003.

Chapter

5

INTERVENTION PROCEDURES

Darcy Umphred, PT, PhD, FAPTA

KEY WORDS

functional training
impairment training
motor programs
sensory retraining

CHAPTER OBJECTIVES

- Differentiate the categories of intervention into practice only, functional training and retraining, impairment training, and hands-on guidance in order to train motor patterns for both balancing impairment problems and functional activities.

- Identify when intervention is not improving stated goals.

- Identify when patient is successfully performing functional activity without assistance or guidance.

INTRODUCTION

Intervention, as defined in the *Guide to Physical Therapy Practice*, is "purposeful and skilled interaction of the PT with the patient/client."[1] Although the definition of intervention continues to define the role of the PT, intervention is intertwined in the role of the PTA. To the PT, intervention incorporates (1) coordination, communication, and documentation of services, (2) patient or client related instruction, and (3) direct patient intervention. Within these 3 categories, coordination of services is the only area that should never be delegated to the PTA. Therefore, the PTA needs to develop skills in communication with the PT, other health care practitioners, the patient, and caregivers. Documentation skills, when appropriately delegated, are a critical form of communication with other individuals on the patient's team and with outside organizations such as accreditation organizations and third party payers. Although reexamination becomes a part of the PTA's delegated responsibilities, it is not within the role of the PTA to interpret the examination results unless the PT has clearly identified a treatment plan that incorporates change in relation to patient test results. It is within the PTA's scope of practice to teach both patients and families functional skills, home programs, and discharge programs only if the PT has taken the responsibility of clearly identifying what those skills or programs are. If the PTA is asked to do an initial exam on the patient and interpret the result, to establish a treatment protocol, or to determine that the patient no longer needs service and write a discharge summary, then that PTA is practicing outside the scope of PTA practice and is placing the patient (consumer of a product) at risk and himself or herself liable. Given the previous scenario, a PTA is being misused and the patient given an incorrect perception of the services being provided. This particular area and the problems it creates is becoming an area for claims denial, malpractice, and consumer fraud. It is the PTA's responsibility to identify his or her scope of practice and skill and never place the patient at risk, even when components of intervention have been delegated. The primary role of the PTA within the therapeutic community is direct intervention with the patient. It is very appropriate to delegate treatment interventions to the PTA when the services of the PTA will positively affect patient progress and when the role of either PT or PTA would, similarly, enhance that progress.

Physical therapy interventions encompass a vast area of techniques that incorporate interactions with the cardiopulmonary, integumentary, musculoskeletal, and neuromuscular systems.[1] Although the specific pathology or disease identified by the physician may fall within one of these bodily system categories, PTs and PTAs do not treat disease or pathology; they treat the functional limitations caused by those diseases or pathologies. For that reason, similar physical therapy techniques may be used for multiple medical diagnoses, or multiple physical therapy interventions may be incorporated into a patient's treatment plan although that individual has one specific disease. In order for the PTA to identify risk factors or contraindication signs exhibited by the patient during an intervention, knowledge of human anatomy, physiology, and disease processes are always a part of a PTA's education. It is the PTA's responsibility to report to the PT any questionable behaviors of the patient at the beginning, during, or at the conclusion of an intervention. If the PTA has any question or concern regarding the health of the patient and/or appropriateness of the intervention itself, that PTA is bound by law and ethics to communicate that concern to the PT as quickly as possible. For that reason, the PTA is often asked to check heart rate (HR), BP, skin color, pain levels, depth and rate of breathing, levels of consciousness, and cognitive response patterns of patients. These assessments become a part of ongoing intervention. Before the patient interventions are delegated, the PT has the legal responsibility to check all contraindications and risk factors to guarantee that the patient can safely receive treatment. Even though this check should make

the PTA feel safe that a patient will not be harmed by intervention, monitoring patient signs is a critical component to maintenance of that safety parameter.

This text discusses clients who have had some form of CNS disease, pathology, or trauma with resultant motor dysfunction of a variety of types. Specific intervention recommendations for specific medical diagnoses can be found in Chapters 7 through 13 of this text. In addition to discussion of specific medical diagnoses and physical therapy interventions, a chapter on cardiopulmonary impact on motor dysfunction will also lead the PTA to avenues of intervention interactions, strategies, and ways to enhance patient performance. The concept of intervention through direct patient contact will be the focus of this chapter.

CATEGORIES OF INTERVENTION

Delegated intervention to a PTA will fall within one of four categories, each category having a slightly different focus. Those categories are (1) functional activity training, (2) impairment training, (3) hands-on guidance by the therapist, and (4) somato-sensory retraining. The first three categories primarily discuss motor dysfunction of the patient, and the fourth category encompasses individuals with sensory or processing problems that result in motor dysfunction. If the goal of physical therapy treatment is purposeful and meaningful functional movement activities, then the ultimate goal of every treatment program should be empowering the patient to achieve independent functional control over movement within the respective environment, whenever possible.

FUNCTIONAL TRAINING

Intervention that focuses on ADLs or leisure time activities, such as group sports (eg, basketball, baseball), individual sports (eg, golfing, swimming, running, fly-fishing), and group or individual physical enhancement activities (eg, martial arts training, water aerobics, treadmill, or elliptical training), fall within the category of *functional training*. When intervention focuses on specific activities, the patient needs practice in order to regain or maintain skill in movement expression as identified by the functional motor strategies needed to perform the activity. If the intervention program goals include performance of any one of these skills, then the functional motor plan is available to the patient and only practice and variance is needed for perfection. In this case, a PT should definitely delegate this activity to the PTA. As the patient improves skill in these activities, delegation may be given to family members or caregivers, when those people are available and willing. Functional training in ADLs includes bed mobility, coming to sit and stand from various surfaces, transferring onto and from various chairs (eg, a w/c or a toilet), transferring into and out of a shower or tub, ambulation on all types of surfaces with various types of visual surrounds (eg, normal lighting, darkened environment, or a moving surround), dressing and undressing, and using adaptive devices (eg, crutches, a cane, or a walker). In a home health environment, the PTA may be asked to do additional functional training such as teaching and practicing bathing, eating, and cooking; however, more often the occupational therapist (OT) and/or a certified occupational therapy assistant (COTA) will be responsible for the patient's practice with these activities. The goal of functional activity training is not to guide the patient with the hands-on skill of the therapist, but rather to guarantee that the patient is performing these activities safely and with repetitive practice. Repetitive and random practice schedules will solidify responses to these activities as automatic, the patient no longer needing to think through the steps of the movement and, instead, performing the activity without effort in a feed-forward program. (See Chapter 3 for practice variations with regard to functional training.) Many times, patients will desire a high level of motor performance as their goal and become very frustrated that the treatment program focuses on activities that individuals assume they can do or should be able to do. For example, if an individual wants to return to fly-fishing at his cabin on a lake, determining how he will get from his cabin to the beach and whether he will sit or stand while fishing will help the therapist communicate to the patient why he is practicing sit to stand and ambulation activities. Once the patient understands that practice will lead to the ultimate goal of fly-fishing, the individual usually becomes a motivated and compliant patient. Functional training should be the ultimate goal of any sequential treatment plan. Understanding the components critical for any functional movement leads to the second category of intervention strategies.

IMPAIRMENT TRAINING

This category is associated with interventions that are system specific and that focus upon a component of a movement that has resulted in dysfunction within the functional activity. There are many subcategories in this area of treatment. Impairments may be the direct result of *musculoskeletal problems* such as ROM limitations, muscle weakness due to disuse, biomechanical malalignment due to joint problems, or leg length discrepancy. A treatment plan with a goal to eliminate these impairments certainly would be well delegated to a PTA.

Similarly, *cardiopulmonary* or *peripheral vascular disease* can create many types of pain, poor endurance to exercise, and even lightheadedness and confusion when the oxygen (O_2) levels drop. For that reason, the PTA will often be asked to monitor breathing, HR, BP, and O_2 level using a finger gauge and pain scales regardless of the medical diagnosis of the patient. If the PTA ever has concerns with this cardiopulmonary/peripheral vascular system, it should be communicated to the PT of record. If that PT is unavailable, concern should be shared with another PT, a nurse, or physician.

Areas of *integumentary* problems encompass medical complications from ulcers, burns, reddened areas, or any unusual reactions of the skin before, during, or following a therapeutic intervention. These impairments are especially important to understand if the patient is being asked to practice specific activities that entail movement across a surface (eg, rolling, coming to sit, or sitting for an extended period of time). Similarly, if a scar limits ROM and thus movement function itself, then interventions that mobilize the tissue using therapeutic modalities to increase tissue elasticity will be delegated to the PTA. The PTA must then be aware that those modalities can also burn the patient, especially if the skin or vascular system cannot accommodate to the modality. Patients with long-term contractures following CNS injury often have skin integrity problems. The skin becomes very fragile and thin and, thus, splits easily if ROM over the joint creates too much stretch at too high a rate. If the skin splits at the joint, it will not only cause pain but also an open wound. The PTA will need to work slowly and pay constant attention to the skin reaction when treating most patients after neurological insults with contractures and limited skin mobility.

Impairments within the *neuromuscular system* include activity states of the spinal motor generators (hyper- or hypotonicity and rigidity), stereotypic or reflexive patterns within functional movement (eg, flexion and extension synergies, reflexive response such as ATNR and STNR, and + supporting reactions), balance problems (eg, sensory input and balance synergy problems), resting fluctuation in motor tonicity (nonintentional tremor), fluctuation in motor tonicity upon purposeful activity (athetosis, ataxia), reaction time to perturbations, rate of movement (how fast or slow the CNS will run a program), cognitive understanding of the task (perception, levels of consciousness, and distractibility), and attitude toward the activity (motivation, levels of emotional stability, and ethnic bias). A brief description and some intervention suggestions will be included within each subsection of this practice pattern.

Range of Motion

In many physical therapy clinics, ROM is delegated to a PTA. When the only limitation is musculoskeletal, the complexity and skill of performing ROM on a patient need not be difficult. When treating a patient with a neuromuscular ROM limitation, a variety of parameters must be considered before delegation. They are as follows. During the ROM, does the joint stay in a correct biomechanical position throughout the range? Is the limitation of range due to hypertonicity around the joint? If so, what muscles are hypertonic and how are they interacting in patterns of movement? With introduction of a rotatory pattern, can the limb be moved into and out of the tightness? What rotatory patterns are limited? If rotation is incorporated into the ROM exercise, does the hypertonicity decrease? If so, does the patient demonstrate joint stabilization, or are muscles around the joint hypotonic? These are questions the PT should consider before delegating this activity. Once the responsibility has been delegated, the PTA should continue to ask these questions. When the range increases and/or the tone around the joint changes, the PTA should report that change to the PT, and potential intervention strategies for impairment training may need modifying. The PTA must always remember to stabilize the joint throughout the motion. The PTA must make sure the pattern of motion used by the patient to perform the activity is normal without substitutions of muscles not normally engaged during the specific motion. The PTA may be asked to instruct the patient to perform the activity within a certain degree of motion and to slowly increase that range as the patient demonstrates normal motor control. If the patient complains of pain, often the cause of pain is malalignment of the joint and can be corrected by moving the joint into a better biomechanical position. As long as the patient is able to correct the joint alignment, then the PTA is impairment training. Once the PTA does the correction for the patient, it is no longer impairment training, but hands-on intervention. Fear of pain during ROM often causes muscle splinting, which leads to incorrect alignment of the joint(s). That fear is often associated with the memory of some other health care practitioner having moved the limb when the patient did not have any control; that movement might then create an initial pain response as well as the memory of the experience. The PTA needs to teach the patient that pain is not okay and that the patient needs to tell the practitioner when it hurts. The PTA must recognize a pain grimace response in addition to requesting verbal communication of pain. If the patient is being assisted through part of the range that may have pain, the patient must trust that the PTA will stop once pain is present. If not, the patient will continue splinting or guarding the joint. Gaining the patient's trust often results in eliminating splinting due to fear of pain and simultaneously causes a gain in ROM.

States of the Spinal Motor Generators (Hyper- or Hypotonicity and Rigidity)

A common impairment seen in patients with CNS damage is an altered state of the spinal motor generators. This altered state can create a variety of movement dysfunctions. When the motor generators are firing at too high a rate, the result will create muscle reactions that are hypertonic and/or reactive to stretch. Usually, when these generators are firing and causing *hypertonicity*, the response is not seen in an individual muscle but is seen in patterns of muscle interactions referred to as synergies. An agonist, or isolated muscle, is naturally linked to other muscles (agonistic synergy) that work closely with a particular muscle to perform specific functional movements. Similarly, if the generators are not firing adequately in a muscle group, then the behavioral response will often be *hypotonicity* within a pattern of movement. Except in specific peripheral nervous system injury or disease, behavior responses are more likely to be seen in patterns. At times, a limb many have a hypertonic agonistic synergy while the antagonistic synergy is hypotonic. If both the agonistic synergy and the antagonistic synergy are hypertonic, then movement in both directions is limited. *Hypertonicity* is an abnormal state of the motor generators and usually follows hypotonicity within muscle groups and instability of the joint. Because of hypotonicity, the body will naturally try to maintain joint integrity and create additional tone in other muscles around the joint structure. Instructing the patient to do slow relaxing rotation away from the tight pattern along with deep breathing often lowers the state of the motor pool and decreases the hypertonicity. The PTA must remember that decreasing hypertonicity does not guarantee stability of the joint or joints or volitional control over movement. Many times, decreasing hypertonicity forces the therapist into a hands-on approach to intervention versus impairment training, due to the decreased state of the motor pool resulting in hypotonicity or weakness. At times, the PT will delegate to the PTA a functional activity within which impairment training and control over specific aspects of a motor program are incorporated. An example of this type of combination would be using a body-weight support harness while having a client walk on a treadmill. The functional activity practiced is walking and varying the rate and incline of the treadmill-walking track in order to accommodate to impairment problems. The motion itself will trigger a stepping program; the PTA should not need to assist in the walking. The body-weight support system eliminates the need for full power and programming for posture and movement during the functional activity. By partially supporting the body weight, the patient is expected to control the entire feed-forward walking program and all its component programs within his or her capable limits. The PTA can change the rate of walking, the power needed to generate force during the walking, the incline or decline of the movement, and other components of walking (eg, hard and soft surfaces of the shoe). All these aspects are considered impairment training because the patient is forced to self-correct the programming within the limits of the impairments. As soon as the PTA needs to guide the movement itself (eg, picking up the foot and placing it in its correct biomechanical position), the body support intervention is not impairment training but would be considered within the third category of intervention. In this third area, discussed on page 62, the PT or PTA needs to use hands-on control to guide motor responses in order to keep the patient within an acceptable parameter of performance. Given the intervention example of body-weight supported walking, the PTA would be delegated both functional and impairment training within the patient's control parameters.

Stereotypic or Reflexive Patterns Within Functional Movement

Patients' movement responses following CNS injury often include stereotypic or reflexive patterns of movement (eg, flexion and extension synergies, reflexive response such as ATNR and STNR, + supporting reactions). These programs are often the only patterns available to the patient's CNS when an external or peripheral stimulus demands or requires a motor response. Similarly, when neuronal loops within the CNS trigger involuntary motor response patterns, the motor system drives those available programs. Thus, individuals in lowered states of consciousness may exhibit hypertonic synergistic patterns of motor responses (eg, extension synergies incorporating hip and knee extension, internal rotation, adduction of the hip, plantarflexion, and pronation of the foot). Most synergies and reflexive patterns are inherent or pre-programmed within the CNS and have been incorporated within early motor development. These patterns reflect combinations of movement patterns in response to demands placed upon the CNS from peripheral input systems and internal feedback loops. Specific reflex responses have been identified in Chapter 4. Specific impairment training techniques that discourage repetitive practice of these stereotypic patterns can be found in Chapters 7, 8, 10, 11 and 12. An easy concept to remember is that the opposite movement pattern from the involuntary pattern is often the solution to gaining or regaining motor control. By activating the antagonistic synergy, the hypertonic

synergy or reflex pattern will often automatically be dampened through the interaction of programs within the CNS. If the patient is able to independently run these antagonistic programs, or components of these programs, then the therapeutic environment is considered impairment training. The patient's CNS must be able to control both agonistic and antagonistic synergy patterns and various combinations of muscle patterns within those synergies to move to functional training. If the patient's motor programming is stuck in one synergy or two stereotypic patterns, the patient will be very limited in responses to the demands of life. These stereotypic patterns often force the biomechanical position of joints to be malaligned, leading to secondary musculoskeletal impairments at a future time. A physical therapy goal will generally encompass reduction of hypertonicity and obligatory responses of stereotypic programs. The PTA needs to remember that the causation of hypertonicity synergies is often instability within joint structures. Similarly, the use of reflexive or stereotypic patterns is the CNS's response to environmental demands, which require gravitational postural responses. In order to empower the patient's CNS to gain or regain the fluid control over multiple patterns of movement, the environment must be modified so that the response can be appropriate to the demand within the environment. This may require environmental adaptation and/or hands-on guidance to guarantee the CNS is in control of the programs, regardless of how limiting that might be early in the therapeutic intervention process. Again, if, by adapting or limiting the environment, the patient is capable of initiating and maintaining a normal movement sequence, then the PTA is impairment training. Once the PTA adds hands-on control of the movement itself, the activity is no longer impairment training and then falls under the next major section within the subcategory of Handling (see page 62).

Balance Problems

Balance, as a functional activity, requires the patient to control all programs needed to either maintain the body's BOS over its COG or to replace the body's COG back under its BOS (Figure 5-1a and 5-1b). Balance training can focus upon maintaining or regaining balance once an anticipated or unexpected perturbation occurs. A perturbation occurs when a directional force causes the body to react in order to maintain or regain balance (COG) over a specific BOS. That BOS may be one foot, both feet, a foot and a knee (one-half kneel), both hips (sitting), or the entire body (the trunk, head, and hips) when a person is lying down and rolling from side to side. The ability to react to the perturbation is based on sensory input from the proprioceptive, vestibular, and visual systems and inherent balance synergy programs (ankle, hip, and

Figure 5-1a. Balance: Maintaining COG within the existing BOS.

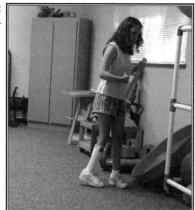

Figure 5-1b. Balance: Replacing BOS back under the COG, stepping.

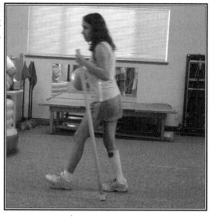

stepping). In addition, when the patient is instructed in the use of a support system (eg, a cane, walker, or transfer bar), a therapist needs to consider the balance within the points of support used by the individual for ambulation or movement from one base to another. Generally, there is a balance aspect to all movement and, thus, a patient will incorporate balance programming as part of the functional activity while moving. Balance impairment training includes creating environments in which the patients will (1) perturb themselves (eg, by weight shifting during reaching), (2) perturb and replace their COG (eg, by stepping or protecting themselves with their arms when falling), and (3) regain balance when an external force, either anticipated (recognized because the perturbation occurs ahead of time) or unanticipated (it just happens), perturbs them during a movement activity (eg, being bumped or shoved by someone else). The PTA is often asked to encourage patients to automatically react to weight shifting during reaching, transferring, and ambulating. The only way those automatic reactions can be observed is when the PTA either distracts the patient's attention during a movement or perturbs the COG without notice.

Resting Fluctuation in Motor Tonicity (Nonintentional Tremor)

Patients with diseases within the basal ganglia or associated pathways often have resting tremors in the hands, tongue, and even the feet. These movements are involuntary, in a specific flowing movement pattern and illustrate a lack of control or inhibition by the CNS to some automatic motor programming. The tremors are exaggerated when the patient has strong emotional reactions to the environment. Often, the tremors can be decreased with slow deep breathing, visualization by the patient of a relaxing environment (eg, picturing a waterfall or watching the wave action of the ocean), and weight bearing of the extremities. Nonintentional tremors usually are not

functionally limiting. The patient must determine whether the movement is socially limiting.

Fluctuation in Motor Tonicity Upon Purposeful Activity (Athetosis, Ataxia)

Patients that have cerebellar problems or motor control problems over certain *motor programs* may have fluctuation of motor tone when moving. If a patient lacks the postural programming to stabilize the joints during movement but has the power and range to generate the movement program, the patient will have problems controlling the rate or speed of the movement and the ability to slow down or reverse the movement during functional activities. The movement often seems too powerful for the activity, and the patient often overshoots the target. The movements themselves are less exaggerated during weight-bearing activities. Thus, patients can practice movement with weighted vests, THERA-BAND (Hygenic Corporation, Akron, Ohio), or theratubing used as resistance and compression to a movement during reaching and the swing phase of gait. If the patients can don the weighted vest or belt themselves and the PTA is to observe and guard during the activity, this intervention would be impairment training. If the PTA needs to apply the resistance and/or compression during a movement, then it is hands-on intervention and not considered impairment training.

Reaction Time to Perturbations

Reaction time to a perturbation is based upon three important aspects of the CNS. First, the brain must receive accurate and nonconflicting sensory information from proprioceptive, vestibular, and visual peripheral receptors. Second, the brain must process this information at various levels, and third, the CNS must select and control the correct motor programs in order to respond appropriately. Thus, the PTA may be instructed in the direction and force of perturbations within specific positions in order to impairment train this function.

Rate of Movement and the Ability to Alter Rate

As individuals grow and learn to control movements, they simultaneously learn to control the rate or speed of that movement. As children learn to walk, they also learn to walk slower and faster. As the rate increases, the walking will turn into running. A PTA may be instructed to teach a patient walking using a walker. Initially, the patient will walk very slowly and should progress to better control and a faster progression. With CNS damage and relearning, often the patient is taught to walk while cognitively thinking about each aspect of the program. Pick up the walker, step with the right foot, pick up the walker, and then step with the left foot. As the patient has never walked with a walker, this is a new motor program. The PTA needs to remember that the patient once had a rate of walking that was normal for that person. It may have been as slow as the movement when using the walker, but more often, it would have been faster. If the PTA needs to impairment train in this area, then the patient needs to practice the movement at various speeds. This impairment training can be accomplished by using a metronome, a forced stepping environment such as a treadmill, or by the PTA actually holding onto the walker and pulling the patient forward to increase the rate of the stepping reaction.

Cognitive Understanding of the Task

There are areas of CNS processing that are not considered motor but directly affect motor performance. Perception, levels of consciousness, and distractibility all affect motor control. The perceptual problems and residual movement dysfunction following CNS damage are huge. The PTA is not expected to evaluate or analyze these problems and their impact on movement. The PT is responsible for clearly describing both the movements and the environment in which the patient is to practice. For example, if a patient overshoots a target and then self-corrects to the target, it is a perceptual problem (praxis). If a patient tries to self-correct the movement throughout a trajectory toward the target, it is a motor control problem (ataxia). That difference needs to be recognized by the PTA, but interpretation of its consequences needs to be determined by the PT. The PT should be told when the patient changes behaviors or motor responses, whether those responses seem better or worse than when first observed. These changes may be due to perceptual learning and improvement or motor control itself, but that analysis, again, is not the responsibility of the PTA.

Attitude Toward the Activity

The patient's emotional system plays a key role in regulation of muscle tone, of compliance to perform the activity, of belief in the importance of the activity and in its relationship to life, and in his or her ethnic bias toward working with you, the PTA. Similarly, the PTA must acknowledge that those four areas affect the motor responses and attitudes of the practitioner. Many individuals, patients, and practitioners radiate tension into their shoulders and necks throughout a stressful day, which can be recognized by a family member at the end of the day. A patient who has motor control problems to begin with will often exaggerate the problems when under pressure or upset. Similarly, when individuals are depressed, their motor system is also depressed and movement is more difficult and tiring. The PTA needs to be aware of the emotional responses of individuals during therapy. Many times, following CNS insults, patients have less control of emotional reactions, thus, they may get angry more easily, cry more often, and laugh inappropriately. Many of these patients recognize the behavior as inappropriate but cannot control the emotional system. It is very important that the PTA create environments within which the patient can develop motor control of both the neuromuscular and the emotional environment. If lack of success in a task creates anger, the PTA may need to provide more successful outcomes of practice versus error recognition by the patient. Understanding the emotional reactions of a patient, the stimulus that triggered that response, and determining whether it helps or hurts the learning is a skill that clinicians need to develop. If, during a transfer, a therapist demands that a patient stand up, the patient may stand because he (1) feels angry, (2) feels disempowered or humiliated (that he is being treated like a child), or (3) just wants the activity to finish, so the therapist will go away. The patient's emotional reaction will create extensor tone, and that tone will help generate the force needed to stand, but teaching someone to stand on top of anger means that every time the individual wants to stand, he will need to be angry. By controlling the noise, distractions, and rate of success or failure, the PTA can allow the patient to practice the movement activities successfully. Once the motor programs are established, reintroducing emotional and perceptual challenges can be integrated into the functional activity as impairment training. The PTA is responsible for carrying out the established program designed by the PT. When the patient is ready or the CNS seems capable of handling additional stress may be recognized by the PTA and that information given to the PT. The decision to change the environment and make it more complex is the responsibility of the PT, unless the PTA has been given clear parameters to identify and document specific changes in behavior and the activity or components to be changed. Patients will go through phases of adjustment to their respective CNS disease or trauma. Similarly, families will be going through adjustments. There is no guarantee that the patient, the family, or the health care providers will be adjusting in a similar manner or time sequence. Thus, the PTA needs to have some understanding of how adjustments or emotional liability affects motor performance. Refer to Chapter 6 for additional information.

HANDS-ON THERAPEUTIC INTERVENTION OR AUGMENTED TREATMENT INTERVENTION

The goals of using the therapist's hands during therapeutic interventions are as follows:

1. To guide or assist the patients during functional movements.

2. To control specific patterns of movement while preventing stereotypic patterns.

3. To give patients the sensory input as feedback for correct movement control.

4. To allow patients to experience the functional movements that will encourage them to move from one spatial position to another.

5. To create a limited environment where patients can succeed at the desired task.

6. To motivate patients by letting them experience some aspect of success and potential accomplishment toward a desired function.

The PTA may be instructed by the PT to teach the patient by verbally describing, visually demonstrating, or kinesthetically handling through a movement. The PT gives those instructions because the best way for the patient to learn has been identified. This is referred to as a learning style. If this has not been identified, the PTA can try instructing the patient using each style or a combination of the three. It is very important that the PTA know his or her learning style because all of us tend to teach through the style with which we are most comfortable. The preferential style of the PTA may not be the best for the patient. It is the responsibility of all health care practitioners to create the optimal environment for learning, which means, initially, to teach through the style of the patient, and then progress to less optimal styles to allow the patient to adapt to the external world.

Handling Techniques

Techniques that are used to guide a movement from one position to another are considered handling techniques. There are many ways to guide or facilitate movement.[2-8] Techniques such as proprioceptive neuromuscular facilitation[2] (PNF) were initially designed to focus on various motor impairments within specific patterns of movement or various diagonal patterns. The focus of this approach is often strengthening muscle groups, increasing range within specific functional patterns, facilitating agonistic and antagonistic patterns to gain coactivation or stability around joints during both weight-bearing and nonweight-bearing activities (closed and open chain activities), and guiding the patient within patterns to move in horizontal (rolling), coming to sit, standing, and ambulating. A PTA may be introduced to these patterns during school, but development of a high level of skill requires additional training and many hours of practice.

The approach that originally used the term *handling techniques* was the Bobath approach[3]: an approach that, within the United States today, has evolved into a methodology known as Neuro-Developmental Treatment (NDT).[4] Although specific aspects of the approach have changed and the theoretical constructs behind the methodology have incorporated more current theories of motor control, motor learning, and neuroplasticity, many of the techniques remain the same.

A PTA will need to learn how to "handle" or guide a patient in performing the following activities:

1. Rolling over or from side to side in bed.

2. Coming to sit from the horizontal position whether on the floor or in bed.

3. Moving over one's BOS in sitting in order to independently sit for reaching, feeding, donning clothes, etc.

4. Coming to stand from both a horizontal position when on the floor or bed (half kneel to stand or squat to stand) or while rising from a chair (partial squat to stand) in order to reach or prior to initiating walking.

5. Patient is unable to perform an activity due to abnormal muscle function (eg, weakness, hypertonicity, or fluctuation in the state of the motor pool).

6. Perceptual/cognitive problems create movement distortions or level of consciousness prevents interactions.

7. When the patient needs to participate in a successful movement response in order to realize potential within his or her motor control system.

Although entire textbooks[5,9,10] discuss specific handling techniques and patterns of movement to be used to assist patients following CNS insult, the PTA is encouraged to watch individuals move, to shut one's eyes, and to feel the movement as the body rolls over, comes to sit, moves in sitting, rises to standing, and

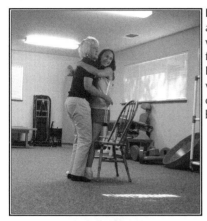

Figure 5-2A. Handling a dependent patient when coming to stand for a transfer: **Incorrect:** therapist is vertical and patient is off vertical and falling backwards.

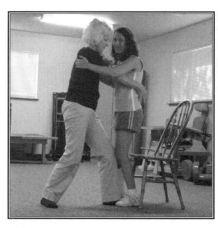

Figure 5-2B. Correct: therapist is slightly off vertical and patient has opportunity to feel vertical or upright posture.

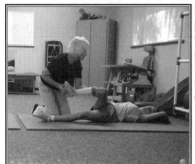

Figure 5-3A. Rolling the patient to the side using the leg or foot as the point of control. Initially handle leg into flexion, slight abduction and external rotation.

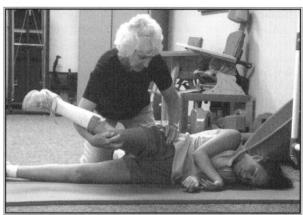

Figure 5-3B. Handle the rotation at the pelvis by maintaining flexion of the hip with slight abduction while guiding into internal rotation.

walks. If a therapist is guiding a patient through a movement, the therapist needs to differentiate feedback that relates to the therapist regarding where the clinician is in space from the feedback that tells the therapist where the patient's body is in space. For example, if a PTA is guiding a patient to standing from a w/c or chair and is guarding the patient by limiting flexion of the patient's knees, then the feet of both the therapist and the patient will occupy space very close to each other. If the therapist is feeling totally stable and vertical, the patient's body cannot be in the same vertical position, and generally, the patient will be leaning backwards and have a sense of falling. If, on the other hand, the therapist feels slightly off balance posterior, then the patient has an opportunity to stand erect. Once the patient is erect, there will be little need to grab the therapist, the patient's biomechanical system will be stacked optimally, the feedback to the patient will be accurate with regards to verticality, and the entire environment will often become more relaxed for both individuals (Figures 5-2A and 5-2B).

Handling techniques are often used to assist a patient to roll over. That patient may be at a low state of consciousness, may have flaccid or hypertonic extremities, may not be able to follow a command, or may not want to move. Generally, it is easiest to assist a patient to roll by handling a LE. If the patient is in supine (on the back) and needs to roll to the side (to relieve body pressure, to change sheets, to prepare to come to sit, or some other functional activity), the

PTA will often handle from one LE. The extremity of choice will be the leg that needs to move in order to attain a sidelying position. That is, if the patient needs to roll to the right, the left leg will need to flex, slightly abduct, and externally rotate initially, followed by flexion and internal rotation to guide the pelvis onto the right side. The opposite would be true if rolling to the left. The specific amount of flexion, abduction, and external rotation needed initially depends upon the patient's muscle tone and ROM. The PTA should guide or control the pelvis at the hip, using the entire leg while moving the leg toward the desired side (Figures 5-3A and 5-3B). The trunk will follow the pelvis either through a body on head or a body on body on head righting reaction.

Handling an individual from sidelying to sit is easily done by applying pressure to the patient's topside anterior iliac crest (AIC) in a downward and posterior direction (Figure 5-4A). The PTA may need to assist the patient's upper body and head. This can be done by supporting the patient from the back, under the bottom side arm (brachial plexus) and head (Figure 5-4B).

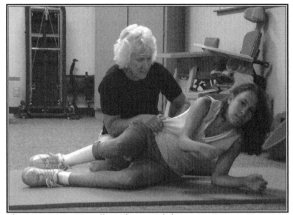

Figure 5-4A. Handling from sidelying to sitting: Pressure is placed in a downward and posterior direction on the topside AIC to guide the topside hip into sitting.

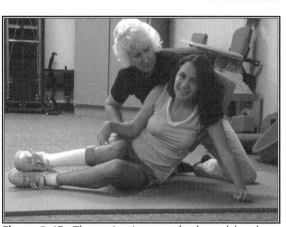

Figure 5-4B. The patient's upper body and head are guided to vertical by supporting the patient's trunk under the brachial plexus and head from the back on the bottom side.

Figure 5-5A. Handling while in sitting: Therapist sitting on a ball while supporting the trunk while placing the arms/shoulder girdle in flexion, abduction, external rotation, and scapular protraction.

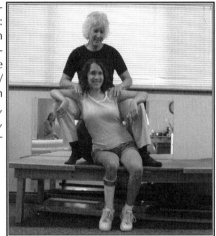

Figure 5-5B. Therapist supporting the patient's trunk with the leg that is kneeling while using the half-kneeling leg to support a shoulder allowing the patient's arm to elevate; externally rotate with shoulder protraction.

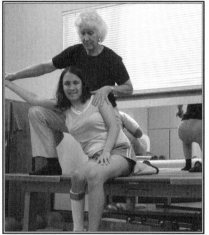

Once the patient is in sitting, a large variety of movement activities can be guided and practiced. The PTA can support the patient from the back while sitting on a ball (Figure 5-5A). In this position, the PTA can control both UEs as well as the trunk to assist in activities such as weight shifting and reaching. The PTA can work on similar activities while in the half-kneel position (Figure 5-5B). The leg that the therapist is using to kneel on can also be used to support the patient's trunk while the half-kneeling leg can be used to direct the patient's UE during reaching and hand to mouth activities. When the therapist is approaching the patient from the front, there are also many patterns that can be facilitated through handling. In Figure 5-5C, the therapist is supporting the patient's arm with a half-kneeling leg. Using the therapist's leg gives the patient a feeling of safety because the arm is resting on a solid body part versus being suspended in space either by the patient's muscle power and ligaments or being held by the therapist. With the therapist's leg supporting the patient's arm, both of

the therapist's hands are free to work on activities such as inhibition of tone in the scapula, shoulder elevation, external rotation, and elbow extension with wrist and finger extension. This UE pattern is usually the antagonistic pattern to that seen in involved UEs of patients following head injuries and strokes. Once high-tone agonistic patterns are relaxed, the PTA can encourage the patient to assist in control over the antagonistic patterns. Ease of movement is the goal, not force production. It would be better to assist the ROM activity while having the patient control or assist as much as possible versus having the patient try so hard that abnormal synergistic patterns of movement are responding in relation to the demand. Remember, movement is effortless. Feel yourself move, and you will recognize how easy it is. The patient should practice that same effortless movement. Handling encourages that practice in a movement controlled by the patient. The entire goal of therapy is always to empower the patient to gain control over all functional activities. Teaching patients to try as hard as they can

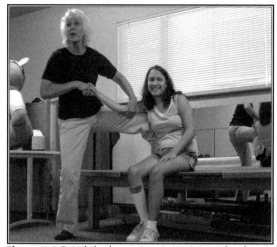

Figure 5-5C. While the patient is in sitting, the therapist supports the patient's involved UE and slowly assists in shoulder elevation, external rotation, and shoulder pro- and retraction.

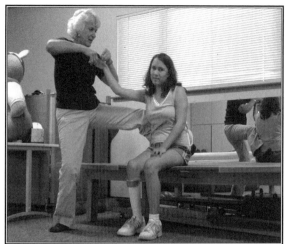

Figure 5-5D. Handling from the front: The therapist handles the patient from the hand and posterior hip. These handling positions should be changed frequently enough to keep the patient from becoming dependent upon the therapists hands.

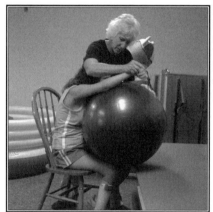

Figure 5-6A. Guiding to stand from the more involved side. The ball is positioned in front of the patient within the patient's lap.

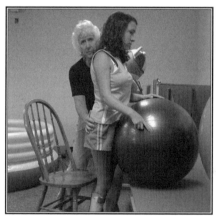

Figure 5-6B. The patient and the ball are guided in order to roll the patient's COG over her feet before bringing her to upright.

will generally create a large amount of hypertonicity and, thus, limit functional control. The PTA can handle the patient's pelvis and pelvic movement by handling the anterior hip through downward and posterior pressure on one side while applying downward and anterior pressure on the opposite posterior pelvic rim. This pressure will facilitate postural extension of the trunk and encourage the patient to sit up and weight shift (Figure 5-5D).

Patients can be brought to standing in many different ways. The patient can be guided to standing from sitting with the therapist guiding from one UE. Usually, the PTA should guide from the more involved UE (Figures 5-6A and 5-6B). If the patient needs maximal assistance to come to stand, then a ball and a high/low mat or table can be used effectively. First, bring the patient forward in the chair. Next, place his UEs over a medium-size ball, which can then be placed on the edge of the high/low mat. Next, bring the patient forward over the ball as the ball rolls onto the mat. The

patient's COG should now be over the feet, with the hips flexed and the trunk supported by the ball. Next, the PTA can press on the high/low mat control device and begin to raise the mat/table. The table will bring the patient to stand in a relaxed manner with maximal support. The arms should remain relaxed in shoulder elevation and scapular protraction. Once the trunk is stacked into a biomechanical position, the PTA may need a counterforce in front of the ball to avoid the ball slipping away from the patient and therapist. Initially, the handling techniques will need to be from the side of the patient. As soon as the patient is relaxed with the trunk resting over the ball with the feet flat, the therapist can reposition his body to the rear of the patient. At that time, the therapist can reach under the patient's upper trunk and guide his upper body toward a vertical posture. Generally, the head will right after the shoulders, and the patient will be standing in a normal upright position. The patient will feel stabilized between the therapist and the ball. Weight shifting can

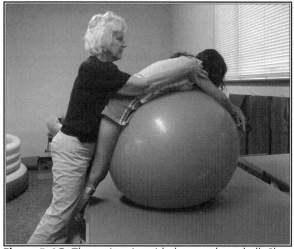

Figure 5-6C. The patient is guided onto a large ball. Slow rocking can be done in this position in order increase relaxation.

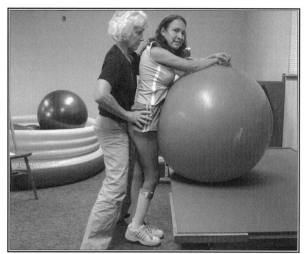

Figure 5-6D. Roll the patient onto her feet while relaxed in order to maintain normal postural extension without causing extensor hypertonicity.

be practiced in order to encourage body support over the feet. If the patient slowly rolls the ball from side to side, forward, and backwards, he will be facilitating his own perturbations for balance and postural reactions. The PTA can also practice partial stand to squat by having the patient or therapist control the table mat's position as it goes up and down. Once the patient can go from stand to sit and back up again, he will usually have the sit to stand pattern within the motor control of his CNS. Therapists often use this same approach on children, using a ball that is large enough to bring the child into standing off the ball (Figures 5-6C and 5-6D).

A PT may ask the PTA to begin ambulation training before the patient comes to standing independently. The PTA must remember that ambulation uses different combinations of motor programs than the sit to stand or stand to sit. The PTA may be asked to stabilize the ankle/knee interactions using an orthotic. Similarly, the PT may want the PTA to instruct the patient in use of either a walker or a cane to assist in balance and stability during gait. It is very important for the PTA to emphasize an erect posture of the patient's trunk and head. If the patient is encouraged to stand and walk on bent hips, the patient will need more power to hold himself upright, will fatigue more quickly, and will limit the type of balance reactions available to the CNS. Additional recommendations for handling children, adolescents, and adults can be found in Chapters 7 though 13.

Use of Assistive Devices While Handling

Body support treadmill training is considered an augmented approach when the therapist or PTA needs to control a motor response, such as placement of the foot during the swing phase. This augmentation is done in order to drive an appropriate motor response and, thus, keep the entire LE within an acceptable parameter of performance during gait.[11-14]

A PTA may use pulleys, theraband, bolsters, wedges, balls, foam, and tapping to limit or encourage specific movement patterns while preventing others. In order for the patient to be considered functionally independent, the PTA and/or PT needs to remove the need by the patient for handling techniques. The continued use of adaptive equipment may allow the patient to be functional without another person assisting, but that equipment often limits the environment within which the patient can function.

Limiting Environmental Parameters and Use of Adaptive Equipment

The PT may ask the PTA to do a home visit in order to determine environmental factors that will limit functional independence. For example, a patient may be able to walk on a hard surface while in the rehabilitation center, but his home may have thick pile carpeting with soft foam support. These two environments are not compatible. Either the patient needs to learn to walk on compliant surfaces while under the care of physical therapy, or the PT needs to recommend that the family pull up the carpet and replace the floor with something that is a noncompliant surface. If the patient needs to stand and take a step or two prior to transferring onto the toilet in his bathroom, then that pattern of movement of stepping, turning, and sitting needs to be the emphasis as part of the intervention program versus transferring on and off a toilet to a chair.

Similarly, if a patient has difficulty rising from a 90 degree angle in sitting, such as from a toilet or lounge chair, a raised toilet seat or a chair that raises the patient to vertical can assist in making the individual more independent within his home environment. The use of adaptive equipment for feeding, long shoe horns for donning shoes, and Velcro (Velcro USA, Manchester, NH) for ties can give an individual more freedom in ADLs. The reality is that even if a patient has the potential and neuroplasticity to regain total independence, priorities must be set by the PT and patient due to limitations in funding and caps on number of visits. Just because the patient is no longer eligible for PT services does not mean he can no longer learn and regain function. It is the PT and the PTA's job to empower that individual to hope. This does not mean unrealistic expectations. On the contrary, it means identifying steps that the patient needs to follow in order to regain functions that are important to that individual. That goal should be the long-term home program, because it should become a part of life activities, not a PT program.

The PTA needs to remember that every time a patient is reinforced by the therapist's voice, feedback is being given to the patient. The use of voice has many effects on the CNS of the patient. A loud voice, unless the patient is hard of hearing, can be perceived as yelling at, or speaking down to the patient. High pitches can become irritating to a patient, where very low pitches can be relaxing. The PTA needs to learn how to modulate the voice to optimize the motor responses of the patient. As the patient regains motor control during intervention, the PTA needs to change the volume and pitch of his voice in order to allow the patient's CNS to practice control under a variety of environmental circumstances.

One very important environmental adaptation for the patient is positioning between therapy sessions. The decision of correct positioning of the limbs and trunk should be a team decision so that consistency is practiced throughout the day. It is very important that the limbs do not hang passively against gravity. This is one of the primary reasons a flaccid shoulder will begin to sublux. The response of the CNS is to create stability, and thus, hypertonicity generally develops. That hypertonicity is in patterns or synergistic programs, and those programs can continue to sublux the shoulder due to asymmetry across the shoulder girdle. Often, some of that subluxation can be prevented by placing pillows under the arm so that the pull of gravity is not vertical. The limb can be placed on a lapboard to support the shoulder. Tape can be used to maintain shoulder alignment. There are many ways to position limbs while sitting and lying down. Pillows, splints, or cones for the hand are often used between therapy sessions. If the PTA is not sure of correct positioning of the patient, asking the PT for suggestions is very appropriate. The PTA needs to remember that no clinician has all the best answers for intervention for each patient. As a PTA, you may find something that works better for the patient. It is your job to show the PT. It is the PT's job to try to figure out why it works.

INTERVENTIONS TO INCREASE SENSORY AWARENESS AND PROCESSING

Following CNS insults, many patients have decreased sensory awareness and/or sensory processing problems. It is the PT's responsibility to evaluate for these deficits, but delegation of training may be given to the PTA. Thus, the PTA needs to be aware of each sensory system and how intervention may increase or decrease input to any one of these systems.

The auditory system was already discussed in relation to use of voice as a therapeutic tool. Similarly, when the PTA demonstrates to the patient, the patient's visual system is engaged in reception and interpretation of the visual array. At times, the environmental input of either or both auditory and visual sensory information may be overwhelming to the CNS and actually decrease function. Thus, the PTA may be asked to initially intervene in a quiet environment in a room where the walls are painted a solid color without pictures or windows, etc. Once the patient begins to improve in motor function, the auditory and visual environments can become more complex and more demanding of the CNS to continue to run appropriate motor programs while the world bombards the brain with sensory information.

Similarly, proprioception and vestibular information can be increased or decreased depending upon the intervention environments created by the therapist. Often, having the patient supine in a quiet environment can lead to a high awareness of proprioceptive information at joints and muscles using assistive motions and joint compression and traction. Once the patient begins to feel those sensations, the PTA can move the patient to more physically demanding environments, such as sitting, and have the patient again be aware of the sensory input. These types of treatment environments would be considered *sensory training* or sensory processing training. They can often be done during the patient's rest periods because they require relaxation and, when accompanied with deep breathing, will often decrease the state of the motor generators, thus dampening inappropriate proprioceptive information from the muscles and joints. Many philosophies and/or intervention suggestions[6,15-18] learned through readings and course attendance emphasize this type of sensory training.

Having patients differentiate sensory objects with vision shielded is a way to help the patient develop or relearn sensory discriminations. Initially, the patient may need to kinesthetically feel and see the object. Then, the object is shielded from sight and the patient asked to recognize what is being felt. That recognition can be through verbal responses or pointing to pictures of similar objects. There is an endless number of ways patients can be taught to process sensory information. Some of those possibilities will be taught while in school, some taught by other therapists in the clinic, some taught in courses, and some discovered by the PTA. This process of learning will continue throughout a therapist's professional lifetime as long as the PTA remains open to learning new skills.

CONCLUSION

Intervention possibilities are numerous,[19] and many are yet to be discovered.[20] As stated previously, the ultimate goal of physical therapy intervention is the patient regaining all movement function as an effortless and enjoyable motor experience. This goal may often be unrealistic given the extent of the lesion, the potential of the patient, and the time available to the PT or PTA for treatment. As a result, decisions need to be made and goals established based upon the specific needs of the patient and family given the environmental restraints of the home, the support systems, the number of visits, the motivation of the patient, and the total health of the individual. The PTA may be delegated many aspects of the intervention program, and the PT may retain certain components. It is the PT's responsibility to delegate appropriately. If the PTA is unsure of the delegated intervention strategies, then the PTA must ask for help. In that way, the PT will develop better communication strategies, and the PTA will develop better intervention skills.

This chapter presented four areas of intervention: functional training, impairment training, hands-on therapeutic or adaptive intervention, and somatosensory input or association training. The ultimate physical therapy goal is functional motor recovery in all aspects of life activities. Although the intervention may need to begin with sensory training and hands-on intervention, the goal is to work to independent functional motor control by the patient. During PT treatment, often specific impairment training needs to be incorporated, such as increasing ROM, decreasing hypertonicity while increasing muscle strength, or increasing respiratory input and exhalation for better oxygenation of the muscle tissues and better endurance, etc. Once a patient can independently run motor programs in a feed-forward fashion, the practice needs to become a life activity in order to retain the skill. At this time, practice needs to be delegated to family, friends, caregivers, and the patient. Transferring throughout the day, brushing teeth, washing hair, and getting from bed to living room to kitchen to outside are an adult's everyday expectations. Generally, if the patient is empowered to learn or relearn those functional skills, the patient will continue to move and practice these skills as part of daily life. If, on the other hand, those activities are thought of as therapy and something that has to be done to get out of the hospital or health care services, then the empowerment of those patients to their own motor potential has not been accomplished, and often, carry-over into life activities is not actualized. As soon as the patient stops practicing, skill can be lost and function decreased. A clinician may find the same patient returning to therapy because he has lost function, but in reality, he has lost or never obtained the motivation to continue what was learned during the initial physical therapy intervention period. There are many additional reasons why a patient may lose function over time. He may become ill and thus loses muscle endurance, and it becomes too hard to do those daily activities. He may have another insult to his CNS or have a progressive problem. None of those medical conditions is within the power of the PT or PTA to control, but helping to empower the patient to realistic possibilities is critical for motivation. It is not acceptable for the daily therapeutic program to be satisfying to the therapist without those feelings of accomplishment extending to the patient. Patients need the feeling of success in order to continue on a road of learning. Empowering the patient to potential is a critical aspect of intervention and certainly part of the PTA's role during intervention. Life changes from day to day, but all of us want to feel that, no matter where we are on this path of learning, we have more potential to learn and grow each day. A patient is no different.

CASE STUDIES

Case #1

Mrs. Jones is a 78-year-old woman who has a history of falling. She does have a history of diabetes and knows she is to drink water once an hour. After MRIs, blood studies, and various other medical examinations, the MD could not make a definitive diagnosis regarding her falling. The patient was sent to physical therapy to determine if interventions might help. Upon the initial visit, Mrs. Jones had a black eye and informed the PT that she had fallen into her closet when she tried to get a shoe. After a thorough balance assessment, the PT determined that Mrs. Jones had all balance strategies, adequate ROM, and knew when she was falling. She used to swim daily with her friends at her senior living inside pool but had stopped after having an episode of pneumonia. During that episode, she stayed at her daughter's apartment next to hers. During that time, she remained in bed the majority of the day for slightly over 4 weeks. She has become very inactive, lives in a small apartment, and only goes out when her daughter takes her to the doctor. She no longer drives, and her daughter does all her grocery shopping. She usually heats a microwave dinner in the evening and has cereal and fruit or cheese for her breakfast and lunch. Her daughter often brings a meal and eats with her. Mrs. Jones is weak, especially in her ankles, knees, and hips bilaterally. That weakness is especially true in her postural muscles in both legs and her back. She spends the majority of the day sitting in her rocking chair watching TV or reading. She has a large pitcher of water by her chair, which allows her to have her hourly glass of water. She also speaks in short sentences. She fatigues quickly during physical activity and has a slowed reaction time to perturbations. The PT has delegated five interventions to the PTA before a reassessment. The PT gave the PTA the following instructions:

1. Have Mrs. Jones practice getting up and down from her chair at least one time an hour by telling her to go to the kitchen and get a glass of water instead of using a pitcher by her chair. Give the responsibility to Mrs. Jones because she is independent in this activity and has walls to stop her falling if she loses her balance.

2. Have Mrs. Jones practice reaching for her shoes and donning them:

   a. First, in sitting from her chair: Session 1.

   b. Second, in standing with a support arm holding onto a table, a chair, or some other stable piece of furniture: Session 2 and 3.

   c. Third, in standing with a shoe directly within her BOS: Session 3 and 4.

   d. Fourth, in standing, have her shoe sequentially farther and farther away from her LOS. Progressing to reaching into the closet by Session 5: progress through this sequence as she increases her tolerance to moving over her center of gravity without falling. She may progress faster or slower depending upon her endurance and fear of falling.

3. Teach Mrs. Jones diaphragmatic breathing:

   a. First, while lying on her bed. Session 1

   b. Second, when standing or walking. Session 2: count the number of syllables she uses in a sentence at the beginning of therapy and at the end. Document and report those numbers to the PT following each session.

4. After you, the PTA, can walk with Mrs. Jones a distance of 25 yards (distance to the mail box and back), instruct the daughter to walk with her mom daily to the mailbox. The daughter should be told that the goal is to increase that distance on a weekly basis. She might walk with her mom to the pool, rest, and walk back. Once she can do that easily, have her mom begin swimming on a daily basis.

Questions

1. Are these interventions appropriate to delegate to the PTA?

2. What clinical symptoms would the PTA want to immediately discuss with the PT?

3. Under which area of intervention does this program fall?

Case #2

Charley is an 8 year old who was diagnosed with cerebral palsy at 3 months of age. His family has been told he has spastic diplegia. He was in therapy as an outpatient in a developmental program until age 5 and now receives physical therapy two times per week while in school. Charley recently underwent heel cord lengthening. The child was placed initially in casts to maintain ROM and allow healing. The casts have now been bivalved and will be used as night splints. The child has now been referred to the outpatient clinic in order to regain functional use of his LEs for gait. The PT has delegated strengthening exercises of the gastroc/soleus muscles to the PTA. The PTA is instructed to do passive stretching to the ankles with a focus of gaining approximately 5 degrees beyond 90 degrees at each session with the goal of gaining and maintaining 110 degrees of ankle ROM for ambulatory activities. The PT also wants the PTA to do strengthening exercises in patterns that encourage the child to break up the extensor synergy (+ supporting reaction) while incorporating ankle function both in weight-bearing and nonweight-bearing. These activities can be encouraged in sit to stand, side-stepping, half kneel to stand, kicking a ball with one foot while maintaining balance and support on the opposite LEs. The PTA is encouraged to play with the child over bolsters, where the child will have to maintain the LEs in external rotation and abduction when coming to stand. The child could be asked to bat a ball, hit a balloon, or catch a ball while increasing the muscle power to succeed at the task.

Questions

1. Are these interventions within the scope of practice of the PTA?

2. How would the PTA document change in range and power of the LEs, and how is that affecting functional behavior?

3. Under which area of intervention does this program fall?

Case #3

The patient is a 28-year-old male who suffered a head trauma following an auto accident 10 days previously. No orthopedic or integumentary problems exist. The patient has a tracheotomy and is intubated for feeding. He lost consciousness immediately, and the paramedics had to resuscitate him following a cardiac arrest. He only was without O_2 for 2 min, and the doctors do not anticipate any severe anoxic injury. The patient was only in ICU for 2 days and has been transferred to a sub-acute rehabilitation unit. The patient is in a persistent vegetative state, considered Level 3 on a Rancho scale. The PT is working with the patient on a ball in vertical in both sitting and kneeling to try to facilitate automatic postural trunk and head control. The PT has delegated ROM exercises to the PTA as well as horizontal rolling and bed mobility. The therapist wants the PTA to encourage rolling by handling from the LEs. Initial handling should begin with the patient in sidelying and facilitate both rolling toward prone and back toward supine. As the patient begins to automatically respond, the PTA is to increase the ROM of the rolling activity with the hopes that the patient will begin to roll. The PT has instructed the PTA to work both in the patient's bed in the morning and on the mat in the PT clinic in the afternoon. Following the PTA intervention, the PT will work on sitting and kneeling, with the PTA assisting by guarding the patient (controlling the roll of the ball) and encouraging interactions with the patient while in the patient's visual gaze.

Questions

1. Are these interventions within the scope of practice of the PTA?

2. What clinical signs would the PTA want to report immediately to the PT?

3. How would the PTA document change?

4. Under which area of intervention does this program fall?

Case #4

Patient is a 58-year-old female who suffered a left CVA 2 weeks ago. She is a CEO of a large corporation and suffered her stroke following a 22-hour air flight. She was returning from a business trip to East Asia. She has minimal speech involvement and has functional motor use of her right UE and LE; however, she has significant loss in sensation. She has normal sensation in her face, trunk, shoulders, and hips but has poor proprioception in her right knee and ankle and no proprioception or tactile sensation in her right elbow, wrist, or hand. She is right-hand dominant. Due to the poor sensation, she is unable to use proprioception to anticipate a pertubation, which could cause a fall in standing or during ambulation. She uses her visual and vestibular system to compensate for poor proprioception, but when distracted in standing or during ambulation, she is slow to react and tends to fall. She has automatic protective extension in a feed-forward UE movement, but without vision, has little idea where her arm is in space or whether her hand is functionally doing anything. The PT has delegated to the PTA various UE sensory awareness exercises with the patient with and without vision. The PT has instructed the PTA to:

a. Have the patient hold various objects first in the left hand and then in the right. The patient is first asked to look at the object while it is in the left hand, manipulate it, and then visualize what it looks like.

b. Have the patient first find an object (spoon, marble, comb, sand paper, cotton, etc) in sand and rice with visual assistance. Then perform the same activity without vision. If she cannot perform this activity initially, tell her what the object is, then have her look at it, shut her eyes, and visualize the form while manipulating it.

The PT was doing sensory awareness retraining first in supine, moving to sitting, and ending in standing in order to facilitate bilateral integration and better somatosensory cortical awareness. Once the patient had some awareness of the right LE, the PT delegated to the PTA bilateral LE weight-bearing activities. The PTA was instructed to:

a. Have the patient practice rocking on her feet visualizing the symmetrical movement at both ankles.

b. Have the patient practice weigh shifting onto and off of the right LE. Then shift to the same activity on the left.

c. Have the patient begin ambulation on a hard surface while visualizing the movement in her right LE. Once she acknowledges that she feels her right LE, the PT should be told in order to begin gait training in various sensory environments.

Questions

1. Are these interventions appropriate to delegate to the PTA?

2. What clinical symptoms would the PTA want to immediately discuss with the PT?

3. How would the PTA document change in the areas of intervention?

4. Under which area of intervention does this program fall?

Suggested author answers are available at www.slackbooks.com/neuroquestions.

REFERENCES

1. *Guide to Physical Therapy Practice.* 2nd ed. Alexandria, Va: American Physical Therapy Association; 2001.

2. Knott M, Voss DE. *Proprioceptive Neuromuscular Facilitation.* New York, NY: Harper and Row; 1968.

3. Bobath B. *Adult Hemiplegia: Evaluation and Treatment.* 2nd ed. London, England: William Heinemann Medical Books; 1978.

4. Bly L. An historical and current view of the basis of NDT. *Pediatric Phys Ther.* 1991;3:131-135.

5. Brunnstrom S. *Movement Therapy in Hemiplegia.* 2nd ed. Philadelphia, Pa: JB Lippincott; 1992.

6. Feldenkrais M. *Awareness Through Movement.* New York, NY: Harper and Row; 1977.

7. Goff B. The application of recent advances in neurophysiology to Miss M Rood's concepts of neuromuscular facilitation. *Physiotherapy.* 1972;58(12):409-415.

8. Johnstone M. *Restoration of Normal Movement After Stroke.* New York, NY: Churchill Livingstone; 1995.

9. Bobath B. *Abnormal Postural Reflex Activity Caused by Brain Lesions.* 3rd ed. Frederick, Md: Aspen Publications; 1985.

10. Bly L. *Baby Treatment Based on NDT Principles.* San Antonio, Tex: Therapy Skill Builders; 1999:1-10.

11. Barbeau H, Visintin M. Optimal outcomes obtained with body-weight support combined with treadmill training in stroke subjects. *Arch Phys Med Rehabil.* 2003;84(10):1458-1465.

12. Hesse S, Werner C. Partial body weight supported treadmill training for gait recovery following stroke. *Adv Neurol.* 2003;92:423-428.

13. Hicks AL, Adams MM, Martin Ginis K, Giangregorio L, Latimer A, Phillips SM, McCartney N. Long-term body-weight-supported treadmill training and subsequent follow-up in persons with chronic SCI: effects on functional walking ability and measures of subjective well-being. *Spinal Cord.* 2005;43(5):291-298.

14. Stein J. Motor recovery strategies after stroke. *Top Stroke Rehabil.* 2004;11(2):12-22.

15. Ayers A. *Sensory Integration and Praxis Test (SIPT) Manual.* Los Angeles, Calif: Western Psychological Association; 1989.

16. Byl NN. Focal hand dystonia may result from aberrant neuroplasticity. *Adv Neurol.* 2004;94:19-28.

17. Byl N, Roderick J, Mohamed O, Hanny M, Kotler J, Smith A, Tang M, Abrams G. Effectiveness of sensory and motor rehabilitation of the upper limb following the principles of neuroplasticity: patients stable poststroke. *Neurorehabil Neural Repair.* 2003;17(3):176-191.

18. Byl NN, Nagarajan SS, Merzenich MM, Roberts T, McKenzie A. Correlation of clinical neuromusculoskeletal and central somatosensory performance: variability in controls and patients with severe and mild focal hand dystonia. *Neural Plast.* 2002;9(3):177-203.

19. Umphred DA, ed. *Neurological Rehabilitation.* 5th ed. Philadelphia, Pa: Elsevier, Incorporated; in press estimated fall 2006.

20. III STEP: symposium on translating evidence into practice. University of Utah, July 15-22, 2005. *Special Editions: Phys Ther.* 2006;86(4,5,6).

Chapter

6

PSYCHOSOCIAL AND COGNITIVE FACTORS AFFECTING THERAPY

Gordon Burton, OT, PhD

KEY WORDS

adjustment
anger
anxiety
denial
depression
disengagement
engagement
hope
hostility
maladaptive
shock
spiritual/spirituality

CHAPTER OBJECTIVES

- Identify six stages of adjustment.
- Identify the difference between engagement and disengagement.
- Develop an understanding of the flexible stages of adjustment.
- Realize that all people are in a state of adjustment, not just clients.
- Recognize that each client is unique and needs to have individualized treatment.

INTRODUCTION

Why do any of us do the things we do? Why do we get up and go through the everyday trials and tribulations that we go through each day? How do we deal with our bodies changing from year to year or decade to decade? How do we deal with the fact that we will all die some day? How do we deal with all of the changes in our lives? How do we deal with functional limitations? How do we deal with disease and pathology?

These are some of the questions that clients may be dealing with on a daily basis, but with a bit of a different slant on the questions. In life, we are all trying to discover our unique purposes and how we are to identify and play roles that match this uniqueness and offer the highest quality in life. Clients try to adjust to life just like therapists. Clients have challenges; some of the challenges are unexpected, and some are not prepared for. Most of us do not think about having an accident and severing our spinal cord, losing some of our brain functions, developing a tumor, or all of the above, but when it happens to us, we have to deal with its reality. "Dealing with it" will be called adjusting or adapting to a disability in this chapter. Some people (clients) adjust or adapt well while others do not, though most people adjust well enough to get by within society. In this chapter, we will discuss some of the highlights of this process, what it means to therapy, and your role as the PTA.

Adjustment is an ongoing process for all of us. We are not suddenly "adjusted" to something. Adjustment is a fluid process that does not flow in just one direction. Family and loved ones often do not go through this process at the same speed or in the same way. Thus, the therapist must always be aware of where each client and each "support" person is at all times within this adjustment process in order to create the best environment and to provide the best intervention. The PTA's role in this process is to make the therapy process progress as smoothly and efficiently as possible.

Each day, you must adjust to successes, failures, accomplishments, and inadequacies; some are consistent failures, and some are consistent accomplishments. A client is no different. Adjustment and adaptation are how one gets through life. We all have limitations that we must adjust to – you will probably never be that ballerina or football star that you would like to be – but we will adjust, adapt, and move on with the process of aging. You may have had friends that never did adjust to not being what they wanted to be and are now angry or dysfunctional because of it. If we do not adapt to life, we become dysfunctional even if we have more life or therapeutic skill potential than others around us do. This may explain why some successful people in high school did not stay successful later in life. They did not adapt to changing life demands.

Some of the keys to facilitating adaptation in the client are to know how that client is unique and to learn that client's adaptation process. Do not try to make each client the same as every other client, and do not force your ways of coping on them. Two case studies in this chapter will help the reader develop both the sensitivity and cognitive understanding of this adjustment process and how it changes as the client goes through life. One case will involve a person who is growing up with a disability, and the other will involve a person who acquired the disability after reaching adulthood.

In this chapter, Sally is a client that was born with CP. She has had to adjust to being "different" all her life, and her "different" is normal for her. She has had to adjust to a society that often does not identify a role for her or has either a negative or an overly positive role that is forced upon her because of her medical diagnosis. Sally can be emotionally damaged by either overly positive or overly negative stereotypes. An example of how an overly positive stereotype may cause problems is when a person is told they must give to society because of a gift of great intelligence. The person may have no need to be overly productive and is criticized or rejected because this potential is not being actualized to society's satisfaction. A negative stereotype may have the same damaging effect by limiting the person's concept of what

could be accomplished, thus preventing that individual from growing and adapting to "be all that they could be." Sally must find her place and use her talents to accomplish what she would like to in life. This goal is difficult for every individual to accomplish, but for a client such as Sally, it may be even harder because she will have some perceived and real motor limitations that may prevent her from accomplishing this goal. Sally may have functional limitations in her upper and lower limbs even with the best of therapy. She has to find ways to accommodate for these limitations in order to prevent them from hampering her love of life. Sally needs to learn how to deal with others and to deal with her physical body in a way that will allow her to adapt to what is needed physically, emotionally, and spiritually. Sally's case study is mentioned throughout this chapter in order to apply components of adjustment and adaptation to her life process.

The second case study used in this chapter involves a young adult male, Fred. Fred acquired a SCI in his twenties. As an adult, he is in the process of adapting his goals and dreams to fit with his new capabilities and limitations following the traumatic injury. A therapist must always be aware of the attitudes of clients toward life activities following and preceding an insult. This event is not all negative since Fred was not goal-directed or focused in his life before the accident. In that respect, Fred may benefit from the structure and guidance he will receive as part of this rehabilitation. He now must deal with the stereotypes and prejudices of others as well as some of the stereotypes and prejudices that he had regarding the disabled before he was injured. He will have to discard some of his old goals or ways of dealing with life activities and challenges but will have an opportunity to focus on what he values as important in his life. This focus can lead to a better life for Fred. Clients have said that "they did not like who they were before their accident, where they were going with their lives and that the disability was a 'god send' to them." (It should be noted that these words were never spoken from a client with a new acute injury but from clients years after their injury). Similarly, clients have communicated that "I had 10,000 opportunities before my injury and I only have 5,000 now but in either case I could only accomplish 1,000 of them either able bodied or disabled."

Roles are the patterns of operating that we go through each day without even thinking. They are how people go through most of life. There are roles for a child, a spouse or partner, a worker, a student, or any other stage or component of life. These roles allow adults to respond as if they were still children interacting with parents. Roles allow each of us to function as a sibling in one situation and a parent in another. Individuals are not cognizant of these roles, but those roles control individual behavior unless each person thinks about her or his behaviors and decides to change them. Roles are very useful in life since, as individuals, none of us have the time or energy to treat each situation in life as a new and novel one. In the case of a new disability, all of our roles must be rethought and reexamined. This process takes time, energy, and a lot of emotional turmoil. Often, the person does not know what the "problem" is.

In the case of a person with an early or congenital disability, such in as our case study of Sally, that person must reexamine the current roles and beliefs in light of changes in function following therapy, deterioration of movement function following a surgery, or simply because role expectations were wrong in the first place. With an acquired disability, such as in the case study of Fred, the person is forced to reexamine all standard roles and change them where appropriate. If the person does not yet know her or his own new abilities and limitations, that person may have a challenge finding and developing "appropriate" new roles. The PTA must be aware of how hard it is for either Fred or Sally to reexamine all that they hold as "true" and, at the same time, deal with the cognitive and physical demands of the medical system and rehabilitation. If Sally were improving in therapy, she may wonder why this therapy was not offered earlier and wonder how many ways her life would have been improved if this had happened when she was younger. She may also feel threatened by her new-found abilities since she may have always used the lack of these abilities as a reason for not engaging in other threatening activities or roles (eg, dating, interacting socially with friends, or assuming gainful employment).

Fred may be experiencing similar emotional reactions as Sally but from another perspective. He may feel that all his abilities are slipping away. He may feel that all he has sacrificed for or delayed gratification for in his life has been wasted. Individuals who have delayed having sex may feel that following an accident such as a spinal injury, they will never know this aspect of life and feel angry about this great loss. Fred may need help in the redirection of his life roles and goals.

Performance is the main goal of therapy and is the main way that a person demonstrates capability. When performance is impaired, the person may be threatened emotionally. When emotionally threatened, performance may be impaired. This is why it is important for the therapist and assistant to always be aware of the client and the client's support systems' unique perspectives on the ramifications of the functional loss and the impairments creating that loss. The emotional system can assist or hinder therapy. Interaction with the staff may be the key to facilitating growth and development of the client with regard to emotional stability and security. The following are some key points for the reader to keep in mind.

GROWTH AND ADAPTATION

The therapist must keep in mind the context from which the client is coming. Just days ago, the client may have been walking around with no major problems and has now suddenly entered the physical therapy setting. The trauma may be multifaceted: (1) the physical trauma that may have occurred to the client, (2) the emotional trauma occurring to the client and the client's support system, and (3) the trauma of each of these bodily systems trying to protect the others. The interaction of these multifaceted components with one's life may lead to post-traumatic stress syndrome. This syndrome usually occurs within the first 6 months following the injury. This syndrome is observed more often in women,[1] but due to cultural barriers, can be hidden with males. The client may blame others, try to protect others, or be so self-absorbed that little else in the world is seen or heard. It may be helpful to get psychological aid for the client early in therapy if this is preventing optimal outcomes or creating obstacles in therapy.[2] It is the PTA's job to develop a trusting relationship with the client. Through this relationship, the client can be helped to focus on the goals of therapy and work on a positive perspective. One error of the medical system is focusing on the disability and pathology and not on the person and the positive capabilities still within the client's grasp.[3] This focus on the negative may cause the client to see only the injury, disease, or pathology and nothing else. In a VA (Veterans Administration) hospital, spouses of people with spinal cord injuries formed a group focusing on why the partners were married in the first place and never looked at the disability as disabling. After a short while, people concluded that they did not marry their spouses for their legs, and the fact that the legs no longer worked was not a major issue after all. This started the decentering from the medical disability model and the focus began being placed upon the people and their future. If we can help clients focus on their function and not their dysfunction, the effect of therapy following treatment will be much better. More work needs to be done to help clients realize their existing potential and to live their lives with the highest quality possible.[4-6] Focusing on how to live, move, and function is one of the keys to helping the client and the family work toward the future.[7] The PTA, under the direction of the PT, must help the client focus on the direction of treatment objectives and must demonstrate how therapy translates into meeting the client's goals.[3] In order to discover the client's true goals, the therapist must gain the trust of the client and establish sound lines of communication. Distrusting health professionals may obstruct the adjustment process and lead to negative consequences.[8] Whenever possible, the client's support system should be enlisted to help establish realistic support for the client and establish goals. It has been found that if the client trusts the health professional, the client will be more compliant and will seek assistance when it is needed.[9]

In the case of Sally, the PT and PTA may work with Sally and her family to see what future goals would be realistic and within the domain of physical therapy. In the case of Fred, the goals may include the accomplishment of previous goals, if they are realistic, or may involve modifying his previous goals with adaptations. This is an issue in therapy for many reasons, but most crucially, when people feel unworthy or disempowered, they tend to perform poorly and have problems with compliance. This reaction may slow or stop the progress of therapy. Helping the client to adapt to "the new body" will help achieve the goals in therapy. Helping clients realize what they can accomplish and "empowering" them with the concept that they can find a way around many barriers and negative situations is a critical aspect of every therapeutic intervention.

Body Image

Body image is an all-encompassing concept that involves how the person and, to some extent, the support system view the person and roles that are expected to be assumed. Many clients experience negative feelings about their bodies and generally negative psychological experiences after injury.[10] Even when clients do not have disfigurements that are readily observable, they often still report changes in body image and negative feelings of self-worth. One issue that may arise relating to body image is sexuality. This concept may take many behavioral forms: flirting, harassment, questions about fertility, or questions regarding whether the client is capable of performing the sex act at all. Flirting may be a sign that clients have had an assault on their femininity or masculinity. By flirting, clients are often trying to determine if they are still seen as a sensual being. In this case, a PTA may let clients down lightly by explaining that dating or flirting with clients is not allowed. This is to ensure that clients do not think that the "turn off" is about their disabilities. Sensitivity should be used because a client could think, "If a medical person finds me repulsive, then no one will ever see me as attractive." It is important for the therapist to try to ascertain the intent behind the behavior. Usually, this can be accomplished by evaluating feelings about the interaction. It is not within the scope of a PTA's duties to determine the stage of adjustment that may be directing client behavior. However, it is within the scope of a PTA's duties to develop caring sensitivity and be able to report to the PT or other health professionals what has been observed

in the client's behavior. If you, as the PTA, do not feel threatened or demeaned when the client is probably flirting, you still must report this to the PT of record. If you feel defensive, demeaned, or very uncomfortable, then you may be experiencing harassment. You should never be harassed on the job, and this client's behavior should be stopped immediately; you must tell the client that the behavior is making you feel uncomfortable and that it should stop now. Again, you should mention this behavior to your supervisor and/or team. If the behavior is considered chronic by the staff, a treatment plan should be designed to stop this behavior. This plan is not the responsibility of the PTA, but carrying out response behaviors to the patient's inappropriate actions is within that scope. It is important, however, to remember that sexual health should not be a neglected area of client treatment. It may take time for the client to ask the appropriate questions.[11]

Questions about any physical performance are within the domain of physical therapy. If the client is asking for information regarding positioning during sex, then this may be brought to the attention of a therapist. If the questions are regarding fertility and the like, these should also be referred to an appropriate medical person. None of these questions should be discouraged or neglected because this area is important for your clients' motivation and sexual health.[12,13] It is important for the PTA to know that in SCI, fertility will generally not be impaired for the female, but issues of lubrication before sex should be addressed by the appropriate person. Males may have erection problems and ejaculation issues, but this can also be addressed by the appropriate person. It is now thought that male fertility issues resulting from a SCI may be dealt with and should not be ruled out.[14-16]

Sally may need to work on body image problems that have resulted from the misperceptions she gained from other people and the media. She may also have learned not to enjoy her body and to deny positive sensations because she has been clinically touched most of her life without regard to her need for privacy.

Fred, on the other hand, may need to talk to other people who have been disabled for a while in order to explore acquired misconceptions and negative stereotypes regarding the impact of disabilities and, specifically, his functional limitations. He may also benefit from practical information that people with similar medical diagnoses can provide.

Family and Client Adjustment

The role of the family must never be forgotten. Though earlier literature hinted that partner relationships may be negatively affected by a member being disabled, this is being questioned in regard to some disabilities, such as adult onset spinal cord injuries.[17] However, pediatric SCI and other disabilities may result in relationship problems.[18,19] It has been shown that adjustment and quality of life can be adversely affected by an inadequate physical environment, thus making the person more dependent. The result of the dependence appears to be poor relationships.[20,21] This can also be seen with the families in which a member has had a brain injury.[22] In studies on muscular dystrophy, it was found that physical dependence is not the only variable that needs to be considered; psychological issues need to be identified and considered as part of intervention.[23,24] According to Turner and Cox, the client and the family need help to work on a number of elements: "to develop new views of vulnerability and strength, make changes in relationships, and facilitate philosophical, physical and spiritual growth."[24] Turner and Cox also felt that the medical staff could facilitate the following: "recognizing the worth of each individual, helping them to envision a future that is full of promise and potential, actively involving each person in their own care trajectory, and celebrating changes to each person's sense of self."[24] Man observed that each family copes differently in relation to a brain-injured family member and that the family's structure should be explored to develop intervention guidelines.[25] It has also been noted that health care professionals should view the situation from the family's perspective in order to approach and support the family's adaptation.[26] This should be done to help the client and the family accept the disability but, at the same time, to help them keep the negative views of society in perspective.[27] In general, it has also been found that family support is a significant factor in the client's subjective functioning[28] and that social engagement is productive.[29]

When dealing with children, it is important to realize that they often feel responsible for almost anything that happens in life (eg, divorce, siblings getting hurt, or general arguments between parents). It is important that the therapist helps the client and the siblings realize that they are not responsible for the client's condition. Part of this magical thinking that often appears is the concept that "bad things happen to bad people;" thus, the child is bad because a bad thing has happened. It is important to be sensitive to this ideation and help dispel this maladaptive thought pattern since it is not true or productive for the client or the siblings and may cause further adjustment problems later in treatment. Siblings of the client should be helped to see their roles as good siblings and should not be placed in the role of caretakers of the disabled sibling. In this way, all children can grow naturally without any one of the children being overly focused upon. At the same time, it is a fact of life that the disabled child will probably need physical assistance, therapy, increased

medical care, and thus, more time devoted to her or him; this is just a fact of life.

It should always be noted by the medical establishment that having a disability is expensive in ways in which they are often not aware. There are the obvious medical costs of therapy, surgery, w/c, or orthoses, but there are other costs such as the possibility of extra cost of transportation, catheters for urination, w/c maintenance, adaptive clothing, and other ongoing costs not covered by most insurance plans. These costs add up and contribute to the emotional costs and demands on the family. Significant others may feel the need to work more to earn the money to cover such expenses, but then that person will not be around to help. This is only one of the many dilemmas that must be dealt with for the support system of the disabled person. The family may be encouraged to contact such groups as the Family Caregiver Support Network (www.caregiver-supportnetwork.org) to get information and assistance with such diverse topics as being a caregiver, legal and financial aid, and communications (this group tends to focus on the adult but may still be a wonderful aid). Such groups will give information to all who need it and help to empower the family. This takes the focus off the medical condition and may help the family to gain a better and more balanced perspective on the condition.

Sally may have to work on skills that will encourage assertiveness and better decision-making. She may need to help her family allow her to be more independent and become more of a risk taker in all aspects of her life.

Fred may need to work on coping skills and strategies that will help him deal with crises. He may have preconceived ideas of the limitations of the disabled that need to be changed.

Stress, Crisis, Loss, and Grief

The adaptation process is one that has been theorized about and speculated upon, and it would appear that the human being is so complex that no two of us react just the same. This is a comforting fact because it means each of us is a truly unique individual. This also means that when you deal with clients, each is unique and is not a diagnosis or a routine entity. To do a good job, you have to listen to their stories, know the context of their lives, know their values, and understand their goals. This is a major undertaking in the context of a treatment session, but it should be your ideal goal for each client. This section will examine some thoughts on how clients adapt to a disability.

After an injury or disabling condition, the client and the family may go through an episode of depression that may interfere with the progress of therapy.[30,31] *Depression* and other inadequate coping modes will impede progress of therapy and decrease levels of life satisfaction for all involved.[2,32] Attempting to help the client and the family avoid depression by keeping them involved in functional and meaningful therapeutic activities is the challenge.[23] The longer the client is in a forced helplessness situation, the more likely it is that the client will feel depressed. Focusing on a positive goal that is relevant to the client and the family may help to keep the client directed towards the future and away from the negative aspects of the situation. If focusing on the client's goals is not enough, other treatment may be needed, and psychiatric assistance may be called for.[33] Acceptance of the disability without surrendering to the condition has been found to be associated with less anger, less hostility, and higher self-efficacy in the individual.[34] *Denial* may work for the very early stages of the disability, but if it lasts, it will hamper the client's progress. A client once explained to me that when he could not do anything, denial was very helpful but that as soon as he could start doing things for himself and others, denial was not at all helpful. Thus, the therapist's job is to help the client defocus from the medical impairment and handicap by focusing on function and the client's goals. If this is done and the focus is on adaptive activities that have meaning to the individual, the client will not experience the role of helplessness and dependence, and quality of life will be maximized.[35-37]

Livneh and Antonak have presented a primer for counselors that can be adapted to assist the therapist in dealing with clients' adjustment to disability.[38] It should always be kept in mind that there is no "normal" or "right" way for a person to go through the adjustment process, and often, we will not see clients long enough to observe all of the stages of adjustment. Remember, there is not a static state of "adjustment" that the person reaches and there remains. We are all in various states of adjustment to life, and clients are no different.

Some of the observed mechanisms that have been noted are *shock, anxiety, denial, depression, anger/hostility,* and *adjustment.* All of these can be seen at some point in the client's life. These aspects of adjustment may be seen at any point of rehabilitation. Even though the client may appear "adjusted" to one aspect of the disability, the same client may be greeted with some new aspect of the disability that he or she may not have experienced before. The client may then go into shock and start adjusting to this aspect of the disability anew. Adjustment is a process, not a place. I have known clients who have been adjusted to their disability for many years but will lose or even gain function over time and must adjust to these changes. This is not a static process.

One aspect that the therapist must watch out for is a form of coping called *disengagement* – this may be denial or avoidance behavior, which can take many forms. It can result in substance abuse, blame, or refusal to interact. Research regarding people with head injuries has demonstrated that if a premorbid coping style for a person was to use drinking or other drugs, the client may revert to these same styles of coping, which can result in poor rehabilitation.[39] It is important to help the client out of this quagmire. The skills of a therapist may not be enough to do this in the short time that the client is in treatment, so a referral to social work or psychiatry may be in order. It is still the therapists' job to help promote *engagement* activities – these behaviors are goal oriented, problem solving, information seeking, and doing things to positively "beat the condition" and demonstrate independence.

Livneh and Antonak promote the following activities for the health professional:

1. Assisting clients to explore the personal meaning of the disability. "Training clients to attain a sense of mastery over their emotional experiences." A way of doing this would be to help the client not to demonstrate emotional outbursts or to help the client look at her or his emotions and to put them into perspective.[38]

2. "Providing clients with relevant medical information. These strategies emphasize imparting accurate information to clients on their medical condition, including its present status, prognosis, anticipated future functional limitations, and when applicable, vocational implications." This may be done by helping the client and family access resources such as Pub Med (pubmedcentral.nih.gov) on-line or helping to find medical references in the library.[38]

3. "Providing clients with supportive family and group experiences. These strategies permit clients (usually with similar disabilities or common life experiences) and, if applicable, their family members or significant others, to share common fears, concerns, needs, and wishes." This can be done in rather unobtrusive ways: scheduling clients with the same disability at the same time so that they meet in the waiting room or while doing group mat activities, or hiring disabled individuals who are health care professionals that can discuss and model positive behaviors and answer relevant questions from the client's perspective. Remember that all clients are potential teachers for you as well as other clients.[38]

4. Teaching clients adaptive coping skills for successful community functioning. "These skills include assertiveness, interpersonal relations, decision making, problem solving, stigma management, and time management skills." This would entail role-playing situations that I have seen happen in the community: an able bodied person asking why the client is

in a w/c, that person preaching to the w/c user because they must have offended God in some way, otherwise the person would not be in a w/c, or telling the client that is such a shame that he or she is disabled because she is so good looking and could have found a man if it were not for the disability. Role-playing can also be used to help a person deal with the possibly awkward experience of going to bed with a new partner and having to explain how to be undressed, what those tubes coming out of the body are for, or what positions are best for someone with this condition.[38]

Sally may work on role-playing in order to develop the skill to ask someone out for a date or to learn to be assertive at the bank or store. Fred may need to work on how to ask for assistance without feeling dependent or how to physically defend himself in the w/c.

Hope and Spiritual Aspects

The process of *hope* can be a generalized and positive force to reduce depression, the sense of powerlessness, and grief.[40] Clients need a realistic sense of hope. The question of what is realistic is always open to interpretation. I had a client with quadriplegia who was a deer hunter. He swore he would go to the mountains in the fall and shoot a deer. All of the staff knew that he was not being realistic, but he came in with venison in the fall from the deer he shot. Another client with quadriplegia lived on the East Coast and said that when he left the hospital, he would drive to the West Coast to live. The staff laughed about this, but sure enough, he was discharged and drove to the West Coast to live. It is hope that keeps most of us going in life. Hope is not always realistic. How many people really believe that they will win the lottery, if not this time, then maybe the next? Sometimes it is this hope that saves us from being overwhelmed by the other realities of life. Try not to take all of the clients' hope away. They may win the lottery, shoot a deer, or drive to another part of the world.

Spirituality is something that provides hope, connection with others, and reason or meaning of existence for many (if not most) people. It is amazing that the medical community has been very slow to accept the power of spirituality since this area gives meaning to so many peoples' lives. Spirituality has been linked to health perception, a sense of connection with others, and well being.[41,42] Anything that helps the client put the disability into perspective and move on with life in a healthy way is good. The western medical system is based on pathology and focuses on that. Physical therapy focuses on doing and behavioral change that is productive. One of the dangers of the medical system is the entrapment in pathology to the point that the client may not see anything but pathology. Spirituality may help the client and the family to see that there is more to life than pathology, stimulate interaction with others, put the disability in perspective, give meaning to life (and the disability), and give the person hope and a sense of well being.[43] This is what we all want for the client and the family.

Sally may benefit from talking to other people with CP that have families, are CEOs of businesses, or are doing whatever they would like to do.

Fred may tap into what his new goals and dreams really were and are in order to see ways to accomplish those dreams.

Cultural Aspects

Culture, subculture, and the culture and beliefs of the client's family are aspects of the client to which the therapist must attend.[44] This concept includes the beliefs about the world and maybe a belief about the cause of the disability or, at least, how the client is viewing the disability. Asking, "why do you think this happened to you?" can lead to a very enlightening experience. "Causes" may range from: "God is punishing me", "I deserved it", or "life is against me." The answer may frame the way that treatment is presented to the client. Using the client's frame of reference may promote trust, mutual acceptance of values, greater compliance with treatment, and a broadening of the therapist's view of the world. One of the great things about therapy is that clients teach us so much about life. Recognizing why a client does something that looks different to us may lead to a key to what that client may need in treatment. It may also help the PTA to see the world from a different perspective. Do not hesitate to let the client know that he or she helped you. Helping others is empowering to the client as well as the therapist.

One example of how the clients' perspective can be very different from the therapist's is if, during treatment, a client says that she is going to die. When presented with the fact that she is in rehabilitation, is not going to die, and is about to be discharged, she falls silent. It is not until the client gets home that the therapist realizes the client was going back to an inner-city situation and that the client's fears of death have merit. Someone who is elderly and very disabled in this area of town is in a life-threatening situation, and she probably *is* going to die (other arrangements are quickly made for her discharge). If the therapist had listened better and knew the client's subculture, this incident could have been avoided. It should be noted that the therapist did try to find out what the client meant. The client thought that it was so obvious (in the client's world) that the therapist's lack of knowledge was a lack of caring for the client's welfare. We should try to avoid this kind of interaction at all costs.

Beliefs and values of cultures and families can play a profound role in the course of treatment. Such things as physical difficulties that can be seen are usually better accepted than problems that cannot be seen, such as brain damage that changes an individual's personality.[45] A person with a back injury may be seen as lazy, whereas a person with a double amputation will be perceived as needing help. At the same time, a person who has lost a body part, in some cultures, may be seen as "not all there" and is avoided socially. Thus, being attuned to the culture and beliefs of the client is imperative in therapy.

Sally will have some of her beliefs challenged. She will need to examine how she thinks about her possible future roles. She may want to examine whether she would like to have children, be a professional woman, or be both. She will have to develop skills that will promote her goals, and she may look to role models that can demonstrate the positive behaviors that are necessary to accomplish these goals.

Fred was very unfocused in his life before the injury and will need help clarifying some of the behaviors that did not work for him before. In doing so, he will have to dispel some of the myths about the disabled that he was taught in his culture. With help, he may be able to see this event as a new beginning that will help him "clean up his act."

Adjustment to disability opens a person to a unique situation and allows him or her to adapt to a changing environment in a productive way. If the person is not able to alter *maladaptive* behaviors and grow in a productive way, the best physical therapy in the world will not be able to make significant progress. We may get a client to do all of the correct exercises and movement patterns but not to be a productive person who enjoys life. The PTA is a significant member of the team who needs to be aware of ways to promote productive behavior that results in a more functional person. It is not the PTA's job to be a psychologist, an OT, or a social worker, but it is important to assist the team and to promote productive behavior and function. The role of psychosocial function is intricately linked to quality of life issues. Movement expresses not only the motor system but is the only avenue that a client can use to express emotions, interact with other individuals, be empowered to bodily functions, and feel good about one's self. The PTAs, as team members and colleagues who are delegated the responsibility of physical therapy interventions, need to identity their own personal beliefs, safety issues, biases, and learning styles and have respect for each patient's uniqueness. With this comprehension incorporated into the behavior of a PTA, the individual will become a much better therapist, will have better compliance from the patients, and will feel more satisfied as a provider of health care.

CHAPTER QUESTIONS

1. What are the six stages of adjustment discussed in this chapter?

2. What is the difference between engagement and disengagement?

3. Is adjustment a static stage that can be reached and maintained?

4. What are the commonalities between client adjustment and PTA adjustment?

5. Why should two clients be treated differently even if they have the same diagnosis?

Suggested author answers are available at www.slackbooks.com/neuroquestions.

REFERENCES

1. Kennedy P, Evans MJ. Evaluation of post traumatic distress in the first 6 months following SCI. *Spinal Cord.* 2001;39:381-386.

2. Kennedy P, Rogers BA. Anxiety and depression after spinal cord injury: a longitudinal analysis. *Arch Phys Med Rehabil.* 2000;81:932-937.

3. Mazaux JM, Croze P, Quintard B, Rouxel L, Joseph PA, Richer E, Debelleix X, Barat M. Satisfaction of life and late psycho-social outcome after severe brain injury: a nine-year follow-up study in Aquitaine. *Acta Neurochir Suppl.* 2002;79:49-51.

4. Ayyangar R. Health maintenance and management in childhood disability. *Phys Med Rehabil Clin N Am.* 2002;13(4):793-821.

5. Kim SJ, Kang KA. Meaning of life for adolescents with a physical disability in Korea. *J Adv Nurs.* 2003;43(2):145-155; discussion 155-157.

6. Stewart DA, Law MC, Rosenbaum P, Willms DG. A qualitative study of the transition to adulthood for youth with physical disabilities. *Phys Occup Ther Pediatr.* 2001;21(4):3-21.

7. Putzke JD, Richards JS, Hicken BL, DeVivo MJ. Predictors of life satisfaction: a spinal cord injury cohort study. *Arch Phys Med Rehabil.* 2002;83(4):555-561.

8. Gullacksen AC, Lidbeck J. The life adjustment process in chronic pain: psychosocial assessment and clinical implications. *Pain Res Manag.* 2004;9(3):145-153.

9. Trachtenberg F, Dugan E, Hall MA. How patients' trust relates to their involvement in medical care. *J Fam Pract.* 2005;54(4):344-352.

10. Taleporos G, McCabe MP. Body image and physical disability: personal perspectives. *Soc Sci Med.* 2002;54(6):971-980.

11. Fisher TL, Laud PW, Byfield MG, Brown TT, Hayat MJ, Fiedler IG. Sexual health after spinal cord injury: a longitudinal study. *Arch Phys Med Rehabil.* 2002;83:1043-1051.

12. Phelps J, Albo M, Dunn K, Joseph A. Spinal cord injury and sexuality in married or partnered men: activities, function, needs, and predictors of sexual adjustment. *Arch Sex Behav.* 2001;30:591-602.

13. Nortvedt MW, Riise T, Myhr KM, Landtblom AM, Bakke A, Nyland HI. Reduced quality of life among multiple sclerosis patients with sexual disturbance and bladder dysfunction. *Mult Scler.* 2001;7(4):231-235.

14. Brackett NL, Nash MS, Lynne CM. Male fertility following spinal cord injury: facts and fiction. *Phys Ther.* 1996;76:1221-1231.

15. Monga M, Dunn K, Rajasekaran M. Characterization of ultrastructural and metabolic abnormalities in semen from men with spinal cord injury. *J Spinal Cord Med.* 2001;24:41-46.

16. Sonksen J, Ohl DA. Penile vibratory stimulation and electroejaculation in the treatment of ejaculatory dysfunction. *Int J Androl.* 2002;25:324-332.

17. Kreuter M. Spinal cord injury and partner relationships. *Spinal Cord.* 2000;38:2-6.

18. Vogel LC, Krajci KA, Anderson CJ. Adults with pediatric-onset spinal cord injuries, part 3: impact of medical complications. *J Spinal Cord Med.* 2002;25:297-305.

19. Evans SA, Airey MC, Chell SM, Connelly JB, Rigby AS, Tennant A. Disability in young adults following major trauma: 5 year follow up of survivors. *BMC Public Health.* 2003;3(1):8.

20. Seki M, Takenaka A, Nakazawa M, Takahashi H, Chino N. Examination of living environment upon return to home for patients with cervical spinal cord injury: report of a case. *Gan To Kagaku Ryoho.* 2002;3(Suppl 29):522-525.

21. Whiteneck G, Meade MA, Dijkers M, Tate DG, Bushnik T, Forchheimer MB. Environmental factors and their role in participation and life satisfaction after spinal cord injury. *Arch Phys Med Rehabil.* 2004;85(11):1793-1803.

22. Kneafsey R, Gawthorpe D. Head injury: long-term consequences for patients and families and implications for nurses. *J Clin Nurs.* 2004;13(5):601-608.

23. Natterlund B, Ahlstrom G. Activities of daily living and quality of life in persons with muscular dystrophy. *J Rehabil Med.* 2001;33(5):206-211.

24. Turner de S, Cox H. Health qualility facilitating post traumatic growth. *Health Quality of Life Outcomes.* 2004;2(1):34.

25. Man DW. Hong Kong family caregivers' stress and coping for people with brain injury. *Int J Rehabil Res.* 2002;25(4):287-295.

26. Taanila A, Syrjala L, Kokkonen J, Jarvelin MR. Child: coping of parents with physically and/or intellectually disabled children. *Care Health Dev.* 2002;28(1):73-86.

27. de Klerk HM. The physically disabled woman's experience of self. *Ampousah L Disabil Rehabil.* 2003;25(19):1132-1139.

28. Koukouli S, Vlachonikolis IG, Philalithis A. Sociodemographic factors and self-reported functional status: the significance of social support. *Health Serv Res.* 2002;2(1):20

29. Mendes de Leon CF, Glass TA, Berkman LF. Social engagement and disability in a community population of older adults. *Am J Epidemiol.* 2003;157(7):633-642.

30. Martz E, Livneh H, Priebe M, Wuermser LA, Ottomanelli L. Predictors of psychosocial adaptation among people with spinal cord injury or disorder. Arch Phys Med Rehabil. 2005;86(6):1182-1192.

31. Bombardier CH, Richards JS, Krause JS, Tulsky D, Tate DG. Symptoms of major depression in people with spinal cord injury: implications for screening. *Arch Phys Med Rehabil.* 2004;85(11):1749-1756.

32. Chan RC. Stress and coping in spouses of persons with spinal cord injuries. *Clin Rehabil.* 2000;14:137-144.

33. Kishi Y, Robinson RG, Kosier JT. Suicidal ideation among patients during the rehabilitation period after life-threatening physical illness. *J Nerv Ment Dis.* 2001;189(a):623-628.

34. Treharne GJ, Lyons AC, Booth DA, Mason SR, Kitas GD. Reactions to disability in patients with early versus established rheumatoid arthritis. *Scand J Rheumatol.* 2004;33(1):30-38.

35. Holmbeck GN, Westhoven VC, Phillips WS, Bowers R, Gruse C, Nikolopoulos T, Totura CM, Davison K. A multimethod, multi-informant, and multidimensional perspective on psychosocial adjustment in preadolescents with spina bifida. *J Consult Clin Psychol.* 2003;71(4):782-796.

36. Voll R. Aspects of the quality of life of chronically ill and handicapped children and adolescents in outpatient and inpatient rehabilitation. *Int J Rehabil Res.* 2001;24(1):43-49.

37. Ville I, Ravaud JF. Subjective well-being and severe motor impairments: the Tetrafigap survey on the long-term outcome of tetraplegic spinal cord injured persons. *Soc Sci Med.* 2001;52:369-384.

38. Livneh H, Antonak RF. Psychosocial adaptation to chronic illness and disability: a primer for counselors. *Journal of Counseling and Development.* 2005;83(1):12-20

39. MacMillan PJ, Hart RP, Martelli MF, Zasler ND. Pre-injury status and adaptation following traumatic brain injury. *Brain Inj.* 2002;16(1):41-49.

40. Lohne V. Hope in patients with spinal cord injury: a literature review related to nursing. *J Neurosci Nurs.* 2001;33:317-325.

41. Delgado C. A discussion of the concept of spirituality. *Nurs Sci Q.* 2005;18(2):157-162.

42. Potter ML, Zauszniewski JA. Spirituality, resourcefulness, and arthritis impact on health perception of elders with rheumatoid arthritis. *J Holist Nurs.* 2000;18(4):311-331; discussions 332-336.

43. Treloar LL. Disability, spiritual beliefs, and the church: the experiences of adults with disabilities and family members. *J Adv Nurs.* 2002;40(5):594-603.

44. Saravanan B, Manigandan C, Macaden A, Tharion G, Bhattacharji S. Re-examining the psychology of spinal cord injury: a meaning centered approach from a cultural perspective. *Spinal Cord.* 2001;39(6):323-326.

45. Brown SA, McCauley SR, Levin HS, Contant C, Boake C. Perception of health and quality of life in minorities after mild-to-moderate traumatic brain injury. *Appl Neuropsychol.* 2004;11(1):54-64.

Chapter

7

CLIENTS WITH CENTRAL NERVOUS SYSTEM INSULT AT BIRTH: CEREBRAL PALSY

Kris Corn, PT, MS, DPT

KEY WORDS

anoxic brain injury
athetosis
cerebral palsy
diplegia
facilitation
handling techniques
hemiplegia
hypoxic brain injury
inhibition
quadriplegia
triplegia

CHAPTER OBJECTIVES

- Introduce the more frequently treated pediatric neurological diagnoses from insults that occur in utero, at birth, or shortly after birth.

- Differentiate between trauma to the CNS in the neonate and acquired trauma after 2 years of age that primarily affects the motor system.

- Present some of the more common characteristics observed in the pediatric neurological patient with the medical diagnosis of CP.

- Introduce handling and treatment ideas for the neurologically impaired child.

INTRODUCTION

PTAs working in the pediatric neurological clinic or hospital will treat a wide and varied population of children who will continually challenge their critical thinking and creativity. When a child's CNS is damaged, there can be one or more systems affected, depending on the location and cause of the insult. PTs and PTAs treat children with movement dysfunction and/or sensory processing disorders in order to prevent skeletal deformities and encourage normal development of motor skills and milestones. Often, insults to the CNS affect postural tone as well as the distal muscle tone, strength, and sensory processing. The postural tone and motor control will influence and be influenced by feedback and feed-forward information from all the sensory systems (see Chapter 3). Some of the more common CNS diagnoses treated in the physical therapy department are CP, genetic disorders, autism spectrum disorders, sensory processing dysfunction, anoxic/hypoxic, and TBI.

For some of these disorders, the causation is clear, while in other CNS dysfunctions, the causation is not well understood or is unknown. It is always helpful to have a clear medical diagnosis, but this is not always possible. In either case, the patient's clinical signs and symptoms (functional limitations) will help the PT

Table 7-1
Areas of Motor Involvement

Area of Central Nervous System Involvement Due to Bleeds or Anoxia

Area of Insult	Cause	Involvement
Periventricular	Central Bleed	Diplegic
Parietal Lobe	Hemispheric Bleed	Hemiplegic
Frontal Motor	Global Ischemia	Quadriplegic
Distal Cortical		Spastic/Multisystem
Cerebellar	Anoxia	Quadriplegic Athetoid
Diencephalon	Total Asphyxia	Ataxic

Classification by Muscle Tone

Pathology	Tone Quality	Impairment
Hypertonic	High tone	Decreased joint mobility and motor control problems.
Hypotonic	Low tone	Increased joint mobility and motor control problems.
Mixed programming	Low-high tone	Increased joint mobility of trunk and neck.
		Decreased joint mobility of the extremities and motor control problems.
Fluctuating programming	Athetoid	Decreased grading of strength/joint ROM, poor stabilization, often normal mobility.
Regulatory inconsistencies	Ataxic	Trunk instability, increased joint mobility, and gait.
In programming		Disturbances in force, rate, timing.

determine the appropriate treatment program for each individual. The PT will then determine what portion of the treatment program will be delegated to the PTA. In some of these medical diagnoses, such as CP and TBI, the specific therapy diagnosis and movement disorder is dependent on the muscle tone and the areas of involvement.

Although physical therapy always considers the medical diagnosis, the PT's function is to treat movement disorders associated with the medical diagnosis (Table 7-1). The classification of muscle tone is beneficial when evaluating and analyzing motor dysfunction and determining appropriate treatment (Table 7-1).

Table 7-2 describes the area or areas of the body involved in the motor dysfunction.

CEREBRAL PALSY

The individual with *cerebral palsy* (CP) incurred damage to the CNS during gestation (prenatal), at the time of birth (natal), or within the first few weeks of life

(postnatal). Basic patterns of motor behavior have not been established at the time of the insult. These basic components of movement are essential in developing normal postural alignment, equilibrium, and protective responses. Reflexive behaviors or stereotypical motor behaviors are repetitively demonstrated and elicited by sensory input or intention. These motor behaviors may become the dominant movement patterns as the child develops, thus considered abnormal and interfering with normal skill acquisition and motor control. Depending on the child's age when the insult occurred and the extent of the involvement, a wide variety of dysfunction in postural control and skill development will be observed.

With or without a formal medical diagnosis of CP, a neonate who has suffered a CNS insult will, within the first few weeks of life, present with far more subtle motor involvement, unless the damage has been fairly severe. The infant's tone may be initially hypotonic, causing decreased head and trunk control. Reflexes are present and may be appropriate based on the infants age or corrected age for those born

Table 7-2
Classification by Areas of Involvement

Medical Classification	Movement Dysfunction
Hemiplegic	The trunk and either both right extremities or both left extremities.
Diplegic	The trunk and LEs have greater involvement than the UEs.
Triplegic	The trunk and three extremities.
Quadraplegic	The trunk and all four extremities.

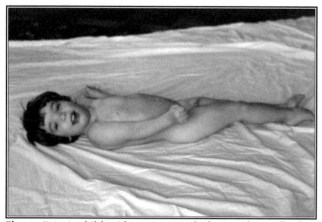

Figure 7-1. A child with severe tonal abnormality will often demonstrate involvement in all four extremities. This child would be considered to have spastic *quadriplegia*.

prematurely. It is essential for the PT to be well appraised of normal neonatal development. It is more common that a child of 12 months or older who is diagnosed with CP is referred for physical therapy because the child has not achieved the normal milestones and appropriate developmental skills (eg, coming to sit or, if placed in sitting, is unable to move independently from the sitting position). Children who are 12 month old should be crawling, pulling to stand, practicing standing balance, or even beginning to take their first steps.[1] (Refer to Chapter 2 for additional information on child development.) Once the PT has evaluated the child and determined what abnormal motor patterns should be eliminated and what normal motor behaviors need to be practiced, the PT will be able to delegate to the PTA the activities that are within the competencies of the PTA.

The older child, between 18 months and 4 years, may have developed compensatory patterns of movement that the PTA will be able to recognize as abnormal movement patterns. The movement may be labored as the child attempts to overcome hypertonicity, asymmetric muscle tone, and decreased postural stability. Repetitive abnormal posturing that accompanies

increased muscle tone will eventually cause contractual deformities of the soft tissues.

Generally, these musculoskeletal problems are first observed in the more involved extremities (Figure 7-1). Without therapy and parental involvement, these soft tissue deformities may cause bony changes, skeletal deformities, and eventual dislocations. Although the hypotonic child does not have to work against increased muscle tone, the child needs to develop sufficient muscle strength and postural control to overcome gravity and be able to come to sit and stand. The hypotonic child generally presents with poor to fair head and trunk control (Figures 7-2 and 7-3). Low tone often causes deformities of the spine due to lack of sufficient symmetric postural control. The PT will differentiate these motor dysfunctions as part of the initial assessment and should continue to evaluate the techniques used and the progress made during each treatment session. The delegation of intervention to the PTA is dependent on the stability of the child's CNS, degree of movement dysfunction, and the involvement of the systems.

The severity of the insult has a significant role in determining the results of habilitation and is extremely important in prescribing the intensity, duration, and type of therapeutic intervention. Children diagnosed with CP are often classified as mild, moderate, or severe. Generally, with appropriate, intensive treatment initiated by 4 to 6 months of age, a mildly involved child will develop sufficient motor control to allow for normal movement patterns, and the moderately involved child will have mild deficits in movement development after physical therapy. The severely involved child can often change, becoming a child with moderate to moderately severe involvement. Although the medical diagnosis of CP is static, the growing and maturing CNS has plasticity, and the motor system will express these motor changes by increased fluidity of movement and skill development if the environment nurtures those movements. In turn, the opposite can occur without appropriate and intensive treatment at an early age. The mildly involved child often develops

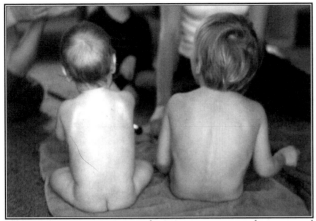

Figure 7-2. Comparison of sitting postures of a normal 6-month-old child to his 2-year-old brother with the diagnosis of spastic *athetosis*: Posterior view.

moderate disabilities, the moderate child develops severe disabilities, and the child who was initially severe often becomes even more involved.

TRAUMATIC AND ANOXIC/HYPOXIC INJURY

This medical diagnosis is generally applied to children over the age of 2 years. Children with TBI and near drowning have one aspect of their CNS involvement in common: both patients have sustained trauma to a nervous system that has already established normal patterns of movement and postural control. Thus, the child will have some knowledge of how to move based on motor memory and motor learning or control up to the age of the insult. This prior learning is often helpful in their treatment, as opposed to the child with CP who has had minimal to no experience developing normal patterns of movement and postural control.

CNS contusions and lacerations of the patient with a TBI can occur with or without skull fracture. Damage can affect any area of the brain, or laceration of the blood vessels supplying the brain can reduce the supply of oxygen to the area of brain. Cranial nerves may be injured, and diffuse axonal injury (DAI) is the most common cause of primary lesions.[2] These injuries may result in coma or a persistent vegetative state secondary to damage as the result of lack of oxygen. These lesions can cause (1) increased intracranial pressure, (2) cerebral hypoxia or ischemia, (3) intracranial hemorrhage, (4) electrolyte imbalance from swelling, (5) secondary infection, and (6) seizures.[3] There are often physiological, cognitive, and behavioral changes after a brain injury along with movement dysfunction. As the child's CNS is adjusting to the insult and changes, the family and their CNSs are also reacting to changes to their family member. The family's input

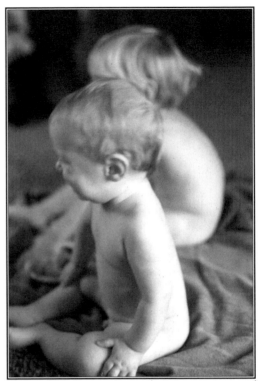

Figure 7-3. Comparison of sitting postures of a normal 6-month-old child to his 2-year-old brother with the diagnosis of spastic athetosis: Lateral view.

to the child with CNS damage can dramatically affect the outcome of therapy.

MEDICAL PROGNOSIS AND OUTCOME

Many of the treatment interventions used for children with CP can be applied to the patient with either contusions or anoxia; however, the outcome may be different based on the neural plasticity and/or prior learning. Although there are many authors who have found that patients younger than age 20 usually recover,[4] this is not always the case. Van der Naalt[5] reports a positive correlation between outcomes of patients with mild to moderate brain injury, lesions seen on CT, and patients with cerebral edema. The Glasgow Coma Scale[6] is a consistent outcome predictor that is used with head trauma and near drowning.

Outcomes for children with CP will vary based on the area of insult, severity, and when treatment is initiated. With early intervention, it is generally possible to improve the functional outcome in mild and moderately involved children. The child with severe disabilities may become less severe and even able to achieve some functional goals. In all cases, physical therapy can make a significant difference in a child's and his family's lives, even if the functional outcomes are limited.

EVALUATION OF THE CHILD WITH NEUROLOGICAL IMPAIRMENT

Initially, the PT takes a thorough history of the pregnancy, labor, delivery, and the child's medical history. It is essential that impairments of all systems be assessed. These would include musculoskeletal, cardiopulmonary, neurological, and integumentary. Specifically, the PT would be assessing muscle tone, muscle strength, joint ROM, tonic neck reflexes, sensory processing of the different sensory organs, patterns of posture and movement, and functional ADLs of the child based on age-appropriate skills. General cognitive and social skills must be noted and considered when assessing the child's overall development.

When evaluating a very young child, it is important for the PT to recognize how rapidly the immature nervous system changes. These children must be reevaluated on an ongoing basis. The PT may ask the PTA to identify changes in order to determine when reassessment is required. Handling and positioning of the child, effectively or ineffectively done, can dramatically affect the child's sensory/motor system and positively or negatively alter his or her motor abilities and skills. Consequently, the PTA must be able to identify the effects of handling, positioning, and other interventions during a treatment session and report to the PT. Feedback from the PTA is essential in determining and identifying the necessary changes needed in the treatment program. Thus, the PTA must be able to differentiate changes in muscle tone, ROM, and the quality and quantity of the movement being facilitated as well as identify the development of functional skills during a treatment session.

During assessment of an older child, the PT must examine the same systems as with the infant; however, contractures, deformities, and diminished motor development will affect motor function at a more complex level of development. From a motor control theory,[3] it is important to determine whether (1) the basic motor patterns are available and appropriately utilized, (2) the appropriate synergies are selected or modified, (3) anticipatory reactions are present if feedback is to be used correctly, and (4) the patient is able to use a variety of motor patterns that match appropriate performance and desired outcomes.

TREATMENT OF THE NEUROLOGICALLY IMPAIRED CHILD

Children with neurological impairment from birth trauma, TBI, or near drowning have or may develop abnormal postural tone that can lead to the development of musculoskeletal complications. The long-term effect of inappropriate movement patterns can lead to catastrophic orthopedic problems in the future. These musculoskeletal impairments generally mean that the sensory/motor system should be assessed and treated early in the child's development. Whatever the cause, children with CP will present with postural tone that is outside the range of normal, either too high (hypertonic) or too low (hypotonic). Tone can also be mixed or fluctuating (athetoid) or ataxic depending on the area of involvement within the CNS.

Postural tone and control is established by the CNS and is responsive to the environment of the child (see Chapter 3). The postural tone controlled from the CNS is influenced by sensory/motor feedback from the various sensory organs and receptors. The environment in which a child is treated will also influence a treatment session. If a child has high tone and the therapy treatment area is noisy and distracting, it will be more difficult to reduce muscle tone. In the case of low postural tone, it may be beneficial to have a more stimulating environment to arouse the CNS.

Gravity cannot be eliminated from life, but the influence can be reduced by the child's position. By placing a child in sidelying as opposed to prone or supine, the influence of the cervical reflexes is reduced. In sidelying, slow, rhythmical, rotational movement of the trunk can further decrease postural tone. This activity can be delegated to a PTA. As tone is decreased, it is then possible to work towards passive ROM of the trunk as well as the extremities. Sitting or standing vertical positions can also help eliminate gravitational effects on the postural system. When the skeletal structures are vertical and properly aligned, this posture promotes appropriate muscle firing, generally causing a decrease in high muscle tone in the spastic muscles and increase in muscle tone in the low-toned child. The reason for this change is that a vertical posture requires less muscle power to hold a head or trunk upright when the COG is over the BOS than when the child is off vertical, and the COG is outside the BOS. Gravitational pull and biomechanics are the causation of these differences.

In this pediatric population, stereotypical posturing and repetitive patterns of movement are observed in the trunk and extremities. These patterns are often due to muscle weakness and the lack of normal postural patterns or motor programs. Initially, the child may present with general hypotonus, but commonly, hypertonus develops, particularly in the extremities, as gravity requires stabilization in order to develop ways to respond to the activity. Extensor tone is generally the first to develop, partially influenced by the CNS and partially by environmental demands such as gravity, positioning, and motivation. If the extensor muscles prevail, the child will be unable to establish midline head control and will become asymmetric, causing shortening of cervical and thoracic spine on one side

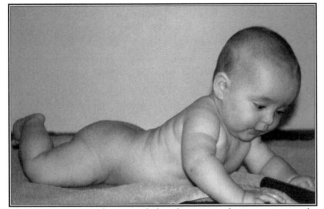

Figure 7-4. Normal postural development of a 3- to 4-month-old child.

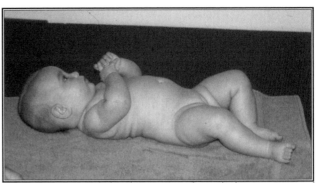

Figure 7-5. Normal development and tonal characteristics of the supine posture of a 3- to 4-month-old child.

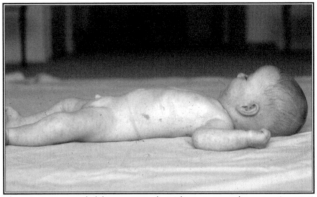

Figure 7-6. A child presented with extreme hypotonia at 6 months old. Although all 4 extremities were hypotonic at this age, he later developed and was diagnosed as a child with spastic *diplegia*.

(see Figure 7-1). This ipsilateral asymmetry generally becomes the side of the body with higher tone. The child with increased extension will usually present with the LEs in extension, adduction, and eventually internal rotation with the feet in plantarflexion. The UEs are more variable in their posturing but are generally dominated by flexion at the shoulder, elbow, wrist, and hand along with ulnar deviation. These patterns of movement are seen in all postures and often intensify as the child works to stabilize the body against gravity. As children repetitively use these patterns for postural control and movement, the patterns become stronger, and it is then more difficult to alter or normalize function. These behaviors are consistent with present theories of motor learning and control (see Chapter 3). The older the child, the more he or she will have practiced and learned stereotypic patterns of movement, making it more difficult to intervene and promote or facilitate normal movement and good postural control.

TREATMENT STRATEGIES

Treatment must be designed to improve movement and postural control, minimize and/or prevent contractures and deformities, improve oral motor function for feeding and prespeech activities, develop attachment to caregivers, and promote social interaction and appropriate responses. To achieve higher functional levels of motor skills, a child must develop levels of competency working against gravity. In the initial stages of normal development, the child works on head control and shoulder girdle development while prone (Figure 7-4) or supine (Figure 7-5), bringing head, hands, and trunk to midline and thereby establishing the basis for postural control against gravity in sitting, standing, and ambulation. When this does not occur and there is insufficient tone

(Figure 7-6) or increased tone (Figure 7-7), then normal development does not occur. As normal trunk and hip strength increase, the child can be placed in sitting (at approximately 6 months old). The infant without insult should sit with an erect spine, gradually gaining strength and stability for postural control and balance (Figure 7-8).

Between 7 and 8 months of age, the able-bodied child develops sufficient strength in the lower trunk musculature and pelvic girdle to allow coming to all fours (Figure 7-9); eventually, they will develop the ability to weight shift and crawl. Ultimately, the goal for all children is the ability to ambulate with a good to normal gait pattern, utilize both hands for playing and learning, and have the postural stability of the trunk, neck, and back of the tongue in order to communicate verbally. Due to the need of the motor system to control walking, balance, and posture simultaneously, early ambulation requires the child to often use one UE to assist (Figure 7-10a and 7-10b). Once those programs become more automatic and variance within all of them under more control by the CNS, the child will shift to two points of support, leaving the UEs free to explore during ambulation. Unfortunately, in children

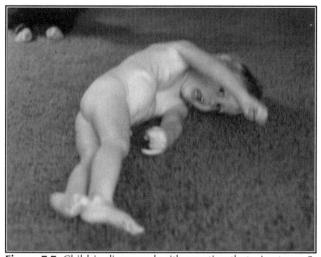

Figure 7-7. Child is diagnosed with spastic athetosis at age 2. Take focus on the rib cage; note the flaring of the rib cage with the retracted sternum.

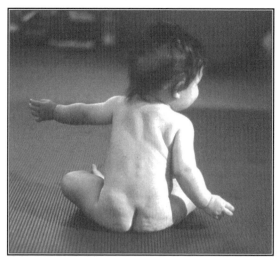

Figure 7-8. Child with normal development by age 7 to 8 months has adequate postural coactivation to allow for balance while her body is in motion. Function requires control of posture, equilibrium, protective responses, rotational forces, and perturbations against gravity while in motion.

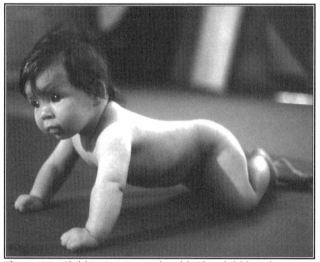

Figure 7-9. Child is 7 to 8 months old. The child has the motor skill to come to all fours and remain in that position. Note that the hands are fists, which is normal when children first get up into this posture. In time, the hands will open and weight bear through the palmar surface with fingers and wrist extended.

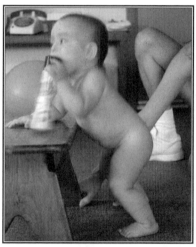

Figure 7-10a. Normal child early standing and cruising between 9 and 12 months. *Side view:* child standing using a hip synergy COG forward requiring upper body support.

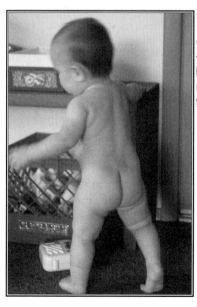

Figure 7-10b. *Posterior view:* same child with weight distributed between lower limbs, but balance strategies still require upper body support: early cruising.

with CP, many of these functional abilities are not possible. The severity and area of trauma to the CNS will be an important factor in the child's motor and cognitive abilities. It has been found, however, that by initiating treatment early, before abnormal patterns of posture and movement become well established and the skeletal system has been adversely impacted, children can gain functional control. Treatment can be effective through handling and positioning, eliminating gravity, and changing postural tone while teaching new patterns of postural control and movement. Listed below are some basic concepts that can help promote improved postural control and movement.

- **Positioning:** to promote symmetry and midline control throughout the body while preventing neck hyperextension, elevated shoulders with adducted scapulae, trunk hyperextension, anterior pelvic tilt, and LE adduction with internal rotation.

- **Therapeutic handling:** to improve tactile, vestibular, proprioceptive, visual, and auditory processing,[3,7-9] assist in normalizing postural tone, develop righting and protective responses, and integrate sensory processing. These *handling techniques* allow the child to practice normal programming and correction of error while the therapist prevents the child from running stereotypic or abnormal patterns.

- **Inhibition and facilitation:** to promote more normal postural tone and encourage better ROM. Generally, the movement will first be inhibitory followed by facilitation into normal patterns of function and movement.

- **Water therapy:** to alter muscle tone abnormalities, decrease the gravitational demands on postural muscles, and decrease resistance of movement of the extremities (ie, bathtub or pool).

- **Oral motor therapy:** to alter the muscle tone (hyper or hypo) of the oral motor structures in order to promote use of the cheek, lips, and tongue for feeding skills and prespeech and speech function.

- **Home exercise program:** to augment clinic-based therapy and empower family, caregivers, and/or the patient. Home programs are used to encourage repetitive practice of normal movement patterns in order to further guarantee motor learning and encourage neuroplasticity.

No matter what a child's functional level, it is critical to teach movement that can lead to function. Thus, it becomes important to know and understand normal movement patterns. The PT and PTA are responsible for helping the child to produce normal movement in order to gain or regain functional control over the demands of life. Life is about movement. There is great joy in being able to move and, ultimately, to move effortlessly, effectively, and efficiently. During treatment, it is important that the PT and PTA strive to reach functional goals. To attain a functional goal, facilitation techniques may be used to promote more normal movement and function for ADLs. Refer to Lois Bly's book *Facilitation Techniques*[10] for examples of how to assist a child in rolling, crawling, and coming to sit or stand and a discussion of the importance of the therapist's handling skills, as it is beyond the scope

of this chapter. As the child matures, adjunct therapies such as horseback riding (hippotherapy), swimming, and skiing are wonderful activities that will help transfer therapy into function along with being normal, fun, and socializing activities.

TESTS USED FOR EVALUATION PURPOSES

Many tests and assessments can be used to determine a child's status. Some are employed to determine the developmental age; others are to establish motor control and function, and still others are to determine the child's neurological status. Some evaluations are administered by neurologists while others are performed in the clinic by the PT. The PTA may be asked to perform and record some of the data collection, but the PT will interpret the findings. Listed below are a few of the more standard assessments used in the clinical setting by the PT:

Prechtl – neurological[11]
Melani-Comparetti – developmental[12]
Brazelton – neonate sensory organization or state of alertness[13]
MIA – movement disorder[14,15]
Bailey – normal development[16,17]
GMFM – functional skills[18]
Pedi – disability inventory[19]
Dubowitz – neurological[20]
Granger – functional evaluation[21]

TREATMENT STRATEGIES THAT MAY BE DELEGATED TO A PHYSICAL THERAPY ASSISTANT

Children with CNS motor dysfunction have postural tone that is either too high or too low. To maximize therapeutic techniques, it is important to first dampen or heighten the postural tone to bring it closer to normal; the techniques employed will then maximize the effects of the interventions. The following are the recommended treatment techniques or positions used by the PT.

Altering Postural Tone

- **Sidelying, sitting, or standing postures:** encourage some internal postural tone or control without a demand causing the CNS to compensate with abnormal tone.

- **Slow, gentle rocking:** with rotation while in sidelying, sitting, kneeling, or standing and with specific emphasis on rotation within the trunk axis.

- **Rhythmic bouncing**: on the therapist's knee or using a ball.

- **Slow movement in anterior-posterior, horizontal, vertical, and inverted postures**: the child may be suspended in the PTA's arms while swinging, or using a hammock, swing, or scooter board.

- **Firm, consistent touch, avoiding intermittent touch**: Firm or maintained touch causes the CNS to adapt while intermittent touch provokes a withdrawal or a protective reaction.

- **Deep pressure through joint structures** (especially the axial trunk): for calming as well as developing postural tone. This can be done manually, using a neopryn vest, or using a weighted blanket. It is very important when using deep pressure through joint structures that the joints themselves are in proper alignment. If the PTA is unsure of that alignment, the PT should be consulted.

- **Inhibition of abnormal patterns of posture using antagonist pattern with rotation**: If the child holds the arm in internal rotation, shoulder and elbow flexion with forearm pronation, wrist flexion, and finger flexion, the pattern that would inhibit that static posture would be shoulder abduction with external rotation, elbow extension, and forearm supination with wrist and finger extension. The rotation (external versus internal, supination versus pronation) is a pivotal component of the child's CNS release of the abnormal posture. The therapist should never try to elicit a release through a quick motion or by use of extreme force. A quick or powerful force elicited by the therapist has the potential of injuring and tearing the child's striated muscle fibers.

- **Facilitation of normal patterns of movement in all spatial postures once postural tone is closer to normal**: These movement patterns must be easy for the child to assist if the therapeutic goal is to have the child's CNS gain control over the movement. It is essential to develop sufficient trunk strength for postural control during both quiet coactivation sitting and standing and dynamic movement in all planes.

Increasing Extensor Tone and Strengthening Muscles for Postural Control

- **Rapid movement using anterior-posterior, horizontal, or angular movement while in prone**: The PTA can hold the child in his or her arms, over a ball, in a hammock swing, or on a scooter board using a slight incline to facilitate automatic postural extension of the head, trunk, and extremities.

- **Facilitation of a biomechanically aligned, upright posture**: accomplished by increasing proprioception input through joint compression down through the trunk with small perturbations. Emphasis must be placed on accurate alignment of the trunk. If the alignment is abnormal, the child will learn that pattern, which has the potential of creating lordosis, kyphosis, or scoliosis in the future. These spinal curvatures are often seen in children with CP and create secondary problems in both the coronary and pulmonary systems.

- **Rapid and irregular bouncing and movement**: while holding the child in your arms, on your lap, on a ball, or in a hammock swing.

- **Weight shifting of the child**: initially on a noncompliant surface, such as a hardwood or linoleum floor, while sitting or standing.

- **Weight shift in sitting or standing on a compliant surface** (ie, dense foam or tilt board): in order to enhance visual and vestibular balance reactions along with postural control.

- **Spinning**: to increase vestibular stimulation for improved postural control (using a hammock or net swing, regular swing, or sit-n-spin). CAUTION: overstimulating a child's system may cause autonomic responses such as vomiting and headaches.

- **Intervention must be balanced with sufficient flexor tone**: after increasing postural extensor tone (short extensor muscles) and muscle strength in a treatment session, to provide stability around the joints and promote movement that is smooth, fluid, and controlled.

Increasing Trunk Flexor Tone and Muscle Strength for Postural Control and Mobility

- **In supine:** bring child's hands to midline or bring child's hands to knees and/or feet. Initially, the child may need assistance, especially with away from shoulder protraction and external rotation.

- **Breast or bottle-feeding**: with the child having proper alignment working towards midline head control with hands to midline.

- **Rolling**: facilitated from supine to side lying to prone with emphasis on trunk rotation and head control. As the neck begins to flex and rotate, the arm on the head side may retract influenced by the ATNR. If the therapist assists the arm into protraction as the neck rotates, often the child will demonstrate some functional reach and/or protective extension.
- **Crawling**: reciprocal hands and knees or hands and feet making sure the trunk flexors are active. The child may be placed on a scooter board to take away a proportion of demands on the postural system while encouraging reciprocal movement of limb patterns.
- **Bouncing the child**: on PTA's knee or on a ball with the child's trunk slightly off vertical in a posterior direction. This encourages head righting while facilitating neck flexion.
- **Swinging**: maintaining flexion and extension for postural control with movement (co-activation) using a hammock or regular swing. Once the child has the ability to functionally control the trunk through postural coactivation of both flexors and extensors, play activities become fun, and the child will often laugh and smile.
- **Spinning**: using postures in greater flexion while maintaining extension for postural control (coactivation) (eg, swing, Sit-n-Spin, rotating chair, and in PTA's arms). Again, it must be stressed that the child should respond positively with motor reactions. If the child is scared, then reduce the speed and observe the reactions.

INHIBITION AND FACILITATION

These are techniques that are utilized together to decrease or increase the sensory motor system output and may be used with the techniques described above. When there is an increase in muscle tone, in a synergy of muscles or a specific muscle, treatment techniques that decrease tone will be required. A description of typical postures of the trunk, UEs, and LEs of a child with CP is categorized with the functional limitations of quadriplegic or diplegic. The children in therapy will present with many of the following postures, but each child presents variations based on the insult and the influences of his or her environment.

Upper Thorax and Upper Extremities

The upper thoracic spine is often extended causing the scapulae to adduct. The shoulder girdle is elevated and protracted, the humerus adducted and internally rotated, the elbow flexed, the forearm pronated, the wrist flexed with ulnar deviation, and the fingers flexed.

Lower Thorax and Lower Extremities

The lower thoracic and lumbar spine are often extended with the pelvis rotated forward; hips are extended, adducted, and internally rotated; knees are extended, and the feet are plantarflexed.

Techniques to Correct These Postures

- Place child in sidelying and gently rock forward and backward, adding passive rotation around the axis of the trunk.
- tone permits within this pattern, bring the LEs into flexion and the UEs into extension.
- Be sure to do this activity to both the right side and the left side.
- Gradually bring the child into supine with the neck in some flexion and bring the arms into adduction in order to abduct the scapulae.
- The LEs are in hip flexion and may be brought out into some abduction and external rotation.
- As the child is able to more easily attain these positions and hold with less assistance, then it may be possible to gradually facilitate movement up towards sitting, over into prone, or into postures requiring the head to come up with support on the forearms (on-elbows).

Presenting the many inhibition and facilitation techniques are far beyond the scope of this chapter. For a more thorough discussion of specific techniques, refer to Bly.[9]

The PTA and PT must always remember that many specific techniques will be taught while in a clinical setting or at continued education courses. Colleagues will find solutions to problems. Being open to listening and watching other therapists who are using techniques that work is a wonderful way to gain additional skills. The answer to every patient problem can be found within the patient. The PTA will inadvertently find solutions to problems, as will the PT. The key is communication with each other. The patient only wants to be empowered to regain the quality of life taken away due to some pathology or accident. The role of the PT and PTA is to help the patient along that path of learning and not become the obstacle to the patient.

CONCLUSION

Today, even children who were traumatized in utero, at birth, or had an insult early in their life will reach adulthood and progress into aging. By doing a Medline search or searching the web, information regarding chronic problems within this population of individuals can be found under the heading "Adults with Development Disabilities." Many of these individuals have or will develop new movement problems or associated organ system dysfunction as they age due to the stress and abnormality of movement and its force on the bones, muscles, nerves, peripheral vascular system, and internal organs. How the PT will approach these new challenges and what will be delegated to the PTA is not known today but will certainly be part of the future when discussing the roles of the PT and PTA in the health care delivery system.

CASE STUDIES

Case #1

TC was born 2 months premature. During labor, his mother experienced a drop in BP. At birth, he was diagnosed with kidney dysfunction, and at 9 months of age, he underwent surgery to correct the problem. At 16 months of age, he was diagnosed with CP, only after his mother repeatedly asked the pediatrician about her concerns. He was first diagnosed with *diplegia*; however, the PT determined that this child's motor deficits included his trunk, both legs, and one arm (*triplegia*). At 18 months of age, he began physical therapy. At the time of evaluation, he lacked adequate head control, had no trunk control, and could not bear weight on his LEs. When placed in standing, his LEs pushed into the support surface, which stimulated the positive support reflex, thereby producing extension, adduction, and internal rotation of the LEs with the feet plantarflexed and inverted. The left UE was held in flexion, and the neck was hyperextended. Following 6 months of treatment, once weekly, and a home exercise program performed daily, he was able to be placed in sitting and maintain this position independently while perturbing his COG during play. He began rolling over in both directions, creeping on all fours, pulling up onto his knees, and began attempts to pull to stand. When he began therapy, there were

minimal vocalizations. Following 6 months of intervention, he had multiple vocalizations and a vocabulary of 30 words due to improved posture and motor control that directly affected respiration, phonation, and articulation.

Physical therapy interventions included the following:

- Altering postural tone.

- Increasing trunk extensor tone for postural control.

- Increasing trunk flexor tone for stability and mobility.

- Repetition of newly acquired motor skills is necessary in order to develop function or motor learning.

- If the child requires immediate intervention and facilitation, the PT may choose not to delegate treatment to the PTA. Once the child begins to demonstrate some internal motor control, the PTA could work on all of the above within that skill, working to the outer limits to allow the child the opportunity to practice, self correct, and develop normal patterns of movement.

Questions

1. What positions or postures would you consider using with TC? Consider that his trunk tone is low while his three extremities demonstrate high muscle tone.

2. Once postural tone is closer to normal and facilitated movement can be freer and easier, would you chose an activity that is gravity eliminated or gravity resisted?

3. Trunk extension must be balanced by trunk flexion. List three ways that you would develop trunk flexion strength.

4. Determine one functional posture in which you would place TC, and explain what activity you would use to encourage repetition.

5. When is it appropriate for the PTA to change or advance the child into new movement patterns?

Case #2

JS and his twin sister were born 1 month prematurely, delivered by emergency cesarean section because his heart rate dropped during his mother's nonstress test. At birth, he weighed 3 lbs, 5 oz, and he sustained an anoxic/ischemic event. He remained in the neonatal unit for 1 month, going home 1 week later than his twin, who had no complications. At 12 months of age, he was diagnosed with CP. He received some therapy initially after he was diagnosed. At 2.5 years, his family moved to another state, where he received physical therapy and ST for 2.5 years. At the time of evaluation, in their new location, he presented with severe motor involvement as well as sensory dysfunction. All sensory systems were involved, which negatively influenced the motor system and caused severe increase in muscle tone, irritability, and fear of movement. Increased muscle tone interfered with all movements of the extremities as well as the oral and facial muscles, impacting eating and sound production for speech. He did not have head or trunk control and could not be placed sitting or standing. He had no speech but communicated with crying.

He received intensive therapy consisting of physical therapy 3 times weekly and speech therapy one time weekly in a private clinic. Emphasis was placed on decreasing his extensor tone, increasing or maintaining ROM, developing postural tone and control, increasing strength, and facilitating normal movement patterns. His motor control improved after 2.5 years of therapy; he was independent in sitting on the floor and in an appropriately fitting chair. He could pull himself to standing and maintain the upright posture to play. He could communicate verbally but lacked sufficient respiratory support for loud sound production. His left UE was used for playing, manipulating toys and objects, and feeding himself, while the right UE minimally assisted. He attended a regular kindergarten with the assistance of an aide. He rode in a therapeutic horseback-riding program once a week, where he gained further strength and postural control. JS's therapy has continued; his therapy will be ongoing until he is no longer making progress towards his goals both medically and educationally. As children grow and mature, it is essential that they receive therapy to help them achieve their full potential.

Questions

1. During JS's initial therapy sessions following the evaluation, the PT could delegate to the PTA incorporating sensory integration activities into intervention and functional skills such as swinging, spinning in a hammock, and bouncing on a ball in prone or sitting.

   What motor behaviors would a PTA be looking for during therapy that would indicate the child is improving?

2. The PTA can work on increasing flexor and extensor postural tone to facilitate head and trunk strength and control. This can be done in sitting while on a hard surface or a ball and progressing to kneeling, half-kneeling, and standing.

   How would the PTA use therapeutic tools such as a ball, bolster, a swing, or one's knee to facilitate this control? How would a PTA progress the child within an identified activity in order for the child to have greater internal control?

3. Between 2 and 6 months of initial treatment, JS's increased tolerance for processing sensory information permitted better organization of the motor system. He was less irritable, less fearful of movement, and he began to develop some head control. He was able to hold his head upright with neck elongation for 30 to 60 seconds. He began reaching for objects with his right UE that previously was held in flexion at the shoulder, elbow, and wrist. At this point in his therapy, the PTA could be responsible for developing strength in the cervical and shoulder girdle musculature to promote good head control. This can be done by placing the child in a mechanically aligned sitting posture both on a hard and a compliant surface. With support on his trunk, weight shift him slowly, causing his COG to shift outside of his BOS (anterior and posterior and lateral). Apply compression down through the shoulders, and then move to the hips. Then use the hips as the pivotal point to cause perturbations. Only perturb the BOS to the limit of the child's ability.

How would the PTA know if the perturbations were too hard? What would the PTA look for in the child's behavior that would suggest the perturbations were creating appropriate learning?

4. During this phase, the PTA could also be responsible for developing head-righting reactions in sitting. Support the trunk appropriately using control from the shoulders, mid-trunk, and hips. Weight-shift him in all planes. The LEs are inhibited from moving into flexion, adduction, and internal rotation during these activities by controlling the legs at the hips and thighs.

What motor behavior by the child would the PTA use to know that the intervention was progressing in a positive direction? Why might noise or sudden movements by other individuals cause the child to lose control?

5. During this phase, the PTA could also be responsible for developing strength and stability of the UEs. While prone in weight bearing, weight shift him initially on fore-arms, and then go to extended arms as strength will permit. Initially, work on non-compliant surfaces on an angle off vertical, and work toward horizontal. As the child's strength and stability improve, move to compliant surfaces.

Identify two motor behaviors exhibited by the child that would help the PTA know the goals of strength and stability of the UEs are being met.

6. During this phase, the PT could increase the respiratory capacity through manual trunk mobilization, and the PTA can be responsible for maintaining the mobility through sidelying and gentle rocking. Then, the PTA can follow with functional activities requiring blowing, sucking, and voicing.

How would the PTA judge whether this goal is being achieved?

7. Between 6 and 12 months of physical therapy, JS's head-righting had emerged and head control was developing. The PTA could be responsible for developing trunk rotation. Rotate the shoulder girdle and/or the pelvic girdle around the vertical axis in sidelying, prone, supine, and sitting postures. Use an activity that requires rotating first to one direction and then to the other. The body will follow the head in a righting reaction, which allows the child to move more freely. Creating an environment where the child is playing will motivate greater self-control and motor learning. For example, place a toy on one side of the child so that he has to reach to pick it up, and then rotate to the other side to complete the activity.

What motor behaviors by the child would clue the PTA that the PT needs to reassess and potentially change the program?

8. During this phase, the PTA could be responsible for developing transition skills from supine to prone to sitting as well as transition through various sitting postures available to him. Postural tone close to normal with proper alignment is necessary in order for movement to occur as fluidly and normally as possible. Guide him with as little or as much assistance as is necessary to help him achieve the movement successfully. As the child improves, slowly reduce the assistance while having the child still succeed at the activity.

Why is the previous sentence a clear indication that motor learning and control is in progress?

9. During this phase, the PTA could be responsible for developing strength and stability of the shoulder and pelvic girdle muscles by positioning in prone on forearms or in weight-bearing on all fours or on hands and feet. Initially, place the child on elbows in prone and weight shift from side to side. The child's head should be stabilized (as if a turtle was poking his head out of a shell). The PTA must make sure the child is not only resting on his joint structure instead of using his own muscle power. When a child only uses positioning to remain on-elbows, it will look as if his head was down in a shell and little postural control will be seen within the shoulder girdle. Once the child can hold with perturbations and begin to weight shift on his elbows, the PTA can use a toy to encourage reaching with one arm while supporting on the other. This activity

can also be done on extended elbows or on all fours.

What would the PTA look for to make sure the child is gaining strength and greater stability?

Suggested author answers are available at www.slackbooks.com/neuroquestions.

Progression of PTA Intervention: Case #2

Once most of these activities are developing and there is increased strength and mobility, the following activities are also delegated to the PTA:

• Increase cervical and upper thoracic muscle strength by placing him:

  a. In prone, on forearms, and while playing and weight shifting.

  b. On extended arms while reaching and playing.

  c. In prone on a scooter board, platform swing, or suspended in PTA's arms while moving him through space.

• Develop trunk-righting responses by:

  a. Rolling in all horizontal position.

  b. Sitting on a lap, ball, or roll as a quiet sitting activity or during play.

  c. Swinging with trunk support. Use an appropriate swing that provides adequate support or, while the child is sitting on the lap of the therapist during the swinging activity, support the child at the pelvis and allow the child to respond to the imposed movements.

  d. Carry him facing away from the caregiver and with his hips on the caregiver's hip, thus encouraging the child to sit up and interact for extended periods of time.

• Develop active trunk rotation around the vertical axis in sitting by having the child:

  a. Swing a bat or racket.

  b. Sit or straddle a roll while reaching and touching his feet or picking up objects off the floor with both hands (to one side and then to the other).

• Teach transitional movements (ie, supine to sit, rolling, all fours, knee standing to half-kneel, coming to standing from the floor or a chair, and facilitating gait by handling at the hips or shoulders):

  a. Supine to sit using diagonal movement patterns, which would be considered a partial rotation pattern from supine to sit.

  b. Moving the child from prone to all fours, handling from the hip. From prone, handling should guide the pelvic girdle back over the knees while encouraging the arms to weight bear.

  c. From side-sit, either have the child come up to or pull to knee standing; weight shift in kneeling. Then rotate the pelvis to encourage one leg to come into half-kneeling. Work or play in half-kneeling so the child weight shifts onto one leg and off the other. Then, have the child come to stand off the half-kneeling leg. Guidance can come from either the back at the hips or the front at the shoulder girdles, arms, or trunk.

• Increase standing balance while engaging the UEs in play by:

  a. Cruising on the furniture or wall

  b. Standing while drawing.

  c. Catching and throwing a ball, frisbee, etc.

  d. Riding a bike.

REFERENCES

1. Adams JH, Graham DI, Murray LS, Scott G. Diffuse axonal injury due to non-missile head injury in humans: an analysis of 45 cases. *Ann Neurol.* 1982;12:557-563.

2. Umphred DA. *Neurological Rehabilitation.* 4th ed. St Louis, Mo: Mosby; 2001.

3. Leahy BJ, Lam CS. Neuropsychological testing and functional outcome for individuals with traumatic brain injury. *Brain Injury.* 1998;12(12):1025-1035.

4. Van der Naalt J, Hew JM, van Zomeren AH, et al. Computed tomography and magnetic resonance imaging in mild to moderate head injury: early and late imaging related to outcome. *Ann Neurol.* 1999;46(1):70-78.

5. Jennet B, Bond M. Assessment of outcome after server brain damage: a practical scale. *Lancet.* 1975;1:480.

6. Kahn-D'Angelo L. The special care nursery. In: Campbell SK, ed. *Physical Therapy for Children.* Philadelphia, Pa: WB Saunders; 1994.

7. Levine MS, Kliebban L. Communication between physician and physical and occupational threats: a neurodevelopmental based prescription. *Pediatrics.* 1981;68:208.

8. White-Trent R, et al. Responses of preterm infants to unimodal and multimodal sensory intervention. *Pediatr Nurs.* 1997;23:169.

9. Bly L. *Facilitation Techniques Based on NDT Principles.* San Antonio, Tex: Therapy Skill Builders; 1997.

10. Bly L. *Motor Skills Acquisition in the First Year.* San Antonia, Tex: Therapy Skill Builders; 1994.

11. Prechtl H. The neurological examination of the full-term newborn infant. 2nd ed. *Clinics in Developmental Medicine.* No 63. Philadelphia, Pa: JB Lippincott; 1977.

12. Stuberg WA, White PJ, Miedaner JA, Dehne PR. *The Milani-Comparetti Motor Development Screening Test: Test manual.* 3rd ed. Omaha, Neb: University of Nebraska Medical Center, Meyer Children's Rehabilitation Institute; 1992.

13. Brazelton TB, Nugent JK. Neonatal behavioral assessment scale. 3rd ed. *Clinics in Developmental Medicine.* No 137. London, England: Mac Keith Press; 1995.

14. Chandler LC. Neuromotor assessment. In: Gibbs ED, Teti DM, eds. *Interdisciplinary Assessment of Infants: A Guide for Early Intervention Professional.* Baltimore, Md: Brookes; 1990.

15. Chandler L, Andrews M, Swanson M. *The Movement Assessment of Infants: A Manual.* Rolling Bay, Wash: Infant Movement Research; 1980.

16. Bayley N. *Manual for the Bayley Scales of Infant Development.* 2nd ed. San Antonio, Tex: The Psychological Corporation; 1993.

17. Black MM, Matula K. *Essentials of Bayley Scales of Infant Development-II Assessment.* New York, NY: John Wiley and Sons; 2000.

18. Russell D, Rosenbaum PL, Cadman DT, et al. The gross motor function measure: a means to evaluate the effects of physical therapy. *Dev Med Child Neurol.* 1989;1:341-352.

19. Haley SM, Coster WJ, Ludlow LH, et al. *Pediatric Evaluation of Disability Inventory (PEDI): Development, Standardization and Administration Manual.* Boston, Mass: New England Medical Center Hospitals and PEDI Research Group; 1992.

20. Dubowitz L, Dubowitz V, Mercuri E. The neurological assessment of the preterm and full-term newborn infant. 2nd ed. *Clinics in Developmental Medicine.* No 148. London, England: Mac Keith Press; 1999.

21. Granger CR, et al. *Guide for the Use of the Functional Independence Measure (Wee FIM) of the Uniform Data Set for Medical Rehabilitation.* Buffalo, NY: Research Foundation, State University of New York; 2000.

Chapter

8

CLIENTS WITH GENETIC AND DEVELOPMENTAL PROBLEMS

Eunice Shen, PT, DPT, MS, PCS

KEY WORDS

developmental coordination disorders
developmental delays
developmental disabilities
Down syndrome
family-centered care
genetic disorders
learning disabilities
mental retardation
mitochondrial disease
muscular dystrophy
osteogenesis imperfecta
pervasive developmental disorder

CHAPTER OBJECTIVES

- To discuss the role of PTs and PTAs when working with children with developmental delays.

- To describe the five developmental skill areas in intervention in which PTs and PTAs provide service.

- To identify signs and examples of developmental delay.

- To describe the most common genetic disorders and the modes of inheritance.

- To identify specific behavior categories and impairments frequently treated by PTs and PTAs.

- To describe components of family-centered therapy for children with developmental delays and genetic disorders.

INTRODUCTION

Normal development is a lifelong process that is a result of the complex interplay of biological, psychological, cultural, and environmental factors[1] (see Chapter 2). One approach to child development tracks development within particular domains, such as gross motor, fine motor, social, emotional, language, and cognition.[2] Within each of these categories are developmental sequences, which reflect positive changes. These categories intertwine throughout life. A deficit in one area may cause secondary complications or impairments within another. Developmental delay is a common problem seen in pediatric physical therapy practice.

What then is developmental delay? Developmental delay occurs when a child has not reach developmental milestones by the typically expected time. Normal developmental milestones are a set of functional skills or age-specific tasks that most children can perform or do within a certain age range. Child development refers to how children perform more complex skills and activities as they get older. Child development is not about growth. Growth implies that the child is getting bigger in physical size. Development refers to the basic functional skill areas discussed in Chapter 2.

The Federal definition of developmental delay is as follows:

"The term child with a disability for children aged 3 through 9 may at the discretion of the State and Local Education Agency (LEA) include a child who is experiencing *developmental delays* as defined by the State as measured by appropriate diagnostic instruments and procedures, in one or more of the following areas: physical development, cognitive development, communication development, social or emotional development, or adaptive development, and who for that reason, need special education and related services."[3]

An understanding of developmental milestones is necessary for those working in pediatrics, whether the professional is a pediatrician, a PT, a PTA, an OT, an OTA, or an early childhood developmental specialist or educator. For parents, it is helpful to use developmental milestones and sequences as a guide to chart the long-range course for their children. These milestones are not recipes for development.[1] The developmental milestones in the first two years of life described by Needlman[2] can be found in Table 8-1. The role of the PTs and PTAs working with children and adolescents with developmental delays will be discussed in this chapter. During the initial examination and evaluation, the PT will document how a child is developing through the patient medical history as well as the developmental history. The verification of developmental delay is, therefore, obtained through an evaluation process. This process includes any combination of the following: observational assessment, standardized development test(s), developmental inventory, behavioral checklist, and parental interviews.[4]

Children and young adults who are developmentally delayed often have other medical problems. These individuals may have any combination of musculoskeletal, neuromuscular, or cardiovascular and pulmonary impairments that affect the normal development of these children.

The PT should document the delays limiting the development of a child. Concerns from the parent(s), caretaker(s), or guardian(s) should also be documented. The therapy plan of care should include the family's goals as well as the therapist's goals. Documentation of disease progression or improvement as well as effects and outcomes of treatment procedures are essential and the responsibility of the PT. Therapists should assess progress, improvement, and functional outcome in a systematic way during and throughout the intervention period. As clinicians, closer attention should be paid to the results of PT intervention. This is the responsibility of both the PT and the PTA. Emphasis

on evidence-based practice challenges clinicians to be professionally astute and responsible for the outcomes of their treatment interventions. When intervention is delegated to the PTA, clear communication needs to be established among the PT, PTA, and family with regards to goals, how they will be measured, and intervention adjustments.

The five development skills areas the PTs and PTAs providing the intervention would be looking at are as follows:

1. **Gross motor:** using large groups of muscle to sit, stand, walk, run, jump, hop, skip, etc; keeping balance; and changing positions.
2. **Fine motor:** using hands to eat, draw, dress, play, write, and do other things.
3. **Language:** speaking and communicating, using body language and gestures, comprehending, and understanding what others say.
4. **Cognitive:** thinking skills and process, learning, understanding, problem solving, reasoning, and remembering.
5. **Social:** interacting with others, cooperating, responding to the feelings of others, and having relationships with family, friends, and others.

Developmental delay can occur in any or all five areas of development. The PTA must remember that progress in one area of development interacts with the other areas. Thus, all changes must be reported to the PT.

The developmental sequences in the gross motor domain, leading from rolling to creeping to walking, are obvious.[2] Difficulties in 1 area, likewise, will affect or influence other areas. For example, if a child is unable to crawl or move around the floor surface, that child may not be able to explore his or her environment. This might limit the child's ability to reach, to explore, or to manipulate toys, thus affecting fine motor skills.

Developmental delay is usually a diagnosis made by a physician. The term *developmental delay* is actually a description of a symptom or sign of a condition rather than a medical diagnosis. However, it is not uncommon to receive a referral for physical therapy intervention from a medical practitioner with the diagnosis of *developmental delay*. An infant's history and physical exam may initially be normal. As each year passes, parents often notice that their child's development is not progressing at the same rate as other children of comparable age. Parents have also reported the reverse scenario during the patient history. Parents can often see problems very early, but a definitive diagnosis may not be made until the child is a few years old because the physician may not want to "label" the child too early or misdiagnose the child. Parents will often be told that the child's delay may be temporary and it

Table 8-1
Developmental Milestones in the First Two Years of Life

Milestone	Average Age of Attainment (mo)	Developmental Implications
Gross Motor		
Head steady in sitting	2	Allows more visual interaction
Pull to sit, no head lag	3	Muscle tone
Hands together in midline	3	Self-discovery
Asymmetric tonic neck reflex gone	4	Child can inspect hands in midline
Sits without support	6	Increasing exploration
Rolls back to stomach	6.5	Truncal flexion, risk of falls
Walks alone	12	Exploration, control of proximity to parents
Runs	16	Supervision more difficult
Fine Motor		
Grasps rattle	3.5	Object use
Reaches for objects	4	Visuomotor coordination
Palmar grasp gone	4	Voluntary release
Transfers object hand to hand	5.5	Comparison of objects
Thumb-finger grasp	8	Able to explore small objects
Turns pages of book	12	Increasing autonomy during book time
Scribbles	13	Visuomotor coordination
Builds tower of two cubes	15	Uses objects in combination
Builds tower of six cubes	22	Requires visual, gross, and fine motor coordination
Communication and Language		
Smiles in response to face, voice	1.5	Child more active in social participation
Monosyllabic babble	6	Experimentation with sounds, tactile sense
Inhibits to "no"	7	Response to tone (nonverbal)
Follows one-step command with gesture	7	Nonverbal communication
Follows one-step command without gesture (eg, "Give it to me")	10	Verbal receptive language
Speaks first real word	12	Beginning of labeling
Speaks four to six words	15	Acquisition of object and personal names
Speaks 10 to 15 words	18	Acquisition of object and personal names
Speaks two-word sentences (eg, "Mommy shoe")	19	Beginning grammaticization, corresponds with 50+ word vocabulary
Cognitive		
Stares momentarily at spot where object disappeared (eg, yard ball dropped)	2	Lack of object permanence (out of sight, out of mind)
Stares at own hand	4	Self-discovery, cause and effect
Bangs two cubes	8	Active comparison of objects
Uncovers toy (after seeing it hidden)	8	Object permanence
Egocentric pretend play (eg, pretends to drink from cup)	12	Beginning symbolic thought
Uses stick to reach toy	17	Able to link actions and solve problems
Pretend play with doll (eg, gives doll bottle)	17	Symbolic thought

Adapted from Needlman RD. Growth and development. In: Behrman RE, Kliegman RM, Jenson HB, eds. Nelson Textbook of Pediatrics. 17th ed. Philadelphia, Pa: Saunders; 2004.

may resolve. Often, delays in medical diagnosing lead to compensatory developmental motor behaviors that lead to secondary complications requiring additional interventions by the PT and PTA.

The American Academy of Pediatrics (AAP) has developed milestones for children from birth through age 5. It is especially important for all therapists and the family to watch for signs of developmental delay during the first 3 years of growth in high-risk infants as well as acknowledge attainment of developmental milestones that are being met.[5] The problems, signs, and symptoms listed in Tables 8-2 and 8-3 are behaviors with which the PT and PTA must be familiar. If a child is not learning a skill that other children of comparable age are learning during a specific period, the PT providing services should let the parent(s) know of concerns and advise them to talk to their physicians. Informing the parents of delays is the responsibility of the PT; thus, if a PTA has concern, those concerns should be shared with the PT. If the PTA provides intervention and recognizes these milestone problems or advances, it is appropriate to discuss it immediately with the PT. A checklist of warning signs of developmental delay in the behavioral, gross motor, vision, and hearing domains can be found in Table 8-4.

Children with developmental delays have a right to an education. The Individuals with Disabilities Education Act (IDEA) is the nation's special education law.[6] IDEA requires states to provide a free appropriate public education (FAPE) in the least restrictive environment (LRE) to all children. Reauthorization of the IDEA 2004 (Public Law [PL] 108-446) preserves the basic structure and civil rights guarantees of IDEA.[6] A significant change in the law concentrates on Part B, which authorizes grants for children with disabilities ages 3 to 21. It contains key provision regarding the structure of special education, related services, and the procedural safeguards that guarantee the provisions of FAPE to children with disabilities. The requirements regarding highly qualified special education teachers became effective immediately upon signature.[6]

Before 1997, the IDEA of 1991 defined children from birth through age 2 as needing early intervention services when diagnosed with a physical or mental condition that has a high probability of resulting in developmental delay or when there are delays in one or more of the following areas: cognitive development, physical development, language and speech development, psychosocial development, or self-help skills.[7] The reauthorization of IDEA in 1997 added that "for children 3 through 9, the state and local education agency may define 'child with disability' as a child who is experiencing developmental delays and needs special education and related services."[8]

CAUSES OF DEVELOPMENTAL DELAY

There are many causes of developmental delay. Genetic defects, complications of pregnancy or birth, and environmental factors are all possible causes. Often, the specific cause is unknown. As children are being monitored for their growth and development, physicians may consider certain diagnoses based on the patterns and changes observed over time.

There is an increasing ability in the area of medicine to find specific causes for developmental delay. If there is no clear-cut etiology in a child's delay, physicians are looking into genetic causes. New syndromes and diagnosis have been made with new technological improvements in testing.[9]

Genetic causes may account for 5% to 25% of children with developmental delays.[10] This includes some children with a normal physical exam or even minimal physical findings. Children are at risk for delays when they are born with a genetic or chromosomal abnormality. An example is *Down syndrome* (DS), which is a disorder that causes developmental delay because of an abnormal chromosome. Congenital malformation, hearing impairment, and growth retardation are some of the associated physical findings and comorbidities that may increase the likelihood of a genetic cause of developmental delay. The PTs, PTAs, and other members of the educational and/or rehabilitation team may often see children with delayed development and those at risk for delayed development in an early intervention program, school setting, or hospital outpatient setting.

GENETIC DISORDERS

A *genetic disorder* is caused by a mutation or change in a gene. Genes are made up of a chemical known as deoxyribonucleic acid (DNA). DNA is actually strings of chemicals that form the codes for the thousands of proteins in the human body. These proteins are used to build cellular structures and carry out the functions of the body's cells. DNA is stored on strands called chromosomes and is usually located in the nucleus of each cell in the body.

Genetic problems occur in several ways: (1) a defective gene is duplicated and passed on to a child, (2) a spontaneous mutation occurs and changes a specific gene's function, and (3) a chromosome may not duplicate itself correctly, causing a partial or complete deletion or addition from the genetic material in the cell.[11] How crucial proteins affect bodily function will be elaborated upon in the section on Duchenne Muscular Dystrophy (page 117).

Table 8-2
Signs of Possible Delay: First Year of Life

Age of Child	Problems Encountered
During week 2, 3, or 4	Sucks poorly and feeds slowly. Does not blink when shown a bright light. Does not focus on and follow a nearby object moving side to side. Rarely moves arms and legs seem stiff. Seems excessively loose in limbs, or floppy. Lower jaw trembles constantly, even when not crying or excited. Does not respond to loud sounds.
By the end of month 3	Still has no moro reflex after 4 months. Does not seem to respond to loud sounds. Does not notice her or his hands by 2 months. Does not follow moving objects with her or his eyes by 2 to 3 months. Does not grasp and hold objects by 3 months. Does not reach for and grasp toys by 3 to 4 months. Begins babbling but doesn't try to imitate any sounds by 4 months. Does not babble by 3 to 4 months. Does not bring objects to her or his mouth by 4 months. Does not push down with her or his legs when feet are placed on a firm surface by 4 months. Has trouble moving one or both eyes in all directions. Crosses her or his eyes most of the time. Does not pay attention to new faces, or seems very frightened by new faces or surroundings. Still has the tonic neck reflex at 4 to 5 months.
By the end of month 7	Seems very stiff with tight muscles. Seems very floppy like a rag doll. Head still flops back like a rag doll. Reaches with one hand only. Refuses to cuddle. Shows no affection for the person who cares for her or him. Doesn't seem to enjoy being around people. One or both eyes consistently turn in or out. Persistent tearing, eye drainage or sensitivity to light. Does not respond to sound around her or him. Has difficulty getting object to her or his mouth. Does not turn his head to locate sounds by 4 months. Does not roll over in either direction (front to back or vice versa) by 5 months. Seems inconsolable at night after 5 months. Does not smile spontaneously by 5 months. Cannot sit with help by 6 months. Does not laugh or make squealing sounds by 6 months. Does not actively reach for objects by 6 to 7 months. Does not follow objects with both eyes at hear ranges (1 to 6 feet) by 7 months. Does not bear some weight on legs by 7 months. Does not try to attract attention through actions by 7 months. Does not babble by 8 months. Shows no interest in games of peek-a-boo by 8 months.
By the end of 12 months	Does not crawl. Drags one side of body while crawling (for over 1 month). Cannot stand when supported. Does not search for objects that are hidden while she or he watches. Says no single word ("mama" or "dada"). Does not learn to use gestures, such as waving or shaking head. Does not point to objects or pictures.

Adapted from American Academy of Pediatrics (AAP), Shelov SP, Hanneman RE, Wray W, Gray A. Caring for Your Baby and Young Child: Birth to Age Five. New York, NY: Bantan Books; 1998.

Table 8-3
Signs of Possible Delay: Second to Fifth Years of Life

Age of Child	Problems Encountered
By the end of 2 years	Cannot walk by 18 months. Fails to develop a mature heel-toe walking pattern after several months of walking or walking on his or her toes. Does not speak at least 15 words by 18 months. Does not use two-word sentences. By 15 months, does not seem to know the function of common objects (eg, brush, telephone, bell, fork, spoon). Does not imitate actions or words. Does not follow instructions. Cannot push a wheeled toy.
By the end of 3 years	Frequent falling and difficulty with stairs. Persistent drooling or very unclear speech. Cannot build a tower of more than four blocks. Difficulty manipulating small objects. Cannot copy a circle. Cannot communicate in short phrases. No involvement in "pretend" play. Cannot understand simple instructions. Little interest in other children. Extreme difficulty separating from mother.
By the end of 4 years	Cannot throw a ball overhand. Cannot jump in place. Cannot ride a tricycle. Cannot grasp a crayon between thumb and fingers. Has difficulty scribbling. Cannot stack four blocks. Still clings or cries whenever his or her parents leave him or her. Shows no interest in interactive games. Ignores other children. Does not respond to people outside the family. Does not engage in fantasy play. Resists dressing, sleeping, and using the toilet. Lashes out without any self-control when angry or upset. Cannot copy a circle. Does not use sentences of more than three words. Does not use "me" and "you" appropriately.
By the end of 5 years	Exhibits extremely fearful or timid behavior. Exhibits extremely aggressive behavior. Cannot separate from parents without major protest. Is easily distracted and unable to concentrate on any single activity for more than 5 min. Shows little interest in playing with other children. Refuses to respond to people in general, or responds only superficially. Rarely uses fantasy or imitation in play. Seems unhappy or sad much of the time. Does not engage in a variety of activities. Avoids or seems aloof with other children and adults. Does not express a wide range of emotions. Has trouble eating, sleeping, or using the toilet. Cannot differentiate between fantasy and reality. Seems unusually passive. Cannot understand two-part commands using prepositions. Cannot correctly give his or her first and last name. Does not use plurals or past tense properly when speaking. Does not talk about his or her daily activities and experiences. Cannot build a tower of six to eight blocks. Seems uncomfortable holding a crayon. Has trouble taking off clothing. Cannot brush his or her teeth efficiently. Cannot wash and dry his or her hands.

Adapted from American Academy of Pediatrics (AAP), Shelov SP, Hanneman RE, Wray W, Gray A. Caring for Your Baby and Young Child: Birth to Age Five. New York, NY: Bantan Books; 1998

Table 8-4
Warning Signs of a Developmental Delay

Behavioral	Gross Motor	Vision	Hearing
Does not pay attention or stay focused on an activity for as long a time as other children the same age.	Has stiff arms and/or legs.	Seems to have difficulty following objects or people with his or her eyes.	Talks in a very loud or very soft voice.
Focuses on unusual objects for long periods of time; enjoys this more than interacting with others.	Has a floppy or limp body posture compared to other children of the same age.	Rubs eyes frequently.	Seems to have difficulty responding when called from across the room, even when it is for something interesting.
Avoids or rarely makes eye contact with others.	Uses one side of body more than the other.	Turns, tilts, or holds head in a strained or unusual position when trying to look at an object.	Has difficulty understanding what has been said or following directions (after the age of 3 years).
Gets unusually frustrated when trying to do simple tasks that most children of the same age can do.	Has a very clumsy manner compared with other children of the same age.	Seems to have difficulty finding or picking up small objects dropped on the floor (after the age of 12 months).	Does not startle to loud noises.
Shows aggressive behaviors, acts out, and appears to be very stubborn compared with other children.		Has difficulty focusing or making eye contact.	Ears appear small or deformed.
Displays violent behaviors on a daily basis.		Closes one eye when trying to look at distant objects.	Fails to develop sounds or words that would be appropriate at her or his age.
Stares into space, rocks body, or talks to self more often than other children of the same age.		Eyes appear to be crossed or turned.	
Does not seek love and approval from a caregiver or parent.		Bring objects too close to eyes to see.	
		One or both eyes appear abnormal in size or coloring.	

Adapted from How Kids Develop. CASRC website. 2005. Available at: http://www.howkidsdevelop.com/developDevDelay.html. Accessed May 6, 2005.

CLASSIFICATION OF GENETIC ABNORMALITIES

Genetic disorders are usually divided into four categories: Chromosomal disorders, specific gene defects or single-gene disorders, sex-linked disorders, and mitochondrial problems.[12] An overview of genetic disorders seen in the pediatric age group can be found in Table 8-5.

Chromosomal Disorders

Chromosomal abnormalities can occur in three different ways: a deviation in the number of chromosomes, an extra chromosome, or a missing chromosome. Chromosomal abnormalities could also involve a missing component or extra portion of a chromosome.[12] Monosomies occur when one of the two paired chromosomes is missing. Children with monosomes rarely survive.[11] Autosomal trisomies occur when there is an extra chromosome in the pair. Children

Table 8-5
Overview of Genetic Disorders Affecting the Pediatric Age Group

Type of Disorder	Characteristic of Disorder	Name of Disorder	Clinical Features
Chromosome Abnormalities	Deviation in number of chromosomes, *47, XY, +21.	Down syndrome (trisomy 21).	Characteristic facial features including flat occiput, flat face; upward slanting eyes; hypotonicity; broad, short feet and hands; protruding abdomen; mental retardation; possible cardiac anomalies.
		Edwards syndrome (trisomy 18).	Small stature; long, narrow skull; low-set ears; hypotonicity; rocker bottom feet; scoliosis; profound mental retardation.
		Patau syndrome (trisomy 13).	Microcephaly; cleft lip and palate; polydactyly of hands and feet; severe to profound mental retardation.
	Deviation in sex chromosomes.	Turner syndrome (XO syndrome).	Congenitally webbed neck; growth retardation; ptosis of upper eyelids; lack of sexual development; congenital heart and kidney disease; scoliosis; low-normal intelligence.
		Klinefelter syndrome (XXY)	Long limbs; tall and slender build until adulthood when obesity becomes a problem (if no testosterone replacement therapy; small penis and testes; low-average to mild mental retardation; tremors, behavior problems.
	Partial deletion syndrome.	Cri-du-chat syndrome (5p-).	High-pitched, catlike cry in infancy; microcephaly; low-set ears; hypotonicity; severe mental retardation; scoliosis; clubfeet; dislocated hips.
		Prader-Willi syndrome (15q-).	Low tone with feeding disorder in infancy; insatiable appetite develops in toddlerhood; moderate mental retardation; hyperflexibility; obesity; characteristic facial features including almond-shaped eyes; and small stature, hands, feet, and penis.
		Williams syndrome (deletion near the elastin gene on chromosome 7).	Characteristic facial abnormalities including prominent lips, medial eyebrow flare, and open mouth; mild microcephaly; mild growth retardation; short nails; mild to moderate mental retardation; cardiovascular anomalies.
Specific Gene Defects	Autosomal dominant.	Neurofibromatosis.	Areas of hyperpigmentation or hypopigmentation of skin inducing "café au lait" spots or axillary "freckling"; tumors along nerves, in connective tissue, eyes, or meninges; macrocephaly; short stature. May have skeletal abnormalities including scoliosis, bowing of long bones, and dislocations.
		Tuberous sclerosis.	Brain lesions causing seizures and mental retardation; skin lesions on cheeks around nose; "café au lait" spots; cystlike areas in bones of fingers; kidney and teeth abnormalities.
		Osteogenesis imperfecta.	Type I: Small stature; thin bones, bowing of the bones; fractures of long bones; hyperextensible joints; kyphoscoliosis, flat feet, thin skin, deafness in adult life; blue sclerae of eyes, blue or yellow teeth.
			Type II: Prenatal growth deficiency; short limbs; multiple fractures; hypotonia; hydrocephalus; frequent early death.
			Type III: Short stature; bowing and angulation of long bones; multiple fractures; kyphoscoliosis.
			Type IV: Osteoporosis leading to fractures; variable mild deformity of long bones; normal sclerae of eyes; may have poor teeth.
	Autosomal recessive.	Spinal muscular atrophy.	Progressive muscle atrophy and weakness; normal intelligence; normal sensation: weakness may begin before birth, in early childhood, or in later childhood.

Table 8-5 (continued)
Overview of Genetic Disorders Affecting the Pediatric Age Group

Type of Disorder	Characteristic of Disorder	Name of Disorder	Clinical Features
	Autosomal recessive.	Sickle cell disease.	A group of diseases characterized by blood disorders related to hemoglobin defects. Mostly seen in people of African or infrequently of Mediterranean descent. Sickle-shaped red blood cells cause anemia and crises of blockages in veins, causing a variety of conditions. These include leg ulcers, arthritis, acute pain, and problems in major organ systems, including the spleen, liver, kidney, bones, heart, and CNS. Children may exhibit weakness, pain, or fever and may have growth retardation.
		Hurler syndrome.	Normal or rapid growth during the first year with deterioration during the second year; coarse facial features characterized by full lips, flared nostrils, thick eyebrows, low nasal bridge, and prominent forehead; still joints; small stature; small teeth, enlarged tongue; kyphosis, short neck; clawhand, hip dislocation and other joint deformities; mental retardation.
		Phenylketonuria.	Children cannot metabolize phenylalanine causing mental retardation, growth retardation, hypertonicity, seizures, pigment deficiency of hair or skin if left untreated. Can be successfully treated by limiting amount of phenylalanine in diet.
Sex-Linked Disorders (all affected are boys, X-linked)		Fragile X syndrome.	One of the most common causes of mental retardation in boys. Characteristic facial features include elongated face, large ears and prominent jaw. Other characteristics include enlarged testicles in adulthood, and prolapse of the mitral valve in the heart. mental retardation is usually in the severe range, sometimes with aggressive behaviors. Some boys will have poor coordination and hypotonia.
	Abnormal gene on X chromosome.	Duchenne muscular dystrophy.	Onset at 1 to 5 years. Progressive, rapid weakness at onset stage; characteristic gait disturbances including toe walking, abducted gait, lordosis, and waddling gait. Progressive weakness leads to w/c use, decreased independence in all areas, and finally death by respiratory or cardiac failure. Loss of ability to walk by age 9 or 10. Death by late teens.
		Lowe syndrome.	Progressive mental deterioration leading to moderate to severe mental retardation, renal dysfunction, cortical cataracts with or without glaucoma leading to blindness later in life, hypotonicity, joint hyperextensibility, growth retardation, large low-set ears, pale skin, and blonde hair.
		Lesh-Nyhan syndrome.	Moderate to severe mental retardation, hypertonicity leading to dislocated hips, club foot, growth retardation, movement disorders including chorea, ballistic movements, and tremor. Self-mutilating behaviors including lip-biting and fingertip-biting characterize this disease.

NOTATION: 46 is the normal number of chromosomes. 47 indicates an extra chromosome present. XY refers to genetic male, +21 refers to the extra chromosome being found on the #21 chromosome.

Adapted from Ratliffe KT. Clinical Pediatric Physical Therapy. St. Louis, Mo: Mosby; 1998:219-274, 230-231.

with trisomy on Chromosome 21, best known as Down Syndrome, are very common and often seen by PTs and PTAs. Trisomy 18 (Edwards syndrome) and Trisomy 13 (Patau syndrome) are also autosomal trisomies and treated by PTs and PTAs.

Incidence of DS increases with maternal and possibly paternal age.[13] Children with DS have varying

degrees of *mental retardation* (MR). They learn more slowly and have difficulty with complex reasoning and judgment.[14] MR has been misunderstood by society and the intellectual potential for children with DS has been underestimated.

Ten features characterizing newborns with DS[15] include hypotonicity, poor Moro reflex, joint hyperextensibility, excess skin on the back of the neck, flat facial profile, slanted palpebral fissures, anomalous auricles, dysplasia of the pelvis, dysplasia of the mid-phalanx of the fifth finger, and simian creases. Delay in the development of normal postural tone is demonstrated by the severe head lag evident when the child is pulled to sit from horizontal and the lack of full antigravity extension noted when suspended horizontally in space.[16] Additional impairments include congenital heart disease, musculoskeletal anomalies, and impairments of the visual and sensory systems. Musculoskeletal impairment often includes increase risk of atlantoaxial dislocation and craniofacial structural abnormality. Trisomy 18 (Edwards syndrome) is the second most common of the trisomies. Again, advanced maternal age is positively correlated. Only 10% of the children with Edwards syndrome survive past the first year of life. These children have more serious organic malformations that affect the cardiovascular, gastrointestinal, urogenital, and skeletal systems. Muscle tone, initially hypotonic, becomes hypertonic as the child ages. However, by preschool and school age, the tone changes back to hypotonicity with joint hyperextensibility.[11] These children are frequently referred to PTs and OTs for musculoskeletal needs, feeding difficulties (poor suck), and developmental delay within a variety of subsystems. Many of the developmental play activities can be delegated to the PTA in order to allow the child additional practice time, some variance in practice for generalizability, and for social development.

Sex Chromosome Disorders

The second most common type of chromosomal abnormalities affects the chromosome pair that directs sexual characteristics. Klinefelter syndrome is the most common sex chromosome abnormality. It is usually not apparent until puberty, when the testes fail to enlarge and gynecomastia occurs. Most males with karotype XXY have normal intelligence, passive personality, reduced libido, and are sterile.

Turner syndrome (XO syndrome) is usually caused by a missing paternal sex chromosome. Characteristics of this syndrome are sexual infantilism, congenital webbed neck, and cubitus valgus. Growth retardation is most noticeable after the age of 5 or 6 years. Referrals to physical therapy are generally due to the skeletal anomalies. These impairments include hip dislocation, pes planus, pes equinovarus, dislocated patella, medial tibial condyles deformity, and deformities due to osteoporosis.

Partial Deletion Disorders

The third type of chromosome disorder is a partial deletion syndrome. The two most common partial deletion syndromes are cri du chat syndrome and Prader-Willi syndrome.

Cri du chat syndrome is also known as the cat-cry syndrome. Approximately 70% of these children are female. Severe MR and associated musculoskeletal deformities are present with both muscular hypotonicity and hypertonicity. Due to the severity of the retardation, a huge amount of repetitive practice in motor tasks needs to occur before the CNS will learn a functional motor program and run it easily upon environmental demand.

Prader-Willi syndrome (PWS) is characterized by obesity, hypogonadism, short stature, hypotonia, dysmorphic facial features, dysfunctional CNS performance, and a compulsive preoccupation with food. The PT will delegate activities to the PTA that increase metabolism to assist in weight control as well as activities that elongate and rotate the trunk to enhance breathing.

Specific Gene Defects or Single-Gene Disorders

A specific or single-gene disorder is a result of a defect or mutation occurring at a single gene rather than the chromosome itself. There are three ways specific gene defects occur: autosomal dominant, autosomal recessive, and sex-linked.

Autosomal dominant conditions require only one mutation to show itself. The term autosomal dominant means that the genetic mutation is on one of the chromosomes that is not sex linked. Only one parent needs to carry the disorder on a dominant gene for the disorder to manifest itself. Three examples of autosomal dominant conditions that have serious neurological consequences and sequelae are *osteogenesis imperfecta*, sclerosis, and neurofibromatosis. Individuals diagnosed with one of these three syndromes often require PT and OT intervention because of musculoskeletal and neuromuscular impairments that lead to functional limitations and delays in normal movement development.

Autosomal recessive conditions require two mutations in order to be manifested. Autosomal recessive means that the disorder is located on the chromosomes of both parents. The recessive gene may remain undetected and recede in the background for many generations in a family. When the person with a recessive gene has a child with another person who has a mutation in that same autosomal gene, the parents will produce a child with the signs and symptoms of the disorder. Examples of autosomal recessive disorders are spinal muscular atrophy, cystic fibrosis, sickle cell anemia, Hurler syndrome, and phenylketonuria.

Sex-Linked Disorders

The sex-linked disorders (X-linked) are passed through the sex chromosomes. The defective gene is carried on the X-chromosome of the mother. Females carrying one abnormal gene usually do not display the trait of the disease because of the dominant normal gene on the other X chromosome from the father. Thus, X-linked disorders affect males and females differently. All individuals affected with an X-linked disorder are boys because they only have one X chromosome. The girl can receive a normal gene from the father's X chromosome. Being a carrier, the girl may pass the disorder to her own female children who routinely show at least some of the disease symptoms. The two most well-known sex-linked disorders are Duchenne *muscular dystrophy* and hemophilia. Fragile X syndrome and Lesch-Nyhan syndrome are also sex-linked disorders. Rett syndrome, an X-linked disorder, is an exception because it affects mostly females. Seizures develop in about 70% to 80% of individuals with Rett syndrome.[12]

Mitochondrial Disorders

Mitochondrial disorders are caused by alterations in the cytoplasmic mitochondrial chromosome. Mitochondria use proteins made by genes in the cell's nucleus. These proteins are imported into the mitochondria.

Mutations can occur in the mitochondrial genes. Mitochondrial disorders affect muscles and the predominant impairments are myopathies. The physical limitation is associated with energy deficits in cells with high energy requirements, such as the nerve and muscle cells. To complicate the matter, not all mitochondrial mutations are inherited. It is important for family planning to know exactly what kind of DNA mutations exist within a family with mitochondrial disorders. There are different patterns of inheritance and implications for the family. The PT should have this history before delegating any intervention to a PTA in order to make sure exercise will not cause additional damage to the nerves and muscle cells themselves.

CLINICAL SYMPTOMS AND BEHAVIORAL DIAGNOSES OFTEN REFERRED TO PHYSICAL THERAPY FOR TREATMENT

The PTs and PTAs should become familiar with the common functional impairments and limitations often found in individuals with developmental delays and genetic disorders. The typical impairments in selected genetic disorders are listed in the Table 8-6.

Specific behavioral categories and impairments frequently treated by PTs and PTAs when providing intervention to these children are identified in the following section.

Hypertonicity

Hypertonicity and spasticity are often used interchangeably; however, they do not have the same meaning. Spasticity is defined as an increased resistance to passive stretch that may be velocity dependent, hypersensitivity to sensory stimuli, clonus, hyperactive deep tendon reflexes, and abnormal posturing or movement of the extremities.[17] The Ashworth scale,[18] modified Ashworth scale,[19] and the Tardieu scale[20] are scales used to measure spasticity. Hypertonicity is defined as stiff and jerky movements that are limited in variety, speed, and coordination.[12] With hypertonicity, there is an increase in connective tissue in the muscle and movements tend to be limited to the middle ranges.

Muscle Tone Abnormalities

Muscle tone is dynamic and influenced by body and head position and by emotional, systemic, environmental, and behavioral factors.[11] When observing tonal characteristics, therapists must differentiate between individuals tending to fix in order to compensate for joint hypermobility versus children that have hypertonia from a CNS problem. The PTA is not responsible for the functional diagnosis of tonal disorders but is responsible for recognizing changes in tone, its effect on movement, and reporting to the PT those changes and how function has been changed.

Delegated Intervention Strategies for Children With Hypertonicity

Hypotonicity

Hypotonicity is often synonymous with low muscle tone. Movements are displayed in the extreme ranges of motion. There are delays in postural reactions and co-activation of muscles around the joint. Locking weight-bearing joints for stability is common and often associated with hyperextensible joints throughout the body. Patients tend to assume position to provide broad BOS to maximize their stability. Children with hypotonia may have floppy joints, poor definition of muscles, hypermobility of joints, and decreased strength and endurance.[11]

Delegated Interventions for Children With Hypotonicity

Contractures and Deformities

Habitual positioning and posturing, as well as increased muscle tone, can result in the development of contractures and deformities. Skeletal anomalies and deformities are associated with many genetic

Table 8-6
Typical Impairments in Selected Genetic Disorders

Genetic Disorder	Hypotonicity	Hypertonicity	Hip Dislocation	Spinal Deformity	Upper Extremity Deformity	Other Deformity	Motor Delays	Cognitive Delays	Cerebellar Dysfunction
Trisomy 21	x			x	x	x	x	x	x
Trisomy 18	x	x		x	x	x	x	x	
Trisomy 13	x	x			x	x	x	x	
Turner syndrome			x	x	x	x			
Klinefelter syndrome						x	x		
Cri-du-chat syndrome	x	x	x	x		x	x	x	
Prader-Willi syndrome	x			x		x	x	x	
Osteogenesis imperfecta				x	x	x	x		
Tuberous sclerosis		x					x	x	
Neurofibromatosis		x		x		x			
Untreated phenylketonuria				x					
Hurler syndrome		x	x	x	x	x	x	x	x
Werdig-Hoffmann syndrome	x			x	x	x	x	x	x
Kugelberg-Welander syndrome	x			x		x	x		
Fragile X syndrome	x			x			x	x	
Lesh-Nyhan syndrome		x	x			x	x	x	x
Hemophilia A					x	x			
Rett syndrome				x	x	x	x		

Adapted from Stuberg WA, Sanger WG. Genetic disorders: a pediatric perspective. In: Umphred DA, ed. Neurological Rehabilitation. 4th ed. St. Louis, Mo: Mosby; 2001.

disorders.[12] Limitations in posture and movement result in the deformities seen in children with genetic disorders and developmental delay. Flexion contractures are often found in both the UEs and LEs. Spinal deformity is also prevalent. Respiratory status is often compromised by chest and skeletal deformities of the spine. Prevention of these deformities often becomes the primary functional goal of the PT and the interventions delegated to the PTA.

Delegated Interventions Regarding Children With Contractures

Mental Retardation

The American Association of Mental Retardation's (AAMR) definition of mental retardation is widely accepted. Emphasis is on adaptive skills and not on an intelligence quotient (IQ) score.

Mental retardation is a disability characterized by significant limitations both in intellectual functioning and in adaptive behavior as expressed in conceptual, social, and practical adaptive skills. This disability originates before age 18.[21]

Many of the old terms used to identify MR are incorporated into frequently used current terms. Delays in achievement of developmental motor milestones are often the first indication of mental retardation.[22] Motor manifestations of certain genetic disorders and conditions often suggest a more global developmental problem.[23] Performance of motor activities may also be affected by a child's intellectual impairment. They may have difficulty following directions and performing motor tasks that have more cognitive components.[24] Although MR is found among the general population of children, the frequency of this problem is more often seen in children with genetic disorders.

Physical Therapy Intervention for Individuals With Mental Retardation

Traditional physical therapy intervention efforts in treatment of children with mental retardation are to limit impairments in musculoskeletal, neuromuscular, and cardiopulmonary functioning with goals directed to reduce functional limitations. Intervention is also focused on preventing and limiting secondary effects of cognitive, communication, and social-emotional impairments resulting from motor disorders and restrictions.[24]

Many treatment activities designed to assist a child with MR may be delegated to the PTA. Repetition of practice will be critical for these children because many cannot use cognition to self-drive motor learning. Practice becomes the major force to motor programming and can provide for the child's needed success as he or she progresses through childhood. Supportive practices for individuals with MR are provided in Table 8-7. The PTs and PTAs should be aware of the child's behavior, both physical and social. Family structure may affect the delivery of PT services. Thus, family concerns and issues should not be ignored. Family members and school personnel can provide information that will help in understanding the child or individual's behavior. A behavioral play may be necessary to implement PT services successfully. Having the parents, guardian, and caregiver involved in goal setting may enhance adherence to the physical therapy program. The PT may delegate most functional movement practice to the PTA. Thus, the PTA may be working on rolling, coming to sit, hand to mouth, sitting, coming to stand, standing, dressing, walking, picking up toys, carrying toys, and other play activities.

Learning Disabilities

The IDEA and the Education of the Handicapped Act (EHA) defined a specific learning disability as "a disorder in one or more of the basic psychological processes involved in understanding, or in using languages, spoken or written, that may manifest itself in an imperfect ability to listen, think, speak, read, write, spell, or do mathematical calculations." The federal definition also includes conditions such as perceptual disabilities, brain injury, minimal brain dysfunction, dyslexia, and developmental aphasia. According to the 34 Code of Federal Regulations 300.7 [c](10), *learning disabilities* do not include "learning problems that are primarily the result of visual, hearing, or motor

disabilities, of mental retardation, of emotional disturbance, or of environmental, cultural, or economic disadvantage."[25]

Physical Therapy Intervention for Learning Disabilities

The PT and PTA are usually not involved unless there is a motor, balance, or age-appropriate motor component to the functional limitation. The following sections will discuss specific disability, diagnosis, and developmental delay and include physical therapy intervention. Supportive practices for children with learning disabilities, mental retardation, autism, and *developmental coordination disorders* (DCD) are listed in Table 8-8.

Pervasive Developmental Disorder

The American Psychiatric Association (APA) defined *pervasive developmental disorder* (PDD) or autism spectrum disorders (ASDs) with five subcategories: autistic disorder, Retts disorder, childhood disintegrative disorder, Asperger disorder, and PDD not otherwise specified. The three qualities (called triad of symptoms characteristic) of PDD are impairment in social interactions; deficiencies in verbal and nonverbal communications; and behaviors that are restrictive, repetitive, and stereotyped.[26]

Physical therapy intervention for PDD is often indicated when the child has:

- Deficits in gross motor skills.
- Poor balance.
- Clumsiness.
- Decreased strength.
- Delay in gross motor skills.

The PT can delegate treatment to the PTA including but not limited to interventions that encompass the entire spectrum of gross and fine motor skills and their respective impairments in strength, range, balance, etc. Treatment can be provided in individual or group therapy sessions. It is important that the individual providing therapy be familiar with the child's behavioral protocol. Limits often need to be set on certain behaviors. The PT needs to provide to the PTA particular consequences for unacceptable behaviors. Behaviors that are to be encouraged need to be identified and procedures established on how these might be accomplished. Each physical therapy program is child specific so there are no specific protocols that have been established regarding physical therapy intervention in children with PDD.

Developmental Coordination Disorders

Past definitions of DCD include clumsiness, developmental clumsiness, and developmental apraxia.

Table 8-7
Supportive Practices for Children With Special Needs

Supportive Practices for Child With Autism	Supportive Practices for Child With a Learning Disability	Supportive Practices for Child With Developmental Coordination Disorders	Supportive Practices for Child With Mental Retardation
Speak clearly.	A child may become easily frustrated or angry because of a long history of failure. Be patient and supportive.	Include other children in the therapy session for peer support.	Keep concepts clear and simple.
Keep instructions simple.	Ask the child to help you understand what kinds of support he or she needs to learn.	Develop and use activities that are cooperative rather than competitive.	Break down activities into small steps.
Try to make sure the child is facing you before talking. This way the child gets visual as well as auditory cues that you are talking.	Allow the child time to process information and generate a response.	Incorporate rhythmic activities into the session.	Ask a child to do only one or two steps at a time.
Structure activities the same from day to day.	Use simple sentence structure if needed.	Use age-appropriate activities to develop specific skills, such as jumprope, hopscotch, and baseball.	Talk to the child. Do not turn to parent or caregiver assuming the child cannot respond.
Prepare the child for changes in routine.	Recognize that the child is not stupid but learns in a different way than other children.	Be aware that the child may have other developmental problems, such as learning disabilities or ADHD, and follow supportive practices for these developmental problems, as well.	Use the same tone of voice you would use with other children of similar age.
Be aware of the child's behaviors and responses to changes in routine and how to handle adverse behaviors.	Ask the teachers or parents for ideas on how to structure therapy sessions, present ideas to a child, or elicit cooperation from a child.		Use visual, auditory, and tactile cues. Demonstrate activity, point to objects, repeat concepts in several different ways so child can understand.
Be patient.			Ask if the child wants help before stepping in.
Encourage verbal and other appropriate responses from the child.			Allow the child extra time to respond. He or she may take more time to organize thoughts or become aware of you.
Involve the child in social situations, even if he or she is reluctant to be included.			

Adapted from Ratliffe KT. Clinical Pediatric Physical Therapy. St. Louis, Mo: Mosby; 1998:219-274, 324-330.

Table 8-8
Clinical Features of Duchenne Muscular Dystrophy With Physical Therapy Interventions by Age of Child

Age	Clinical Features	Physical Therapy Interventions
Birth to 2 years	May learn to walk late.	Monitor developmental and functional skills, strength, and ROM.
3 to 5 years	Falling; toe walking; clumsiness; reluctance to run; hypertrophy in calves and deltoids; weakness of neck flexors, abdominals, and shoulder and hip extensor muscles.	Teach family ROM of gastrocsoleus and tensor fascia latae groups, positioning, and general exercise program, such as swimming. Monitor strength and ROM.
6 to 8 years	Toe walking, lordosis, lack of reciprocal arm swing, cannot climb stairs without support, easily tired, limited ambulation distance, walks with wide-based gait, trendelenberg, cannot rise from floor without help.	A general exercise program such as swimming. Monitor strength and ROM; consult with family and school on how to modify activities to avoid fatigue; develop standing and walking program; teach breathing exercises; consult with physical education instructor for the ROM program in school; prescribe night splints for ankles; monitor spinal alignment.
9 to 11 years	Walks with braces; may undergo tenotomy surgeries to prolong ambulation or surgery to stabilize scoliosis; respiratory insufficiency; beginning scoliosis; if no surgery or braces, may lose ambulation skills.	Fit and prescribe KAFOs; prescribe and teach to use rollator walker, parapodium, or reciprocating gait orthosis; develop program to integrate walking into school activities; intervention before and after surgery for strengthening and gait training; breathing exercises; manual w/c for longer distances with appropriate seating and positioning supports; consider motorized scooter for independent seated mobility; provide ROM, positioning monitor scoliosis, and limb contractures.
12 to 14 years	Loss of ambulation skills, increasing respiratory difficulty; obesity; increasing contractures at hips, knees, ankles and elbows; progression of scoliosis; osteoporosis; dependent transfers; increasing need for assistance in ADLs.	Continue with standing program as long as possible; manage obesity and contractures; power w/c for independent mobility; instruct family and school on use of mechanical lifting device (Hoyer or other); recommend commode chair, shower chair, other equipment, as needed; work with teacher and other team members to develop positioning in classroom and access to computer to facilitate academic work.
15 to 17 years	Dependent in many ADLs, possible need for assisted ventilation, increased respiratory compromise.	Adapted equipment to assist with ADLs including a ball-bearing feeder; develop regular schedule and method for pressure relief, and monitor skin; adapt power or manual chair for mechanical ventilation, if indicated; teach family assisted coughing, breathing, exercise, and postural drainage; monitor respiratory function, consider mechanical or power-control bed; comfort mattress, such as air flow or alternating pressure pad; work with child, family, and team to assist in planning or vocational goals for child.
18+ years	Need for assisted ventilation, dependence in all ADLs, death comes after a period of declining respiratory function.	May need to adapt controls of power chair to sip and puff or other control that is accessible to individual with DMD, skin care, management on contractures, positioning, consultation regarding access to higher educational or vocational activities, provide support to individual and family, provide family information about accessible transportation for family and/or child.

Adapted from Ratliffe KT. Clinical Pediatric Physical Therapy. St. Louis, Mo: Mosby; 1998:219-274, 243.

DCD is associated with learning disabilities, sensory integration problems, and minimal brain dysfunction (MBD). DCD is diagnosed when motor coordination is markedly below expected levels, significantly interferes with academic achievement or ADLs, and is not due to known physical disorders.[27] DCD represents a cluster of characteristics affecting around 5% of the regular school-aged population.[27] Etiology is unknown. Abnormal gross and fine motor coordination and expressive speech problems are present. Movement is the primary focus on these nonprogressive motor abnormalities seen in childhood.

Physical Therapy Intervention for Developmental Coordination Disorders

The PTs can use their knowledge and background in motor development to examine, evaluate, and plan intervention programs for individuals with DCD. The PT should identify the motor impairments and functional limitations that prevent the child from achieving at school and in ADLs. Intervention to prevent or minimize the functional and societal limitations can be provided by either the PT or PTA. Deficits in gross motor skills are often the primary reasons for referral to physical therapy. A child who has the ability to perform gross motor skills, but is lacking in the quality of movement, may have difficulty receiving PT services. The educational and medical systems make it more difficult to justify services for children who have fine motor deficit. Both the PT and PTA function as members of the comprehensive school team needed to manage DCD, and thus, the role may become more consultative than direct hands-on intervention. The PT may provide direct consultation to the classroom teacher and aides as well as the adaptive physical education teacher on gross motor play and activities.

The PTA may be asked to monitor the changes in these children and report that information to the PT. The PTA may also be asked to assist the teachers and classroom aides in order to clarify specific motor play activities. When the PTA is in the classroom, the PT may ask the PTA to make sure the play activities are facilitating the movement behaviors that will lead to functional improvement. Consultation may also be provided regarding sitting and standing postures; positioning while on the floor, in a classroom chair, or in a w/c; and handling techniques to improve normal tone and the emotional organization of the child's CNS. To optimize performance in the classroom, the PT may be asked to consult on school equipment to determine the proper type of chair to sit on and the appropriate desk height. The PTA may be asked to observe the child in the classroom and provide assistance to the teacher in order to help guarantee the equipment is being used appropriately.

Developmental Disabilities

Developmental disabilities are a diverse group of severe chronic conditions that are due to mental and/or physical impairments. People with developmental disabilities have problems with life activities such as language, mobility, learning, self-help, and independent living. Developmental disabilities begin anytime during development up to 22 years of age and usually last throughout the person's lifetime.[28,29]

The term *developmental disabilities* is used in many school districts and states in the United States. This term is generally used to identify the more severe, chronic, and medically involved children. Substantially, a positive response to these criteria limits function in three or more of the following areas: self-care, receptive and expressive language, learning, mobility, self-direction, capacity for independent living, economic self-sufficiency, and results in a need for individualized, interdisciplinary services for extended duration. Included under the category of developmental disabilities are autism, CP, epilepsy, MR, severe emotionally handicapped, and certain sensory and language disorders.[11,28] The severity of the diagnosis and conditions usually require indefinite assistance in major life activities. Milder forms of the diseases and conditions are generally not considered developmental disabilities.

SPECIFIC GENETIC OR INHERITED DISEASE TREATED BY PHYSICAL THERAPY

The remaining section of this chapter will discuss medical diagnoses caused by genetic disorders. Clinical features and physical intervention by the PT and appropriate delegation to PTA will be described. The PT and PTA play an important role in facilitating independence and continued activity in the home and workplace. Sequential PT intervention progression of a child that has any one of the various medical diagnoses classified as genetic or developmental disabilities will vary child by child as well as change as the child ages. Clinical features and physical intervention by the PT or delegated to a PTA will depend upon many variables. The PT and PTA play an important role in facilitating independence and continued activity in the home and workplace. Therapy programs for each child should be individually tailored to meet the child's functional needs and should be comprehensive, coordinated, and integrated with educational and medical treatment plans.[30] Parent and sibling needs should also be considered when establishing these treatment plans. Documentation by both the PT and the PTA of effective intervention will be crucial to evidence-based management of these children throughout their lifetime.

This section will help the PTA understand the sequential progression of a child from birth to the age of adulthood when medically diagnosed with a genetic or inherited disease. The specific medical problem and level of PT intervention will be introduced and changed according to the child's specific functional needs and age-appropriate activities. The PTA is reminded that these specific problems have great variance and the PT is responsible for making

Table 8-9

Signs and Symptoms of Spinal Cord Compression as a Result of Atlantoaxial Dislocation

Areflexia
Babinski
Brisk deep tendon reflexes
Clonus
Changes in gait
Extensor plantar reflex
Headaches
Heel cord tightness
Incoordination
Increased muscle tone
Limited cervical motion
Neurogenic bladder (incontinence or retention)
Neck pain
Spasms of neck muscles
Scissoring posture
Sensory changes
Torticollis
Vertigo
Weakness

Adapted from Gajdosik CG, Ostertag S. Cervical instability and down syndrome: review of the literature and implications for physical therapists. Pediatr Phys Ther. 1996;8:31-36.

sure the PTA has the necessary understanding to deal effectively with any intervention delegated.

The Patient With Down Syndrome

Trisomy 21 is the most common of the three types of DS. Ninety-two percent of children with DS have an extra chromosome on the twenty-first pair.[11] Incidence of DS rises with increasing maternal age.[12,31] A child born with DS is usually recognized by the medical team in the delivery room. The clinical features are easily identified across ethnic backgrounds, race, and gender. Confirmation of diagnosis is by a blood test called chromosomal karyotype.

Clinical Features Seen in Children With Down Syndrome

A child born with DS has a flat facial profile. There is an upward slant to the eye, a short neck, abnormally shaped ears, white spots on the iris of the eye (called Brushfield spots), and a single deep transverse crease on the palm of the hand. Some individuals with DS may not possess all these features. More prevalent associated medical disorders include congenital hypothyroidism, hearing loss, congenital heart disease, and vision disorders. MR is present in all children with DS. Most have IQs that fall in the mild to moderate range of MR. Atlantoaxial instability (AA), malformation of

the upper part of the cervical spine under the base of the skull, is very common in DS. Increased incidence of anomalies of osseous and ligamentous structures of the cervical spine lead to AA. This instability can predispose individuals with DS to subluxation and spinal cord compression and impingement. Thus, the PT should rule out AA before delegating intervention to the PTA. Yet, knowledge and close monitoring of the common signs and symptoms of AA instability is important for the PTA. Parent education with regards to issues of AA instabilities, signs, risk, and activities to avoid is also very crucial. Table 8-9 identifies the signs and symptoms of spinal cord compression resulting from AA dislocation. Signs of numbness and tingling sensation require medical attention immediately.

The PTs and PTAs working with DS individuals should be aware of treatment activities that put undue stress on the cervical spine. PT treatment should avoid exaggerated neck flexion, extension and rotation positions, and forceful twisting and turning of the head. Joint approximation or compression of the cervical spine should be performed cautiously and gently. Care should be taken in placing the DS child in an inverted position to avoid the risk of falling on the head. Physical activity that places the neck out of risk for trauma is critical.[32] The PT needs to inform the PTA of any precautions, and the PTA needs to report back to the PT if any problem presents itself during intervention. Many children will attend programs that require the PT to participate in an individualized family service plan (IFSP) or individualized education plan (IEP). Motor skill development should be addressed in the IFSP or IEP process and monitored regularly by the PT for progress. A general criteria to measure and monitor progress in the child with DS is to observe if the child is displaying more physical skills at home, in his or her neighborhood, and at school.

Physical Therapy Intervention Strategies for Child With Down Syndrome Related to Specific Stages of Development

Newborns born with DS have hypotonia or poor muscle tone. This tone affects the child's head and trunk control. Both deficits along with a large protruding tongue affect normal feeding. Children with DS are delayed in their general development. Most of the research over the past 20 years suggests that the average onset of walking for children with DS is about 24 months.

The primary goal parents or care providers have for their children who are delayed and nonambulatory is for them to walk. Therapy interventions for infants and children with DS have been based on assumptions that providing motor activity in excess of or more appropriate than that which is experienced naturally in the home will aid in development.[33] These assumptions are validated by research in motor learning, motor control, and neuroplasticity (see Chapter 3).

Children with DS who experienced early intervention programming show that early intervention group subjects have significantly higher scores on measures of intellectual and adaptive functioning than did children in the comparison group.[34] Children receiving early intervention had beneficial effect and were provided a foundation for subsequent learning and development. However, as these children age, learning and development progress has been shown to decline.[35,36]

Interventions that promote postural reaction in infants with DS enhance motor milestone development.[37] Because children with DS may vary in perceptual motor performance, intervention in the motor domain should be varied according to the child's performance profile.[38] When designing rehabilitation programs for children with DS, Uyanik et al[39] suggested that all treatment methods (ie, sensory integrative therapy and neurodevelopmental therapy) should be applied in combination and should support each other according to the needs of the DS child.[39] Many of the specific interventions can be easily delegated to the PTA.

Newborn/Infancy Stage

PT services are important to help the growing child with DS avoid developing abnormal compensatory movement patterns. The following four factors affect how the child with DS will move and explore the environment: hypotonia, ligamentous laxity, decreased strength, and short arms and legs, which make sitting and climbing activities difficult.

Goals of PT are to develop skills that follow developmental sequences, such as rolling and coming to sit. Teaching handling and carrying techniques is also important. Therapy can work to increase motor expressions of interactions. Head turning to parent's voice or turning to a toy or brightly colored objects are ways to encourage these interactions. A PTA should be very comfortable in handling children to facilitate normal movement as well as playing with the children to encourage appropriate movement responses within identified learning environments.

The Role of the PTA

During the newborn and infancy stages, the PTA can play a key role in working with the family and early intervention providers on handling and carrying mechanics, positioning, gross motor, developmental and play activities to encourage development. The use of equipment, such as treadmill training,[33,40] should first be identified by the PT, but the training of the parents for a home education program (HEP) can be delegated to a PTA who has the skill and understanding

of the intervention protocol. It is important for physical therapy to participate in integrating and coordinating services with other disciplines (eg, occupational therapy), speech, and education that are involved in the child's care. Thus, the PTA's observations during interventions need to be communicated with the PT on a regular basis to guarantee that the PT service is consistent with expectations of other professionals and the family.

As stated earlier, each state has their PT practice act and guidelines on personnel working in an early intervention program. PTAs may be employed by agencies providing early intervention services to children who are not school age. There should be a PT in those programs to evaluate the child and to appropriately delegate and supervise for PTAs.

Toddler and Preschool Stage

Children with DS have developmental delays in all areas and compensatory movement patterns frequently observed. It is not uncommon to see them sitting with trunk rounded and tilted pelvis. Many children stand with a lordosis (stomach out and back arched). Standing and walking with hips in external rotation, knees stiff, and feet flat and turned out are also observed. Many children with DS will be referred to physical therapy because of these gait problems. The PT may ask the PTA to assist the child in walking while holding the child at the pelvis in order to force more internal rotation and shifting of the weight forward on the feet to prevent locking of the knees. The child may also need to wear foot orthosis as part of the treatment intervention. The PT should instruct the PTA in proper use of the orthoses, and then the PTA can teach the parents, when appropriate.

Families often expect walking to become a primary goal. Physical therapy services will be directed toward prewalking skills and advanced gait skills. Prewalking skills include activities that require pulling to tall kneeling, pulling to stand, and squat to stand activities. Advanced gait skills would include stair activities, walking on uneven surfaces and on different terrain, running, jumping, and kicking a ball. Again, the PT can delegate many of these activities, especially if the primary goal is repetition of practice to promote normal movement.

Although the PT needs to work with the staff in an early intervention program or preschool program to establish and facilitate group activities that will benefit the child or children with DS in their development, running the groups can be delegated as long as the PTA feels comfortable with the specific goals and interventions identified for each child. The PTA can be the primary treating therapist to provide the therapy for gross motor activities, and the prewalking and gait activities. These programs can be carried out on a daily or biweekly basis, in a group setting or in individual treatment sessions. The use of goals related to language, fine motor skills, and socialization incorporating the context of gross motor activities is essential.

School Age and Adolescent Stage

Children and adolescents with DS are less active and spend more time indoors. Thus, due to inactivity, many tend to become overweight. It is important to emphasize physical fitness and exercise programs during this stage. Referral and access to community recreation programs (eg, Gymboree, dance, gyms, the YMCA, and city parks) is essential. Participation in afternoon and weekend programs will enhance and develop strength, balance, speed, and endurance.

The PT's role may be to provide consultation to the school team and to the after school program in which the child with DS may be a participant. The PT and PTA may provide more direct services if the youngster has a medical condition that requires surgery and postoperative physical therapy is indicated. As mentioned earlier, the instability of the atlantoaxial spine should be monitored. Signs of spinal compression can result in spastic hemiplegia, spastic triplegia, or spastic quadriplegia. When working on activities with the child with DS, if any of these signs or symptoms develop, the PTA should immediately notify the PT and stop the intervention.

Due to concerns about the sedentary status of many children with DS, efforts should be made to produce a more active program in the school setting. Here, the PT may choose to have the PTA work closely with the teaching staff, primarily with the teacher's aide or the adaptive physical education personnel. The PTA does not need to do additional therapy for these children, but the PTA can be creative, plan, and promote healthy activities to encourage participation. Group activities are ideal to promote fitness and peer interactions.

Adult Stage

Life expectancy has increased for individuals with DS. Many young adults with DS live with their elderly parents. Transition plans can assist adults with DS to live in semi-independent housing situations. It is important that these young adults learn skills that would increase independence in life skills, especially as their parents age and develop health problems themselves. PTAs may be working in group homes or centers that provide activities for adults with DS. Physical fitness and promotion of healthy activities will remain important throughout their lives. When performing a systematic and well-designed aerobic training regimen, adults with DS demonstrated improvements in ventilation.[41] Structure and repetition of practice, such as aerobic rowing training, encourages both exercises endurance and work capacity as well as bringing fun and pleasure to the young adult with DS.[42] As part of the aging process, Alzheimer's disease may be a problem for adults with DS. Concerns with balance and falls will necessitate learning safety strategies as well as staying physically fit.

The Patient With Osteogensis Imperfecta

Osteogenesis imperfecta (OI) is a skeletal disorder of remarkable clinical variability.[43] OI occurs in approximately 1:5,000 to 1:10,000 individuals of all racial and ethnic origins.[44] OI is a rare genetic disorder characterized by bones that break easily and often from little or no apparent cause. OI is a spectrum of diseases that results from deficits in collagen synthesis. It can be a dominant or recessive inherited disease or occur as a mutation.

There is no effective therapy to cure OI. Treatment strategies by the physicians were primarily on conservative and surgical intervention. With new forms of pharmaceutical intervention emerging, it is important for the PT and PTA to document outcomes of standing and walking in a multidisciplinary approach to rehabilitation.

PT prognosis depends on the number and severity of symptoms. Due to the great clinical variability associated with OI, it is difficult to predict which children are at particular risk for significant disability. The type or severity of OI is the most important clinical indicator of the ultimate ability to walk.[43] The early achievement of motor milestones contributes to the ability of independent walking when the type of OI is uncertain. The goals of rehabilitation for infants and children with OI are as follows:

- To promote the acquisition of gross motor development.
- To facilitate all safe forms of active movement.
- To maximize functional independence.
- To improve quality of life.

Young children and adolescents with OI more clearly perceive their physical limitations, while children in the elementary school age group often are resistant to restriction in athletic competition.[45] The PTA needs to always consult with the delegating PT when the PTA questions that the child may be trying to perform at a level that will be injurious to his or her body. Walking is a major emphasis for parents of OI children. Outcomes are complicated by fractures and surgeries.

Children with OI may present with bowing of their legs, muscle weakness due to disuse, hip flexion and external rotation, and feet in equinas. Spinal deformities and vertebral compression may also be present.

A combination of these problems may limit the acquisition of gross motor skills as well as the PT's decision to delegate intervention to the PTA. All therapists need to be aware that parents and caregivers might be fearful of handling their child. These caretakers may also be overly protective and fearful of potential fractures.

Infancy Stage

The PT will generally provide PT services due to the medically fragile condition of the infant. The PTA may not have a direct role during this age. Parent education is most crucial during early infancy. PT intervention is directed towards encouraging handling and carrying techniques to promote bonding. The PT will instruct the parents in handling and carrying techniques during positioning, bathing, dressing, and feeding, which should be reviewed and monitored. The PTA can be very effective in reinforcing those motor skills. Safety precautions to prevent fractures must be reviewed and understood by all the therapists working with children with OI.

Positioning in sidelying will prevent occipital flattening, torticollis, and frog-leg postures of the hips. This can be recommended during the waking hours. To reduce the risk of fractures, parents can be shown how to gently range the UEs and LEs without using aggressive movements or force. Quick, jerky movements should always be avoided. Infants should be supported properly when being moved or positioned. The baby crib and play pen should be well padded. A slight bump may cause a fracture. Splinting the extremities is sometimes necessary. Mobility aids such as a well-cushioned and covered stroller to transport the infant can prevent injuries or fractures. Another strategy to prevent fractures is to recognize signs of fractures. An infant who cries when being handled or moved may have a fracture, and immediate medical attention is necessary.

Toddler and Preschooler Stage

Primary impairments of bone fragility, joint laxity, and reduced muscle strength will affect movement and locomotion at this age. A secondary impairment of disuse and muscle atrophy is osteoporosis. Thus, emphasizing to the family that play must be fun but not rough is important. During the crawling stage, any means of locomotion should be encouraged.

The ability to reciprocate crawl is not crucial for weight-bearing in standing or for eventual ambulation. If a child can scoot, combat crawl, or reciprocal crawl, he can explore the environment and assist in transfer skills. Play and socialization for all children is important. In children with OI, both play and socialization may be limited and hampered when there is a lack of mobility or weight-bearing ability.

For this and other reasons, children with OI may attend an early intervention program and interact with PTAs working within that environment. Due to a higher incidence of fractures secondary to their medical diagnosis, it is more likely that these children may receive PT services in an outpatient hospital or rehabilitation center, another frequent work environment for a PTA. Due to fractures and muscle weakness, aquatic therapy may be recommended. The PT can work on strengthening the LEs through resistance and assistance of water. Water also is a means to provide weight-bearing in a protected environment. Aquatic therapy may also improve cardiovascular fitness.[11,46]

At the beginning of the preambulation and standing period, the PT may have the PTA provide direct services for safe weight-bearing. Protected weight-bearing is provided with the use of LE splints or bracing. Standing frames and tables or supine standers may be used to encourage weight-bearing with support. The PTA will encourage correct handling and positioning techniques by showing families and school staff how to move the child with proper support in order to reduce the risk of fractures. The PTA can also monitor brace and splinting wear. Any problems observed (eg, pain, redness, pressure areas, skin breakdown or sores from orthotics and splint wear) should be reported to the PT and/or physician immediately. Many children with OI have surgeries to prevent fractures on long bones in the legs. The doctor will place a rod in the femur or tibia to provide mechanical support of the body weight during weight-bearing activities.

Following surgeries or fractures, knee ankle foot orthosis (KAFOs) are prescribed to provide protection, support, and facilitate weight-bearing activities. Walking is encouraged as a therapeutic exercise and for mobility. Weight-bearing activities can take place in the pool postoperatively and on land.

After surgery, when the child with OI returns to the school setting, the PTA can practice strengthening activities, weight-bearing activities, and gait training. The child will have bracing and adaptive equipment to aid in ambulatory activities. If the child is not an ambulatory candidate, the PT should evaluate mobility skills. Manual or powered w/c training for mobility may be indicated and taught by the PTA.

School Age and Adolescent Stage

As in the toddler and preschool age groups, frequent hospitalizations due to fractures are a reality for the school age and adolescent group. Surgeries and bracing are the primary rehabilitation intervention. PT intervention is similar to that described for the previous age groups. Preventing hip flexion contractures and strengthening hip extensors and quadriceps is important. When a child improves in hip extensor and quadricep strength, an ankle foot orthosis (AFO) may be prescribed and the KAFO may no longer be indicated. The PT can delegate to the PTA protocols for fitness programs that will improve flexibility, endurance, and strength.

The Role of the PTA

The PTA in the school setting will play a very active role in providing PT services for a child with OI. Teaching mobility skills will be very important.

For the ambulatory child, the PTA will be teaching the child to put on and take off his braces and to use the braces for standing and gait activities. For the nonambulatory child or the child who only ambulated at home, the PTA will be teaching w/c mobility, manual or powered, which will enable the child to access the school campus and community.

A PTA may be asked to monitor an adolescent child in the school setting. Monitoring is recommended to ensure that the durable medical equipment (ie, w/c, ambulatory equipment, or orthosis) is maintained in good condition for safe use. Working with adaptive physical education personnel on fitness activities can also be beneficial. The PT and PTA can provide valuable assistance by referring the adolescent and his family to community resources for both recreational and fitness programs.

Adult Stage

Most adults with OI use a manual or power w/c for community mobility. Those who remain a household ambulator may use assistive devices. Once an individual with OI reaches adulthood, the only time a therapist is asked to work with that individual is following another fracture or surgical procedure. Treatment strategies should focus on improving functional ability in the individual. That functional training may be delegated to a PTA in a variety of clinical settings.[47]

The Patient With Duchenne Muscular Dystrophy

Duchenne muscular dystrophy (DMD) is the most common fatal genetic disease of childhood. It is the most devastating of the dystrophies because there is no known cure. It affects all ethnicities, races, nationalities, and socioeconomic groups. DMD affects males, as it is an X-linked disease. It occurs in 1 in 3,500 boys worldwide.[48,49] The gene for DMD is found on the X chromosome. It is identified as depletion of a large protein called dystrophin. Dystrophin strengthens muscle, and without it, the cell membrane becomes permeable, and the muscle cell eventually dies. Overuse of the muscle will increase its metabolism and the rate of cellular death. Thus, therapists need to balance muscle activity to avoid disuse with overuse and muscle damage.

Clinical Features

DMD is characterized by rapidly progressive muscle weakness. Enlargement of muscles and pseudohypertrophy of the calf are most noticeable. The Gower sign is a distinctive behavior of boys with DMD. The Gower sign describes how a child with DMD gets up from the floor surface to standing because of pelvis and trunk weakness. When on the floor surface, the child with DMD would start in an all fours position, resting on his elbow. Next, the child would extend his legs one at a time until they are upright, but with his hands still on the floor (toe-touching posture). He then will use his hands and crawl up on his legs to come to a full standing position.

Children with DMD show early signs of muscle weakness. They begin walking relatively late in childhood and develop a waddling type gait due to hip and knee instability or postural control. They have difficulty getting up from the floor surface and climbing stairs. Typical weakness begins and progresses from the proximal to distal muscle groups. Children usually lose their ability to walk by their preteen years. Other self-help skills are lost progressively. Death occurs by late teens or twenties by respiratory or cardiac causes. There is no recipe for PT intervention. The PTA should think of management of the disease process through maintaining functional control rather than treatment to eliminate dysfunction.

Infancy to Preschool Stage

A child with DMD is not medically diagnosed until he is in his preschool years and begins to demonstrate the typical motor dysfunction of the disease. The signs are subtle and a slight delay in developmental milestones makes early medical diagnosing difficult. The infant may also be described as slightly hypotonic. Children who are identified early usually have a sibling or family history of DMD, which makes the physician more suspicious of the problem. The Gower sign can appear at as early as 15 months and would give an indication of the disease being present.

Preschool Stage

During the early years, when the DMD child is still walking, intense one to one therapy is not necessary. Stretching for tight muscles described in this section can be done as a home program. Families and school staff should be encouraged to maintain and promote activities. DMD is usually identified and diagnosed between 3 to 5 years of age. Impairments demonstrated are muscle weaknesses in the proximal areas (neck flexors, abdominals, intrascapular, and hip extensor muscle groups). ROM limitation is usually not evident before 5 years of age. Gastrocnemius and tensor fascia latae muscles are usually the first to be tight. Lordotic posture increases with age, and winging of the scapula becomes more pronounced as postural muscle groups are lost.

PT intervention goals are directed toward teaching family members ROM and general strengthening exercises. Unfortunately, there is a lack of research of what kind of PT services and how much is ideal for DMD. DMD is known to show fragile muscle membranes. Extra stress on these membranes may tear the membranes, damage muscle cells, and hasten muscle degeneration.[50] Although the literature is inconsistent with regard to whether controlled and modified strength training can improve functional skill in child with DMD,[51] the use of high resistance training is contraindicated with a rapidly progressive disorder such as DMD. Ansved[51] recommends that exercise regimens should be commenced in the early stage of the disease, when there is still a substantial amount of trainable muscle fibers. Delegation of the training is appropriate as long as the PTA does not push the child to fatigue and helps the child learn and recognize limitations within muscle groups before fatigue.

Children with DMD can be referred to exercise programs such as swimming and walking instead of weight lifting in order to maintain cardiovascular health.[52] A certain amount of weight bearing will head off the development of bone-weakening disorders, including osteoporosis. Keeping joint ROM supple will prevent development of contractures commonly seen as the DMD disease progress.

The Role of the PTA

In a preschool setting or outpatient center, it is appropriate for the PT to delegate to the PTA a program of ROM and general strengthening exercises through functional movement. While the child is still ambulatory, formal exercises are not necessary. Teaching and monitoring home programs to maintain ROM of the hips and ankles are important. Teaching the child to self-range during functional activities helps maintain elongation as well as prevent functional limitations.

School Age Stage

This will be a very difficult period for the primary caregivers. Initial symptoms of the disability start to occur. The child with DMD will be clumsier and fall more frequently. The challenge of keeping up with peers during playtime and recess time will become more evident. Gait deviations such as waddling gait and toe walking will become more visible. The child with DMD will be increasingly hesitant to participate in some activities if they are difficult to perform or if the child is uncomfortable or afraid of falling.

The Role of the PTA

As the symptoms of DMD progressively manifest themselves during this age, the PTA will have an increasing role in the treatment of a school-aged child with DMD. Due to increased toe walking, passive ROM exercises on a regular basis will be important and this should be done as a home program. Once the medical practitioners prescribe bracing, the PTA can help develop strategies to help the child be more independent when putting on bracing and can do guided practice when walking with his new equipment. Mental practice of the physical activity can help the child program the CNS without fatiguing the peripheral musculoskeletal system.

Children get bored with routine ROM and strengthening exercises. If there is a swimming pool in the school setting, pool therapy could be a fun strengthening activity while using different strokes can provide active ROM. Otherwise, a referral to local community centers for swimming would be beneficial. The PTA can also provide play activities and strategies that will help strengthen muscles during play. Coactivation activities (eg, forming bridges, fishing and pulling small weights, abdominal curls, and quad sets) could be arranged into a more fun routine such as dance or music therapy. It is important for the PTA to communicate regularly with the delegating PT and other team members in the school setting. Any changes in the child's condition or equipment needs should be reported to the PT. This is especially true when current activity causes increased fatigue.

To maintain standing and ambulation skills, the orthopedic surgeon may release tight musculatures in the hips and ankles. The goal of postoperative care is to get the child back up to standing and walking to maintain strength and function. The medical practitioner would prescribe bracing and a standing program to increase weight bearing in a standing frame or device. Tecklin[53] recommends 3 to 5 hours per day of standing and/or walking. For the child with DMD who no longer ambulates, Tecklin recommends that an hour of standing with support would be beneficial. It also helps to avoid bone density loss.[54] After the PT develops the classroom program for standing, both the PT and PTA can teach the school staff to carry out the daily standing program. The PTA can be delegated to monitor the standing program for adherence and document endurance and ability to maintain ambulation. Brace wear should also be monitored and ROM maintenance documented.

For the ambulatory child, the PTA can design walking programs as part of the therapy program. Walking to and from therapy, around the school playground, or to and from lunch or specific classes can be varied throughout the school week.

Adolescent Stage

The adolescent period marks a time of significant disability regression. Walking is lost as a means of mobility and the adolescent enters a w/c stage. Contractures make it difficult to ambulate and affect w/c transfers. There is also increasing difficulty with ADLs. Sleeping is also affected by the difficulty or inability of the adolescent with DMD to move, turn, or roll by him- or herself. Respiratory compromise occurs with decreasing pulmonary capacity due to weakening of respiratory muscles.

The role of the PT and PTA is to help the adolescent and family manage mobility problems as deterioration occurs. Respiratory muscles are affected in DMD and in many forms of muscular disease, such as Spinal Muscular Atrophy. The PT will need to instruct the family and care providers in chest percussion and gravity drainage to loosen and mobilize mucus in the airways of individuals with DMD. The PTA may be instructed to do these procedures within the school environment. Deep breathing and coughing techniques need to be taught and practiced. Diaphragmatic breathing, purse-lip breathing, and breathing exercises using the spirometer are therapeutic methods to help improve breathing patterns, and the practice can be monitored by the PTA.[55-57] During the adolescent period, most children and families choose not to progress to this step.

Technology to aid in mobility, self-care, and enabling vocational, educational, and recreational pursuits is key to providing the best quality of life for a person with DMD. Frequent monitoring of physical function, pulmonary function, living a healthy lifestyle, and a proactive management of lung and orthopedic complications are key in providing the longest possible life for the individuals with DMD.

The Role of the PTA

The PTA can assist the PT in any of the interventions previously mentioned. The PTA can be invaluable in providing power w/c mobility training, monitoring the use of splints and braces in implementation of a standing program in the classroom, and conducting breathing exercise groups to help improve pulmonary function. Working with families and care providers would include teaching positioning, lifting and transfer skills, pressure care for weight-bearing surfaces in sitting, and breathing activities. The PTA should encourage activities that the DMD individuals can continue to perform in arts, reading, computer games, and educational programs as well as table games such as checkers, chess, and board games. No profession can cure this disease, but therapy can help maintain function and emphasize and encourage positive management of the disease process to promote a better quality of life.

The Patient With Mitochondrial Disease

The expanding clinical spectrum of *mitochondrial diseases* is becoming clearer.[58] All patients with mitochondrial disease have nervous system involvement.[59] The most frequent neurological manifestations were abnormal muscle tone, seizures, extrapyramidal movements, and autonomic dysfunctions.

Myopathies, regardless of their varied etiologies, are associated with muscle damage and often associated with other organ system involvement causing physical impairment.[60] The resulting physical impairments affect mobility, ADLs, communication, and cardio respiratory fitness, and a reduced quality of life results. Functional impact depends on several factors: type of myopathy or disorders, extent of clinical involvement, duration of disease, time to diagnosis and treatment, rate of progression, and response to medical management. The overall goal of rehabilitation is to enhance function and the quality of life, especially for those with progressive diseases.[61]

Since many of the infants and children with mitochondria disorders referred to physical therapy are developmentally delayed and nonambulators, the PT must focus on the management problems associated with lack of mobility. Positioning, handling, and carrying principles and treatment ideas described with the DS and DMD patients can be applied and modified for the mitochondrial disorders. W/c mobility and a positioning device will most likely be indicated early in the child's life.

FAMILY-CENTERED CARE

Family-centered service is both a philosophy and an approach to service delivery that is considered to be among the best practices of early intervention and pediatric rehabilitation.[62] Research evidence shows strong support for family-centered service in promoting the psychosocial well-being of children and their parents and leads to an increased satisfaction with service delivery. The family-centered philosophy is based on the belief that all families are deeply caring and want to nurture and support their children.[63] Care provided is built on collaboration. In *family-centered care*, families are involved at all levels of care.

Thomas and Johnson shared 6 family roles that families may assume over time as their child's needs change.[63] These roles are as follows:

1. Families as experts in the care of their children.

2. Families as coordinators of their children's care.

3. Families as consultants and advisors.

4. Families as teachers of professional.

5. Families as providers of support.

6. Families as advocates and visionaries.

Understanding and respecting the roles of the parents enhances the collaboration efforts. As professionals, the PT and PTA need to learn how to enable and empower families to choose roles that are meaningful to them, their child with special needs, and with their families.

An important part of treatment planning is effective goal setting. In order to maximize treatment outcomes, the PT should identify patient goals and objectives after the patient examination.[4] It may be the PTA's responsibility to provide intervention that will guide the child and the family toward those goals and objectives.

Cultural and ethnic values, perception of disease, and the disease process itself are often missing links in developing a treatment plan that will have a more favorable outcome. Demographic changes anticipated over the next decade magnify the importance of addressing racial or ethnic disparities in health and health care.[64] Family constellation, family support and network, and community resources all affect delivery of services. Minority health and health disparities exist in the United States.[65] Cross-cultural competence is important in professional and interpersonal interaction and an area in which every service provider should be educated initially and throughout his or her career. This competency should incorporate values, behaviors, and attitudes that occur across all groups.[66]

For PTs and PTAs working with children with disabilities, it is important to know and understand federal, state, and local laws, rules, regulations, and guidelines that govern the services provided in the educational setting. Those working in an educational environment see the natural environment the children are facing daily while attending school. In working with school staff and family members, therapists strive to help make life better for these children and their families. Working as a team member may include planning the incorporation of handling techniques and positioning of adaptive equipment into the daily environment. Additionally, using creativity and exploring a variety of options for intervention that can be fully included in the home and school setting may be of benefit to individuals with functional limitations.

CONCLUSION

In summary, it is important to consider interpersonal and communication styles of the therapist with the families. Families need to be involved. Respect for the family and their understanding of their child must be interwoven with every therapeutic session. No one providing service should speak in a condescending manner nor demonstrate aversion toward people who are of different cultural, educational, religious, or socioeconomic backgrounds. As health care professionals, the PT and PTA need to try to provide information and possibly respond to questions families may have about the disease process and prognosis. If a PTA is asked a question that is beyond the scope of practice to answer, he or she should either refer the family to the PT or let the family know that an answer will be provided, but the question needs to be discussed with the PT. The specific role the PTA plays in providing service to these children will be based upon many variables, which have been presented throughout this chapter. By working together to provide family-centered care, the PT and PTA can help provide a better quality of life for these children and their families.

REFERENCES

1. McConnaughey F, Quinn PO. Your baby's development. In: Stray-Gundersen K, ed. *Babies With Down Syndrome*. 2nd ed. Bethesda, Md: Woodbine House; 1995.

2. Needlman RD. Growth and development. In: Behrman RE, Kliegman RM, Jenson HB, eds. *Nelson Textbook of Pediatrics*. 17th ed. Philadelphia, Pa: Saunders; 2004.

3. Rules and regulations. *Federal Register* [online via GPO access]. 1999;64(48):12421,12439. Available at: http://www.ed.gov/legislation/FedRegister/finrule/1999-1/031299a.html. Accessed November 17, 2005.

4. *Guide to Physical Therapist Practice*. 2nd ed. Alexandria, Va: American Physical Therapy Association; 2001;81:S31-S738.

5. American Academy of Pediatrics (AAP), Shelov SP, Hanneman RE, eds. *Caring for Your Baby and Young Child: Birth to Age 5*. New York, NY: Bantam Books; 1998.

6. Individuals with Disabilities Education Act (IDEA). Public Law 108-446. Available at: http://www.cde.ca.gov. Accessed May 4, 2005.

7. Effgen SK. The educational environment. In: Campbell SK, ed. *Physical Therapy for Children*. Philadelphia, Pa: WB Saunders; 1994.

8. Szklut SE, Breath DM. Learning disabilities. In: Umphred DA, ed. *Neurological Rehabilitation*. 4th ed. St. Louis, Mo; Mosby; 2001.

9. Macmillan C. Genetics and developmental delay. *Semin Pediatr Neurol*. 1998:5(1):39-44.

10. Curry CJ, Stevenson RE, Aughton D, Byrne J, Carey JC, Cassidy S, et al. Evaluation of mental retardation: recommendations of a consensus conference: American college of medical genetics. *Am J Med Genet.* 1997;72(4):468-477.

11. Ratliffe KT. *Clinical Pediatric Physical Therapy.* St. Louis, Mo: Mosby; 1998:219-274, 313-347.

12. Stuberg WA, Sanger WG. Genetic disorders: a pediatric perspective. In: Umphred DA, ed. *Neurological Rehabilitation.* 4th ed. St. Louis, Mo: Mosby; 2001.

13. Harris SR, Shea AM. Down syndrome. In: Campbell SK, ed. *Pediatric Neurologic Physical Therapy.* 2nd ed. New York, NY: Churchill Livingstone, 1991.

14. Kozma C. What is Down syndrome. In: Stray-Gundersen K, ed. *Babies with Down Syndrome.* 2nd ed. Bethesda, Md: Woodbine House; 1995.

15. Hall D. Mongolism in newborn infants. *Clin Pediatr.* 1978;5:90.

16. Cowie VA. *A Study of the Early Development of Mongols.* Oxford, Mich: Pergamon Press; 1970.

17. Haley SM, Inacio CA. Evaluation of spasticity and its effect on motor function. In: Glenn MB, White J, eds. *The Practical Management of Spasticity in Children and Adults.* Philadelphia, Pa: Lea and Febiger; 1990.

18. Lee K, et al. The Ashworth scale: a reliable and reproducible method of measuring spasticity. *J Neurol Rehabil.* 1989;3:205-209.

19. Bohannon RW, Smith MB. Interrater reliability of a modified Ashworth scale of muscle spasticity. *Phys Ther.* 1987;67(2):206-207.

20. Boyd RN, et al. Validity of a clinical measure of spasticity in children with cerebral palsy in a double-blinded randomized controlled trial. American Academy of Cerebral Palsy Portland. *Dev Med Child Neurol.* 1998;40(suppl 78):7.

21. American Association on Mental Retardation (AAMR). The AAMR definition of mental retardation. Available at: http://www.aamr.org. Accessed May 6, 2005.

22. Chinitz SP, Feder CZ. Psychological assessment. In: Molnar GE, ed. *Pediatric Rehabilitation.* 2nd ed. Baltimore, Md: Williams and Wilkins; 1992:48-87.

23. Nomura Y, Segawa Y. Characteristics of motor disturbance in rett syndrome. *Brain Development.* 1990;12:27-30.

24. McEwen I. Mental retardation. In: Campbell SK, ed. *Physical Therapy for Children.* Philadelphia, Pa: WB Saunders; 1994.

25. National Dissemination Center for Children with Disabilities (NICHCY). *Learning Disabilities Fact Sheet 7.* Washington, DC; 2004. Available at: http://www.nichcy.org. Accessed May 14, 2005.

26. American Psychiatric Association (APA). *Diagnostic and Statistical Manual of Mental Disorders: DSM-IV-TR.* 4th ed, text revision. Washington, DC: APA; 2000.

27. David KS. Developmental coordination disorders. In: Campbell SK, ed. *Physical Therapy for Children.* Philadelphia, Pa: WB Saunders; 1994.

28. National Center on Birth Defects and Developmental Disabilities. What are developmental disabilities? Available at: http://www.cdc.gov/ncbddd/dd. Accessed May 14, 2005.

29. Developmental Disabilities Assistance and Bill of Rights Act (DD Act) of 2000. Public Law 106-402. Available at: http://www/txddc.state.tx.us/council/definition/asp. Accessed May 10, 2005.

30. Michaud LJ. Committee on children with disabilities: prescribing therapy services for children with motor disabilities. *Pediatrics.* 2004;113(6):1836-1838.

31. Cuckle HS, Wald NJ, Thompson SG. Estimating a woman's risk of having a pregnancy associated with down's syndrome using her age and serum alpha-fetoprotein level. *Br J Obstet Gynaecol.* 1987;94:387-402.

32. Gajdosik CG, Ostertag S. Cervical instability and down syndrome: review of the literature and implications for physical therapists. *Pediatr Phys Ther.* 1996;8:31-36.

33. Ulrich DA, Ulrich BD, Angulo-Kingler RM, Yun J. Treadmill training of infants with down syndrome: evidence-based developmental outcomes. *Pediatrics.* 2001;108(5):E84-91.

34. Connolly BH, Morgan S, Russell FF. Evaluation of children with down syndrome who participated in an early intervention program. second follow-up study. *Phys Ther.* 1984;64(10):1515-1519.

35. Connolly B, Morgan S, Russell FF, Richardson B. Early intervention with down syndrome children: follow-up report. *Phys Ther.* 1980;60(11):1405-1408.

36. Connolly BH, Morgan SB, Russell FF, Fulliton WL. A longitudinal study of children with down syndrome who experienced early intervention programming. *Phys Ther.* 1993;73(3):170-179.

37. Haley SM. Postural reactions in infants with down syndrome: relationship to motor milestone development and age. *Phys Ther.* 1986;66(1):17-22.

38. Spano M, Mercuri E, Rando T, Panto T, Gagliano A, Henderson S, Guzzetta F. Motor and perceptual-motor competence in children with down syndrome: variation in performance with age. *Eur J Paediatr Neurol.* 1999;3(1):7-13.

39. Uyanik M, Bumin G, Kayihan H. Comparison of different therapy approaches in children with down syndrome. *Pediatr Int.* 2003;45(1):68-73.

40. Ulrich BD, Ulrich DA, Collier DH, Cole EL. Developmental shifts in the ability of Infants with down syndrome to produce treadmill steps. *Phys Ther.* 1995;75:14-23.

41. Tsimaras V, Giagazoglou P, Fotiadou E, Christoulas K, Angelopoulou N. Jog-walk training in cardiorespiratory fitness of adults with down syndrome. *Percept Mot Skills.* 2003;96(3[pt 2]):1239-1251.

42. Varela AM, Sardinha LB, Pitetti KH. Effects of an aerobic rowing training regimen in young adults with down syndrome. *Am J Ment Retard.* 2001;106(2):135-144.

43. Englebert RHH, Uiterwaal CSP, Gulmans, VAM, Pruijs H, Helders PJM. Osteogenesis imperfecta in childhood: prognosis for walking. *J Pediatr.* 2000;137(3):397-402.

44. Byers PH, Steiner RD. Osteogenesis imperfecta. *Ann Rev Med.* 1992;43:269-182.

45. Cintas HL, Siegel KL, Furst GP, Gerber LH. Brief assessment of motor function (BAMF): reliability and concurrent validity of the gross motor scale. *American Journal of Physical Medicine and Rehabilitation.* 2003;82(1):33-41.

46. Bleakney DA, Donohoe M. Osteogenesis imperfecta. In: Campbell SK, ed. *Physical Therapy for Children.* Philadelphia, Pa: WB Saunders; 1994.

47. Englebert RH, Uiterwaal CS, Gerver WJ, van der Net JJ, Pruijs HE, Helders PJ. Osteogenesis imperfecta in childhood: impairment and disability: a prospective study with a 4-year follow-up. *Arch Phys Med Rehabil.* 2004;85:772-778.

48. Moser H. Duchenne muscular dystrophy: pathogenetic aspects and genetic prevention. *Human Genetics.* 1984;66:17-40.

49. Mostacciuolo ML, Lombardi A, Cambilla V, Danieli GA, Angelini C. Population data on benign and severe forms for X-linked muscular dystrophy. *Human Genetics.* 1987;75:217-220.

50. Sarnat HR. Neuromuscular disorders. In: Behrman RE, Kliegman RM, Jenson HB, eds. *Nelson Textbook of Pediatrics.* 17th ed. Philadelphia, Pa: Elsevier Science; 2004.

51. Ansved T. Muscle training muscular dystrophies. *Acta Physio Scand.* 2001;171(3):359-366.

52. Bar-Or O. Role of exercise in the assessment and management of neuromuscular disease in children. *Med Sci Sports Exerc.* 1996;28(4):421-427.

53. Tecklin, JS. *Pediatric Physical Therapy.* 2nd ed. Philadelphia, Pa: JB Lippincot; 1994.

54. Thompson CR, Figoni SF, Devocelle HA, Fifer-Moeller TM, Lockhart TL, Lockhart TA. Effect of dynamic weight bearing on lower extremities bone mineral density in children with neuromuscular impairment. *Clinical Kinesiology.* 2000;54(1):13-18.

55. Watts N. Improvement of breathing patterns. *Phys Ther.* 1968;48:563-576.

56. Kigin CM. Breathing exercises for the medical patient: the art and the science. *Phys Ther.* 1990;70:700-706.

57. Adkins HV. Improvement of breathing ability in children with respiratory muscle paralysis. *Phys Ther.* 1968;48:577-581.

58. De Vivo DC. The expanding clinical spectrum of mitochondrial diseases. *Brain Dev.* 1993;15(1):1-22.

59. Nissenkorn A, Zeharia A, Lev D, Watemberg N, Fattal-Valesvski A, Barash V, Gutman A, Harel S, Lerman-Sagie T. Neurologic presentations of mitochondrial disorders. *J Child Neurol.* 2000;15(1):44-48.

60. Hicks JE. Role of rehabilitation in the management of myopathies. *Curr Opin Rheumatol.* 1998;10(6):548-555.

61. Gropman AL. Diagnosis and treatment of childhood mitochondrial diseases. *Curr Neurol Neurosci Rep.* 2001;1(2):185-194.

62. King S, Teplicky R, King G, Rosenbaum P. Family-centered service for children with cerebral palsy and their families: a review of the literature. *Seminars in Pediatric Neurology.* 2004;11(1):78-86.

63. Thomas J, Johnson BH. Family roles: the most relevant aspect of family-centered care. In: Wallace HM, Biehl RE, MacQueen JC, Blackman JA, eds. *Mosby's Resource Guide to Children With Disabilities and Chronic Illness.* St. Louis, Mo: Mosby-Year Book, Incorporated; 1997.

64. Betancourt JR, Green AR, Carrillo JE. Ananeh-Firempong O 2nd. Defining cultural competence: a practical framework for addressing racial/ethnic disparities in health and health care. *Public Health Rep.* 2003;118(4):293-302.

65. Fowler K. PTs confront minority health and health disparities. *PT Magazine.* 2004:42-47.

66. Lynch EW. Developing cross-cultural competence. In: Lynch EW, Hanson MJ, eds. *Developing Cross-Cultural Competence.* 3rd ed. Baltimore, Md: Paul H Brooks Publishing; 2004.

Chapter

9

CLIENTS WITH SPINAL CORD INJURY

Claire Beekman, PT, MS, NCS

KEY WORDS

autonomic dysreflexia
crede
paraplegia
sacral sparing
tetraplegia

CHAPTER OBJECTIVES

- Explain the difference between a complete and incomplete traumatic SCI.

- Define sacral sparing.

- Define the motor level and sensory neurologic levels of injury.

- Discuss the common characteristics of the clinical picture of a person with SCI.

- Define autonomic dysreflexia, and discuss why it is a medical emergency and what the PTA should do when it occurs.

- Identify complications that may occur with a SCI.

- Discuss why pressure sores occur in people with SCI and how they can be prevented.

- Identify and discuss the purposes of physical therapy for people with SCI.

- Discuss physical therapy interventions used by PTs and PTAs working with people with SCI.

INTRODUCTION

Traumatic SCI occurs when an external force, such as fracture of the vertebrae or penetration of an object, causes stretching, bruising, laceration, or compression to the vulnerable spinal cord. Primary damage is the result of mechanical injury to the neurons. Secondary damage takes place due to multiple biochemical and histological changes, which occur over days and weeks following injury.[1] This cascade of destruction, which occurs in the area of injury and surrounding areas of edema and necrosis, is considered a primary focus of laboratory and clinical treatments to limit the extent of spinal cord damage.[1]

Physical therapy for individuals with a SCI begins in the acute hospital setting, once the site of injury has been stabilized, and continues throughout the inpatient and outpatient rehabilitation settings. Some individuals may also receive physical therapy at home. Individuals with a SCI may require physical therapy years after the injury due to complications or when new impairments or functional limitations occur due to other pathologies. PTAs are important members of the rehabilitation team working with individuals following a SCI. Their role includes assisting the PT in providing select interventions for people with SCI, performing tests and measures appropriate for the patient population, and providing patient and family education in all types of practice settings until the client has reached his or her maximum functional abilities. Examples of the types of interventions, tests and measures, or patient and family education a PTA may provide are discussed throughout this chapter. Good communication between the supervising PT and the PTA is imperative when dealing with patients with SCI to ensure the appropriate progression of the therapy program.

EPIDEMIOLOGY OF SPINAL CORD INJURY

Incidence

The estimated incidence of SCI in the United States (US) is 40 cases per million population or 11,000 new cases per year. The number of people who have SCI in the US today is thought to be approximately 240,000 people. SCI affects primarily young Caucasian men. Over 80% of people with SCI are men, and over half of those affected are from 6 to 30 years of age; 11% of people are over 61 at the time of injury.[2]

Causes

The most common cause of SCI is motor vehicle accidents (41%), followed by falls and acts of violence, primarily gun shot wounds. In the past 25 years, the proportion of injuries due to motor vehicle crashes and recreational sporting activities has decreased while that due to falls has increased. The number of injuries from acts of violence peaked in the 1990s and has decreased since then.[2] Preinjury use of alcohol is reported at an alarmingly high 96% of people sustaining a SCI.[3]

Life Expectancy

Life expectancy has increased in recent years, but it is still somewhat lower than for people who have not had a SCI. Mortality rates are higher in the first year following injury than in subsequent years, particularly in severely injured people, such as those with high *tetraplegia*.[2]

DESCRIBING THE NEUROLOGICAL INJURY

Level and Extent of Injury

A lesion to the spinal cord affects the transmission of sensory information to the brain and motor information to the periphery. Each spinal nerve root innervates a precise area of the skin called a dermatome and a group of muscles called a myotome. By precisely documenting sensation and muscle strength, the clinician can identify whether an injury is complete or incomplete and establish the neurological level of injury (Figure 9-1). Specific criteria described by the American Spinal Injury Association (ASIA)[4,5] are used to make these determinations. Use of these criteria assures that professionals who work with people with SCI will speak a "common language," that outcomes of research will be comparable, and that functional predictors can be developed.[4,5]

Complete Versus Incomplete Injury

An incomplete SCI is defined by the presence of *sacral sparing*, which is partial or complete preservation of motor function, sensory function, or both in the S4 and S5 spinal segments of the cord. Anal sensation and voluntary contraction of the external anal sphincter indicate sensory and motor incomplete injuries. Based on sensory and motor evaluation, 1 of 5 ASIA impairment scales is assigned, A, B, C, D, or E.[4,5] (Table 9-1). With an incomplete injury, motor function below the injury can vary, depending on the severity of the injury. Muscles a few levels below the level of injury can be weak or less than fair plus (F), but this is not considered to be an incomplete injury unless the lowest sacral segments are also spared. In patients with a complete injury, a zone of partial preservation (ZPP) may exist. This identifies the most caudal segment with some sensory or motor function. For example, if a patient's injury is classified as C5, ASIA A, but he or she has impaired sensation to T1, then T1 is said to be the sensory ZPP.

Level of Injury

The *level of injury* describes the patient functionally in that it refers to the segmental neurological level of the spinal cord where function remains, rather than to the vertebral level affected. Specific segments of the cord innervate specific muscles. For example, the musculocutaneous nerve innervates the biceps brachii and is composed of nerves from C5 and C6 roots. C5 nerves innervate a sufficient number of motor units so that a person with a C5 lesion has F strength in the biceps bilaterally. Motor level of injury is determined by the last nerve root that innervates key muscles at F strength, providing that the muscles innervated at the levels above are of Normal (N) strength.[4,5] Sensory level of injury is determined by the last nerve root at which sensation is normal. People with SCI may have different injury levels on the right and left sides of the body.

Tetraplegia Versus Paraplegia

The preferred nomenclature to describe a person with four extremities affected by SCI is *tetraplegia*, a term that has replaced *quadriplegia*. The extent of

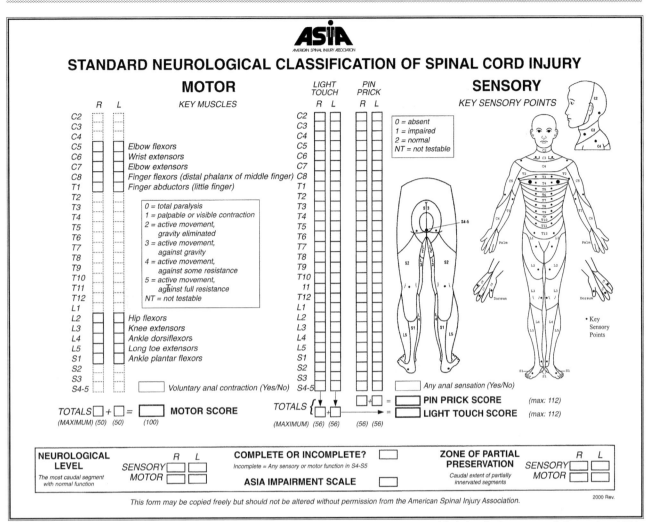

Figure 9-1. Worksheet to consistently document motor and sensory impairments, establish level of injury, and determine ASIA impairment scale in persons with SCI. (Reprinted with permission from *International Standards for Neurological Classification of Spinal Cord Injury*. Chicago, Ill: American Spinal Injury Association; revised 2002.)

Table 9-1
American Spinal Injury Association (ASIA) Impairment Scale

A = **Complete.** No sensory or motor function is preserved in the sacral segments S4 and S5.

B = **Incomplete.*** Sensory but not motor function is preserved below the neurological level and includes the sacral segments S4 and S5.

C = **Incomplete.*** Motor function is preserved below the neurological level, and more than half of the key muscles below the neurological level have a muscle grade of less than 3 (Grades 0 to 2).

D = **Incomplete.*** Motor function is preserved below the neurological level, and at least half of key muscles below the neurological level have a muscle grade greater than or equal to 3.

E = **Normal.** Sensory and motor function are normal.

*Must have sensory or motor function in S4 and S5. In addition, the individual must have either voluntary anal sphincter contraction or sparing of motor function more than 3 levels below the motor level.

Adapted from *International Standards for Neurological Classification of Spinal Cord Injury. Chicago, Ill: American Spinal Injury Association; revised 2002.*

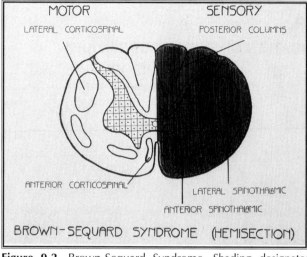

Figure 9-2. Brown-Sequard Syndrome. Shading designates area of injury on this schematic cross-section of the spinal cord. Complete hemisection results in loss of ipsilateral motor function and proprioception and contralateral light touch and pin prick sensations below the level of injury. (Printed with permission from Rancho Los Amigos National Rehabilitation Center, Downey, Calif.)

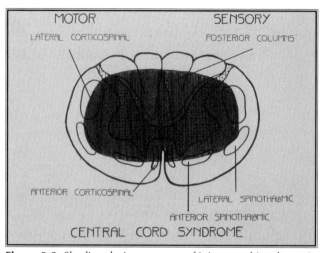

Figure 9-3. Shading designates area of injury on this schematic cross section of the spinal cord. Greater involvement of the UEs than the LEs occurs because neurons within each tract are organized by cervical, thoracic, and lumbar regions with the cervical ones being more central. (Printed with permission from Rancho Los Amigos National Rehabilitation Center, Downey, Calif.)

involvement in the UEs in the person with complete tetraplegia can vary from loss of slight finger motion in the person with a C8 injury to complete loss of UE use in people with C1 to C4 injuries. T1 is the first level of injury at which the person is said to have *paraplegia*; in paraplegia, the UEs are not affected.

Reflexic Versus Areflexic Injury

Most spinal cord injuries are considered to be *reflexic*, or upper motor neuron lesions, because the spinal cord is a part of the CNS. Symptoms of a reflexic injury include spasticity, hypertonicity, and pathologic reflexes. *Areflexic* injuries, or lower motor neuron injuries, are seen when the damage is to peripheral nerves (eg, the cauda equine) or following infarct to the cord. The clinical picture of an areflexic injury includes flaccidity, atrophy, and absence of reflexes. Areflexia also occurs during the period of spinal shock that follows anatomic or physiologic transaction or near transaction of the cord.[1] During spinal shock, a transient suppression of reflex activity occurs below the injury. Proposed explanations for this phenomenon include decreased excitability of the spinal neurons, decreased descending facilitation, and increased spinal inhibition.[1,6]

Special Kinds of Spinal Cord Injury

Damage to specific areas of the spinal cord results in unique sensory and motor clinical pictures. Several clinical syndromes have been described as follows.

Brown-Sequard Syndrome

Brown-Sequard syndrome results from a hemisection of the spinal cord. Because various sensory and motor tracts cross at different levels of the cord, a characteristic clinical picture is seen – contralateral loss of pain and temperature sensations, ipsilateral loss of proprioception, and ipsilateral spastic motor paralysis below the level of injury. A pure injury is rare, but a person can exhibit sensory and motor loss that approximates this distinctive pattern (Figure 9-2).

Central Cord Syndrome

Central cord syndrome is seen primarily in older people with cervical spondylosis and hyperextension injuries. The person with a central cord syndrome has greater involvement of the UEs than the LEs because of the nature of the injury and the location of the tracts to the arms being more central than those innervating the legs[7] (Figure 9-3).

Anterior Cord Syndrome

Anterior Cord Syndrome designates an injury in which the anterior portion of the spinal cord is damaged more than the posterior portion. In the person with this syndrome, the most dorsal tracts, which carry proprioception, are spared, while the most anterior tracts, which carry motor function, are affected to a variable extent.

Cauda Equina Syndrome

Cauda Equina Syndrome occurs with injury to the lumbosacral nerve roots within the neural canal.

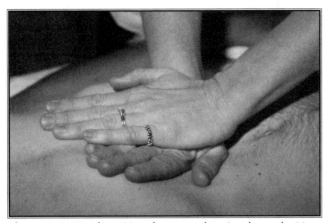

Figure 9-4. Hand position for manual assisted cough. Note how fingers are below the xiphoid process and overlapped to localize force. The patient's head is to the left.

Because the cauda equina is part of the peripheral nervous system, an areflexic motor injury is seen.

CLINICAL PICTURE OF SPINAL CORD INJURY

Although the clinical picture varies from person to person, depending on the level and extent of injury, the following specific characteristics are common.

Motor Loss

Motor loss below the level of injury may be complete or partial. Based on the segmental innervations of the muscles, ASIA has chosen key muscles to represent each of the neurological levels.[4,5] A list of the muscles representing each neurological level is provided in the Standard Neurological Classification of Spinal Cord Injury worksheet (see Figure 9-1). These muscles can easily be tested while keeping the patient in a supine position, which allows evaluation of patients who have an unstable spine or may be unable to assume a sitting position during the acute period following injury. The PT may ask the PTA to perform follow-up manual muscle tests of select muscles during the individual's rehabilitation.

Involvement of Respiratory Muscles

With injuries above L1, some or all of the respiratory muscles will be affected. Forced vital capacity (FVC) and inspiratory capacity (IC) increase with descending SCI level, down to T10.[8] In able-bodied people, inspiration is carried out by a combination of the diaphragm (innervated by C3 to C5) and intercostal muscles (innervated by T1 to T11). Intercostal muscles are also used, as are abdominal muscles (innervated by T8 to T12) in forced breathing and for coughing. The neck muscles (innervated by C2 to C4) are quiet in able-bodied people but active in people with cervical injuries.[9] When patients lack adequate diaphragm function, they must receive complete or partial mechanical ventilation. At least initially, the patient who lacks abdominal muscles will have a nonfunctional cough. Because he or she is unable to generate a cough force sufficient to raise secretions, assistance in maintaining a clear airway will be required by means of tracheal suctioning, manual positive pressure insufflation,[10] or manual assistance for coughing[11] (Figure 9-4). Respiratory complications are common in people with both cervical and thoracic-level injuries.[12]

Sensory Loss

Sensory loss occurs in a dermatomal pattern. For ASIA testing,[4,5] sensation includes light touch and pin prick and is tested in the specific areas identified on the worksheet (see Figure 9-1). Sensation is graded as normal, impaired, or absent. When the patient is unable to discriminate between sharp and dull input at a given dermatome, sensation for pinprick is considered absent. Proprioception is also tested and graded. The results of proprioception tests help predict functional outcome since patients with impaired or absent proprioception will have difficulty controlling extremity movement, even with good motor function. With a complete injury, all sensation is lost below the level of injury. The PT may ask the PTA to repeat select sensory testing for individuals with an incomplete SCI.

Spasticity

Spasticity is seen in the majority of people with SCI after the period of spinal shock, which lasts a variable amount of time after injury.[6] It affects skeletal muscles as well as muscles of the bowel, bladder, and sexual organs. The extent of spasticity and the muscles affected varies; it may be minimal or it may interfere with function and sitting position. Some people are able to use their spasticity to assist them functionally. Spasticity is often increased by irritants, such as a full bladder, pressure sores, or urologic infections. Treatment with medications (eg, baclofen) may be required to reduce interfering spasticity.

Bowel, Bladder, and Sexual Dysfunction

The majority of people with SCI lose total or partial voluntary control of bowel and bladder function. The nature of the bowel and bladder dysfunction will be determined by whether the injury is reflexic or areflexic and whether it is complete or incomplete. People who lack volitional bladder control will require retraining or implementation of a compensatory voiding program. Methods of voiding urine include using an indwelling, condom, or suprapubic catheter;

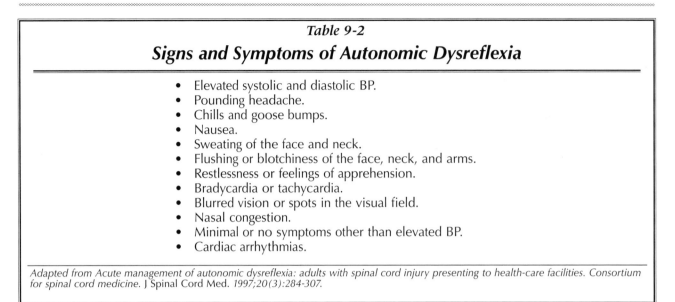

Table 9-2
Signs and Symptoms of Autonomic Dysreflexia

- Elevated systolic and diastolic BP.
- Pounding headache.
- Chills and goose bumps.
- Nausea.
- Sweating of the face and neck.
- Flushing or blotchiness of the face, neck, and arms.
- Restlessness or feelings of apprehension.
- Bradycardia or tachycardia.
- Blurred vision or spots in the visual field.
- Nasal congestion.
- Minimal or no symptoms other than elevated BP.
- Cardiac arrhythmias.

Adapted from Acute management of autonomic dysreflexia: adults with spinal cord injury presenting to health-care facilities. Consortium for spinal cord medicine. J Spinal Cord Med. 1997;20(3):284-307.

intermittent catheterization; or performing a maneuver called *crede*, in which pressing on the bladder forces urine out. People who lack volitional bowel function may experience incontinence and will require retraining of bowel function and elimination.[13,14] Males with reflexive motor function are able to achieve a reflexive erection either spontaneously or by stimulation but are unable to ejaculate. Most men with areflexic injuries are unable to have erections or ejaculate. Women's menstrual periods may stop for up to a year following SCI,[2] but after that time, normal cycles usually return. Women are able to become pregnant following SCI.

Autonomic Dysreflexia or Autonomic Hyperreflexia

Autonomic dysreflexia (AD) is a total body sympathetic nervous system response to noxious stimuli, which may be observed in people with spinal cord lesions above T6.[15] Noxious stimuli from spinal segments S2 to S4, which include bladder distention, bowel impaction, pressure sores, catheter irritation, LE hamstring stretching, tight clothing, a restrictive leg bag strap, or medical tests (eg, intravenous pyelogram (IVP) or barium enema), can trigger this sympathetic response.[15,16] Signs and symptoms of AD include increased BP; pounding headache; sweating, flushing, or blotchiness of the face; chills; and blurred vision (Table 9-2).

An example of how this can occur with bladder distension is as follows.[15] Normally, as the bladder fills, it stretches. Stretch receptors in the bladder are activated and transmit impulses to the sacral portion of the spinal cord. From there, the impulses ascend in the spinothalamic tract and synapse in the sympathetic chain ganglia. This stimulation of the sympathetic nervous system causes a sympathetic response, which includes blood vessel constriction and increased BP. This increased BP is sensed by the baroreceptors in the carotid sinus, and a message is sent to the vasomotor center in the brain stem via the glossopharyngeal nerve. In people whose spinal cords are intact, the vasomotor center, in turn, sends a message down the cord to the sympathetic ganglia reporting that the BP is high and triggering a decrease in the sympathetic vasoconstrictive response. In people with damaged spinal cords, the impulse from the vasomotor center is unable to travel normally down the cord. The message does not reach the sympathetic ganglia, and the BP remains high.[15]

During an episode of AD, arterial BP may reach extremely high levels, may be prolonged, and may cause a cerebral vascular accident (CVA) and death.[15,17] Because acute elevations of BP represent an immediate threat to the patient's life, AD is considered a medical emergency.[17] The source of the irritation which caused AD must be identified and eliminated.[15-17] Immediate treatment measures by the PTA would include the following: monitoring the BP; loosening tight clothing or constrictive devices (eg, a binder, stockings, or leg strap); getting the patient into the sitting position; making sure urine flow is unimpeded; and notifying the PT, nurse, and MD. All facilities that treat people with SCI should establish procedures for dealing with this emergency and staff who can respond with the appropriate course of action. The person with SCI must also recognize the importance of treating AD immediately and must be able to instruct others on how to help. In some facilities, patients receive written instructions for what to do should AD occur at home. AD can sometimes be prevented by careful attention to bowel and bladder training, skin care, and by attention to clothing, catheters, etc. If elimination of the precipitating cause is not sufficient to reduce the BP, treatment with an antihypertensive drug will be required.[15-17]

Psychological Reaction to Loss

During the initial period following SCI, patients go through a series of adjustment phases of loss and grieving similar to those described by Kubler-Ross for people who are dying.[18] Patient responses to SCI can vary greatly and may include anger, depression, withdrawal, and having unrealistic expectations. Personnel can support the patient by understanding this process and helping him or her move through these phases by gaining independence and continuing to modify goals as progress is achieved.

Pain

Pain is a common finding in people with SCI and is a barrier to rehabilitation and quality of life. The reported incidence is about 65%, with about 30% of the people with SCI reporting severe pain.[19,20] Research into pain following SCI has been limited by lack of consistent pain classifications and inability to identify the mechanisms involved with the development of this pain. A recently proposed classification[19,20] identifies two types of pain: (1) nociceptive pain, of which musculoskeletal pain is an example, and (2) neuropathic pain, which may be located above, at, or below the level of injury. *Musculoskeletal pain* is related to mechanical instability, inflammation, muscle spasm, and overuse of muscles and joints[20] and is described as dull, aching, and movement-related.[19] It often involves the shoulder or wrist.[21-23] Transcutaneous electrical nerve stimulation (TENS) can be effective in reducing musculoskeletal pain.[20] *Neuropathic pain* has a different quality from nociceptive pain. It is described as sharp, stabbing, burning, or electrical pain and is associated with a painful, hypersensitive response to normally non-noxious stimuli.[19,20] The mechanism of neuropathic pain is not known, but is thought to be related to damage to neurons within the spinal cord that transmit pain sensation.[20] Chronic neuropathic pain can be incapacitating, and conventional medical management is frequently not effective. Treatment with a combination of medications and modalities may be required.

Complications

Orthostatic hypotension is a drop in BP that can occur the first time the patient with SCI tries to sit or stand. Loss of the LE muscle pump can cause pooling of the blood in the legs and abdomen, with resultant reduction in the amount of blood reaching the brain. The patient becomes dizzy. An abdominal binder or corset and elastic stockings are used to substitute for lost muscle tone. Orthostatic hypotension usually resolves over time, although it may persist for 10 to 12 weeks or longer.[6] Use of a tilt table, recliner w/c, or medication may be required to help the patient adapt to the upright position.

Deep vein thrombosis (DVT), a blood clot in a vein (usually of the leg), is associated with being inactive or on bed rest. DVT is of medical concern because the clot could become dislodged, travel to the lungs, and cause a pulmonary embolus, which could be fatal. DVT is treated medically with anticoagulants or, if anticoagulants are contraindicated, with an inferior vena cava filter.

Common *concomitant injuries* include fractures of the extremities and brachial plexus, abdominal, and brain injuries. Brain injuries occur in more than 50% of people with SCI.[24] Brain injuries affect the person's ability to undergo rehabilitation and may impact the ability to learn and to deal with the complex emotional adjustments placed on him or her after SCI.[24]

Another complication is *heterotopic ossification* (HO), an abnormal overgrowth of bone in the joint space and around the joint, which occurs with an incidence of 10% to 20%.[25] Common signs and symptoms are decreased ROM, localized swelling, and pain. The PTA who works with the patient daily on functional activities and exercise may be the first person to note these changes. In people with SCI, HO occurs within 3 months of injury, is associated with spasticity, and most often affects the hip. It may not be visible on x-ray until the bone becomes mature. Treatment is ROM to the affected joint, use of medication (typically etidronate),[26] and if necessary, surgical removal of the bone.[25]

Decreased bone mineral density (BMD) occurs following complete SCI, and people with paraplegia and tetraplegia exhibit similar changes. BMD declines significantly during the first 3 months following SCI and reaches a loss of about 37% by 16 months.[27] Once BMD has decreased 37%, the fracture index has been exceeded, and the person is at risk for fractures.[27] People with SCI should be aware of this late-occurring risk, and the PTA must exert caution when working with these people. Despite caution, fractures may occur during transfers or as the consequence of a fall, unusual movement, or LE passive ROM.

Another problem that occurs as a result of sympathetic nervous system dysfunction is *impaired temperature regulation*. The patient may complain about being cold and require warmer clothing. In the heat, however, the patient will be unable to sweat below the level of injury and can be at risk for heat stroke due to difficulty cooling the body.

Problems associated with normal aging, such as musculoskeletal[28] and cardiovascular changes,[29] are magnified in people with SCI.

RECOVERY FOLLOWING SPINAL CORD INJURY

Knowledge about the prognosis for neurological recovery following SCI allows the physician to counsel patients about the time during which recovery occurs and probable functional outcome. Studies have shown that neurological recovery is not related to gender, race, type of fracture, mechanism of injury, or timing or type of surgical procedures.[30] Rather, the most important prognostic variable is completeness of injury. Improved outcomes are seen in younger patients and those with a central cord or Brown Sequard syndrome, both incomplete injuries.[6,31] Although controversy surrounds the administration of high-dose steroids in the period immediately following injury, their use is not currently recommended.[30,32]

Functional Motor Recovery

Motor recovery is the principal determinant of a patient's functional capabilities[33] and the primary determinant of motor recovery is completeness of injury at 1 month. Most motor recovery occurs within the first 3 months, and only a very few people have experienced a late conversion from a complete to an incomplete injury. Key muscles that are innervated at 1 month following injury usually recover to a grade of F or greater, while those which are graded at zero are unlikely to recover to a functional level of F.[33,34] Patients with complete injuries are unlikely to walk at a community level,[34] although they may walk with orthoses for exercise. A higher percentage of patients with incomplete injuries are likely to be community ambulators—76% of patients with incomplete paraplegia and 46% of those with incomplete tetraplegia.[34]

TREATMENT

Stabilization of the Spine

Emergency personnel, both paramedics and emergency room staff, must evaluate the extent of the person's injury, while taking measures to save the person's life. This includes utilizing medical treatments to stabilize the person's vital signs.

If the spine is unstable due to a fracture or dislocation of the vertebrae or disruption of ligaments, stabilization of the spinal column is required. Stabilization of the bones assures that loss of nerve function is minimized and that alignment and integrity of the spinal column is ensured. At the scene of an accident and before vertebral stabilization, care is taken to prevent movement of the neck or back, which could cause further damage to the spinal cord. Late symptoms of

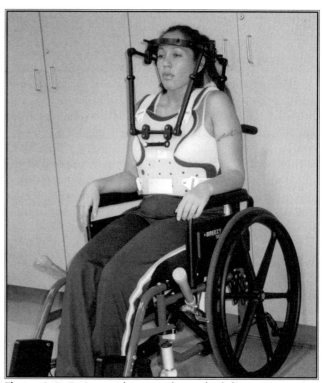

Figure 9-5. Patient with cervical vertebral fracture immobilized in a halo vest.

cervical instability include pain and tenderness at the site of the fracture or injury, increased radiating neck and arm pain, and increased loss of sensation or strength. When the patient reports symptoms of this nature, treatment must be stopped and the PT and physician notified immediately.

Decades ago, patients were placed in Stryker or Circle-Electric beds for 12 weeks or more until the vertebral fracture healed. This meant prolonged periods of bed rest, which delayed rehabilitation and resulted in harmful sequelae. Today, depending on the type of injury, the spine may be stabilized surgically by use of an orthosis or by both means, and the patient is quickly allowed out of bed to begin rehabilitation.

A halo vest (Figure 9-5) or collar (Figure 9-6) for neck injuries or a thoraco-lumbo-sacral orthosis (TLSO), also called a body jacket (Figure 9-7) for thoracic and lumbar injuries may be applied. This is like putting a fractured arm in a cast to immobilize it. The length of time the patient wears the device and restrictions on movement and activities during the time of healing depend on the type of fracture and stabilization, how well the fracture heals, and the protocol of the physician and facility. The PTA must look for and pay close attention to any restrictions listed in the medical record.

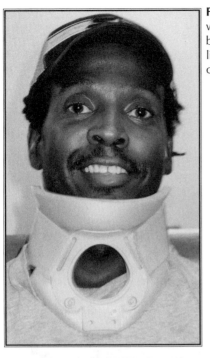

Figure 9-6. Patient with cervical vertebral fracture immobilized in a Philadelphia collar.

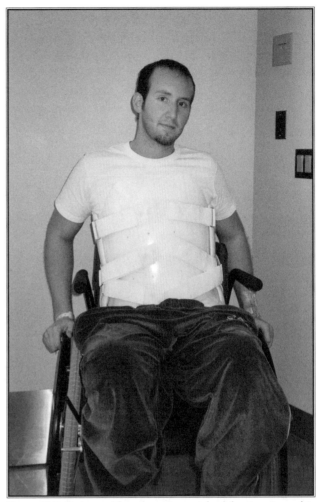

Figure 9-7. Patient with a thoracic vertebral fracture immobilized in a thoraco-lumbo-sacral orthosis (TLSO).

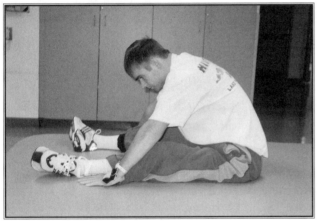

Figure 9-8. Patient with C6 tetraplegia. One hundred degree straight leg ROM minimizes stretching of the back muscles when the patient leans forward to perform functional activities in the long sitting position.

Physical Therapy Interventions

Prevent Deformity and Maintain Range of Motion

Positioning, passive ROM exercises, and use of orthoses or splints can prevent loss of mobility in extremity joints. This is especially important when the person is unable to move his or her extremities or when an imbalance between agonist and antagonistic muscles occurs because of level of injury or hypertonic muscles. For example, the elbow of the person with C5 tetraplegia tends to be flexed because the biceps brachii muscle is innervated, but the triceps brachii is not. Splints can help hold the elbows in extension when the person is not using his arms for functional activities. In people with cervical injuries, the shoulders are particularly vulnerable to developing limited ROM and associated pain. Close attention to maintaining ROM, especially abduction and external rotation of the shoulder and interventions to reduce pain, such as heat, cold, or TENS are important to prevent a disabling pain cycle.

All joints should be kept mobile. Care should be taken to avoid inadvertently overstretching the back extensor muscles, which can occur when the person with tight hamstring muscles leans forward with the knees straight in the long sitting position (Figure 9-8). If the trunk muscles are overstretched, the trunk will tend to elongate during transfers, making it more difficult to clear the buttocks. People with complete SCI who will be doing activities in long sitting (eg, dressing, scooting, and self ROM) need 100 to 110 degrees of hamstring range, as determined by flexing the hip with the knee straight (straight leg raise). Because this stretch is more effective when done relatively slowly

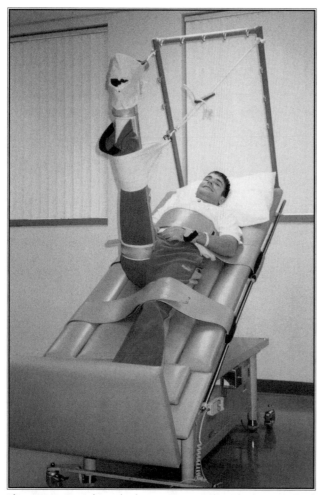

Figure 9-9. Stretching the hamstring muscles. The bar attached to the top of the tilt table has eye bolts across the top and along the sides for attaching clips. A knee cage holds the knee extension while the leg is raised and held by slings and ropes, which are adjusted to also hold the leg in neutral abduction/adduction.

and with the pelvis stabilized as much as possible in supine, a device such as the one in Figure 9-9 may be used. Initially, physical therapy personnel will need to provide passive LE ROM. People with adequate UE function can learn to do their own passive LE ROM, typically with the assistance of a strap.

People with tetraplegia who lack triceps function need full elbow extension and wrist extension to lock the elbows for functional activities (eg, transfers and sitting balance). Because of the shape of the ulna and distal humerus, passive stretching of the elbow may cause soft-tissue damage. Use of a resting splint can help maintain full ROM.

PTAs play an active role in providing interventions to prevent deformity, increase or maintain ROM, and in performing goniometric measurements to demonstrate progress. They may also be involved in

Figure 9-10. The PTA assists the patient to maintain a forward trunk position while performing UE strengthening exercises. The patient is performing "reverse dips" to strengthen the elbow and shoulder extensor muscles.

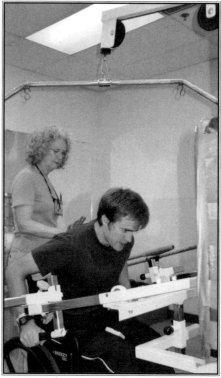

teaching the individual and family members how to perform stretching and ROM.

Strengthen Weak Muscles

Muscles that are innervated below the level of injury will lose function or be weak. In addition, diminished muscle strength and endurance are associated with bed rest, which is common after injury. Muscles with remaining function must be strengthened by progressive resistive exercise to provide the maximum strength possible for performing functional activities (Figures 9-10 and 9-11). In people with complete SCI, the UE muscles must substitute for those lost in the LEs for transfers and w/c propulsion. Specific muscles most vulnerable to fatigue during w/c propulsion are the pectoralis major, supraspinatus, middle and posterior deltoid, subscapularis, and middle trapezius.[35] People with tetraplegia are at greater risk of shoulder pathology because their UE muscles are weaker than those of able-bodied people and people with paraplegia,[36] and activities such as grooming will require different patterns of muscular activity than those used by able-bodied people.[37] People with incomplete injuries require strengthening of LE muscles, as well (Figure 9-12). The PTA will need to perform periodic manual muscle tests of specific muscles in order to modify the patient's exercise program and determine when advancing the functional program is warranted.

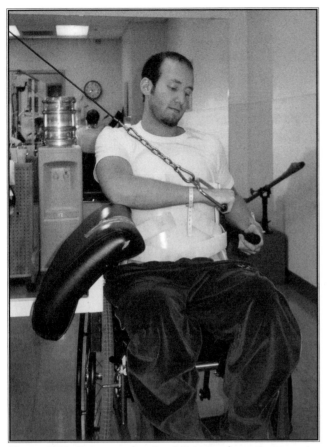

Figure 9-11. Patient performing UE internal rotation exercise with weights. The patient lacks lower trunk musculature and uses his left arm to help stabilize his body while performing the exercise.

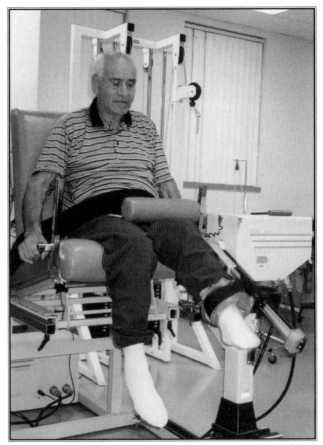

Figure 9-12. Patient with incomplete tetraplegia performing strengthening exercises for the quadriceps muscle on an isokinetic exercise machine.

Develop Endurance

Endurance training is aimed at improving muscular performance and aerobic capacity, in order to improve the efficiency of mobility and improve overall health. Disproportionally high rates of cardiovascular disease and hypertension occur in people with SCI compared with able-bodied individuals.[2,29] Some people have difficulty maintaining an ideal body weight because of limited ability to exercise. Endurance can be achieved by weight training with low weights and high number of repetitions, use of an UE ergometer or similar device, and w/c propulsion, all of which are interventions appropriate for the role of the PTA.

Respiratory Program

People with thoracic-level injuries initially demonstrate lower respiratory measurements than able-bodied people. Respiratory function returns to able-bodied levels when they undergo UE muscle training.[38] The respiratory program for people with cervical-level injuries focuses on interventions for developing strength and endurance in the respiratory muscles; maintaining rib cage mobility, and learning assisted cough, bronchial hygiene, and postural drainage for home use. Specialized voluntary breathing techniques, such as neck breathing[39] or glossopharyngeal breathing (GPB),[40] may be taught to ventilator-dependent people. High compliance to a structured inspiratory training program, using diaphragm weights (Figure 9-13), or an inspiratory muscle trainer, 15 to 30 min per day for 8 weeks, has been shown to result in increased vital capacity (VC) and measures of inspiratory capacity.[41-43] Lerman and Weiss describe a variety of respiratory exercises that can be incorporated into a respiratory program, including breath holding, taking triple breaths for rib cage expansion, and neck exercises.[44] Exercises can be made more difficult by increasing resistance, increasing the time that the exercise is performed, and changing the patient's position.

Weekly monitoring of VC is used to assess patients' progress and modify the respiratory program, as needed. VC is greater in people with cervical injuries in supine[7] and greater in people with lower injuries in sitting. Use of a consistent position allows for more

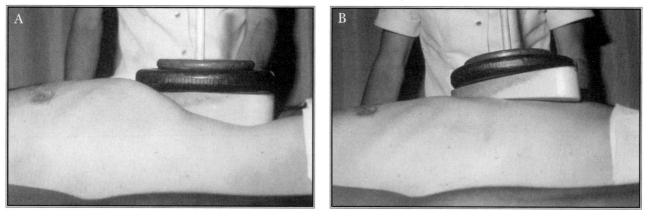

Figure 9-13. Diaphragm strengthening. Resistive strengthening exercises of the diaphragm. The triangular weight pan is designed to fit in the area below the xiphoid process. Note position of the diaphragm (A) before he takes a breath and (B) after he inspires. The patient's head is on the left.

accurate assessment of respiratory function. A corset can assist with respiration when the patient is sitting, as it helps substitute for the abdominal muscles and improve the lung volume. People with C6 injuries may have a VC of 20% to 30% of normal initially, but typically have a VC of 65% of normal at more long-term follow-up.[45]

PTAs working in rehabilitation settings serving patients with SCI may be actively involved in providing all of the interventions discussed above, including testing VC.

Learn Functional Skills

The person with a complete SCI or residual impairments from an incomplete SCI will need to perform functional activities in a modified manner. The extent of independence achieved and the way in which these activities are performed will depend on the level and completeness of injury. Functional activities include bed mobility and transfers; sitting pressure relief; eating; grooming; dressing; bathing; hygiene; assuring adequate bowel and bladder function; driving, walking, and moving around in the community; and meal and home management activities. See Table 9-3 for a summary of select activities for given levels of SCI, and refer to the Consortium for Spinal Cord Medicine publication *Outcomes Following Traumatic Spinal Cord Injury: Clinical Practice Guidelines for Health-Care Professionals* for more detail on expected outcomes.[46] Patients with C6 injuries will use a tenodesis grip to manipulate objects. Tenodesis is passive closing of the fingers when the wrist is actively extended. When practicing mat activities, like propped sitting, care must be taken to maintain finger flexion needed for a tenodesis grip. Patients who have F biceps but lack shoulder strength may be fitted with mobile arm supports (MAS) (Figure 9-14). This device attaches to the w/c to help

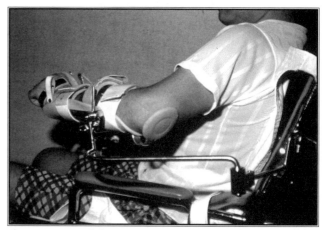

Figure 9-14. Mobile arm support (MAS) attaches to the back post of the w/c to assist with shoulder flexion and abduction. Functional arm use can be achieved with the patient with weak elbow and shoulder muscles.

support the shoulder while the patient bends his or her elbow for activities such as eating and combing hair.

PTAs play a key role in providing functional training interventions and assessing the current level of assistance required by the patient with a SCI. It is important that the PTA know expected functional activities for the different levels of SCI, identify his or her own limitations in providing these interventions, and determine when to ask the PT to reassess the patient. Interventions designed to address all of the functional skills discussed below are appropriate for the role of a PTA.

Bed mobility

Bed mobility consists of rolling, scooting, moving up and down in bed, balance activities, coming to sitting (Figures 9-15A to 9-15D), long and short-sitting balance (Figure 9-16) LE management, and self-ROM.

Table 9-3
Select Functional Outcomes for Persons With Complete Spinal Cord Injury

SCI Level	Muscles Present*	Transfer Type	Functional Capabilities	Wheelchair Type
C1 to C3	Scalenes. Partial SCM, trapezius.	Mechanical lift. Dependent.	Mouthstick activities. Sip and puff, possibly chin control or mouth joystick for ECUs. Power assisted pressure relief.	Power w/c with recliner or tilt-in-space. Sip and puff, chin, or mouth control joystick.
C4	Diaphragm (partial). SCM, Upper trapezius.	Mechanical lift. Dependent.	Mouthstick activities. Sip and puff, mouth, or chin-control joystick for ECUs. May use MAS.	Power w/c with recliner or tilt-in-space with sip and puff, chin, mouth, or possibly head control joystick.
C5	Diaphragm. Deltoid. Biceps.	Mechanical lift. Dependent, possibly assisted sliding board.	Self feeding, light grooming, light functional activities, computer use with wrist and hand orthoses. Forward pressure relief, possibly with loops.	Power w/c with recliner or tilt-in-space with hand control, possibly, in mid-line.
C6	Radial wrist extensors. Pectoralis major, clavicular portion.	Sliding board, with assistance or independently; possibly depression.	Rolling, coming to sit, dressing, grooming, scooting, short and long sitting balance. Forward pressure relief. Drive car with assistive devices.	Power upright with hand control, possibly ultralight manual with friction rims.
C7	Triceps. Wrist flexors. Finger extensors. Pectoralis major, sternal portion. Latissimus dorsi.	Depression; may require a sliding board.	Rolling, coming to sit, dressing, grooming, sitting balance, w/c into car. Depression or forward pressure relief.	Ultralight manual w/c, possibly with friction rims; possibly power w/c.
C8	Finger flexors.	Depression.	Depression pressure relief. Independent functional activities except floor and stairs.	Ultralight manual w/c.
T1	Intrinsic muscles of hand.	Depression.	Same as C8.	Ultralight manual w/c.
T2 to L1	Increasing innervation of intercostals, trunk flexors and extensors.	Depression.	Ambulation with RGOs and UE assistive devices, for exercise only. Modified independent for all functional activities except floor and stairs.	Ultralight manual w/c.
L2	Quadratus lumborum. Hip flexors.	Depression.	Ambulation with KAFOs or RGOs and UE assistive devices for exercise only. Modified independent for all functional activities.	Ultralight manual w/c.
L3	Quadriceps.	Stand or squat pivot.	Ambulation with AFOs and UE assistive devices. Modified independent for all functional activities.	Typically still requires light weight or ultralight manual w/c.
L5	Ankle dorsiflexors. Knee flexors. Hip abductors.	Stand pivot.	Ambulation with AFOs. May not require UE assistive devices. Modified independent for all functional activities.	May require a w/c for long distances.

Table 9-3 (continued)
Select Functional Outcomes for Persons With Complete Spinal Cord Injury

SCI Level	Muscles Present*	Transfer Type	Functional Capabilities	Wheelchair Type
S1	Plantar flexors. Hip extensors.	As able-bodied.	Ambulation with no orthoses or UE assistive devices. Independent for functional activities.	May be modified independent for bowel and bladder care. No w/c.

AFO = ankle foot orthosis
KAFO = knee ankle foot orthosis
RGO = reciprocating gait orthosis
SCM = sternocleidomastoid muscle
ECU = environmental control unit
MAS = mobile arm support
Modified independent = independent with adaptive equipment

Guidelines may require modification for cardiovascular, musculoskeletal, neurological, or other problems
*New muscles at each level are in addition to previously-innervated muscles. Underlined muscles are ASIA key muscles for that level.[4,5]

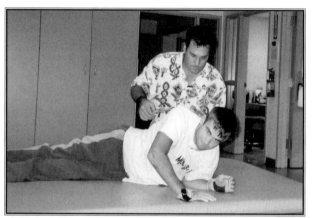

Figure 9-15A. Patient with C6 tetraplegia practicing coming to sit on the mat. The patient rolls to his side and the PTA assists him to initiate the sitting movement.

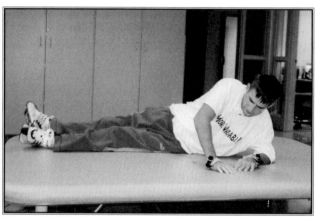

Figure 9-15B. The patient moves his arm up on the mat in preparation for pushing to sitting.

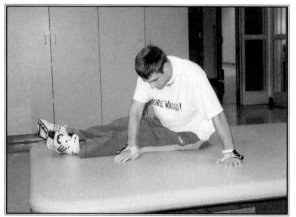

Figure 9-15C. The patient continues to move his arms around in front of him until he is sitting upright.

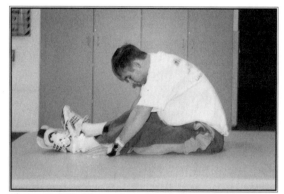

Figure 9-15D. The patient then independently comes to sitting.

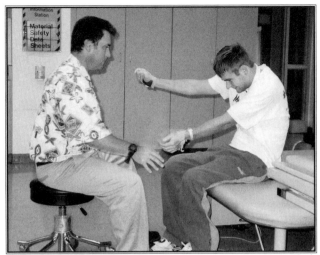

Figure 9-16. Patient with C6 tetraplegia practicing sitting balance with the PTA.

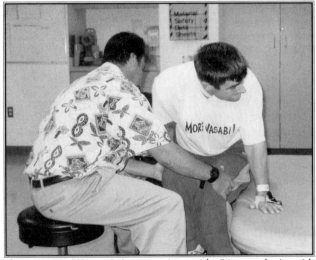

Figure 9-18. PTA assisting a patient with C6 tetraplegia with depression transfer to the w/c. Note how the patient turns his head to the left, as he lifts his body to facilitate movement of his buttocks to the right and onto the w/c.

Transfers

Transfers allow the person to move from place to place, including to or from a lower or higher surface. For the person with high tetraplegia, a dependent transfer or use of a mechanical lift will be required. A sliding board can assist people who have weak arms. A depression transfer is used by people with stronger arms. A depression transfer is accomplished when the person straightens his or her elbows, depresses the shoulders, lifts the buttocks off the supporting surface, turns, and moves onto a nearby surface (Figures 9-17 and 9-18). A stand- or squat-pivot transfer is used by people with sufficient motor function to take weight on their LE. Transfers to all surfaces are practiced, including a mat, bed, toilet, w/c, tub, car, the ground,

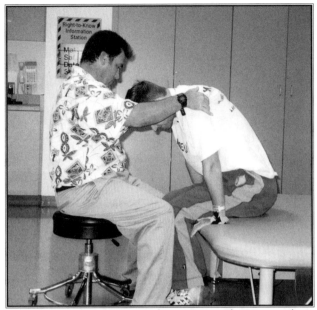

Figure 9-17. The PTA spots the patient with C6 tetraplegia practicing a depression lift on the mat. Skill in performing a depression on the mat will make transfers easier to perform.

and other sitting surfaces. The PT or PTA must be skillful in assisting the patient during the transfer, and the patient must have confidence in the person assisting. Initially, the patient may fail to lean far enough forward or move his or her shoulders and head enough to transfer efficiently. Details of how to perform functional activities for people at varying levels of injury can be found in the book *Spinal Cord Injury: Functional Rehabilitation*, by Somers.[47]

Wheelchair Mobility Training

W/c mobility training involves learning to maneuver in tight spaces; over uneven terrain, like gravel or grass; over a threshold; up and down ramps; through doors; and backward, forward, and to the sides. A person who uses a manual w/c learns how to navigate curbs, go up and down stairs, and get from the ground to the w/c (Figures 9-19A to 9-19F), in addition to those skills learned by all w/c users. The wheel position, including its location forward or backward, the angle of the seat, the amount the wheels flare out (camber), and the person's position in the w/c, are important in maximizing the efficiency of w/c propulsion. A person in a manual w/c learns to perform a *wheelie*, balancing on the large wheels while tilted backward. Patients can practice this while attached to an overhead safety cord or being spotted by the clinician. The surface the person pushes on affects velocity, with tile being easier than carpet. In a manual w/c, a person with higher injury levels pushes at slower speeds and travels shorter distances than a person with lower levels of injury. People with C6 tetraplegia are so limited by UE

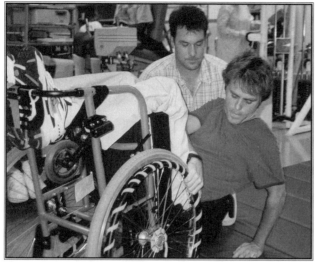

Figure 9-19A. PTA assisting a patient in practicing floor to w/c transfers. Patient is lowered to the floor from his w/c.

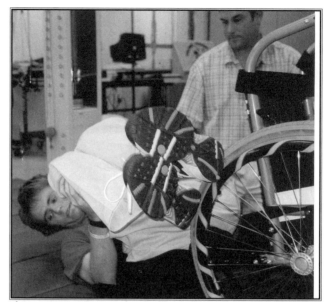

Figure 9-19B. Patient then rolls his legs to the side and away from the w/c.

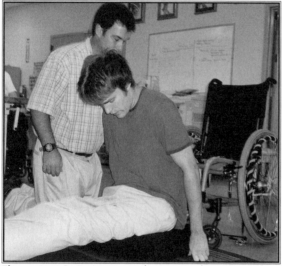

Figure 9-19C. Patient puts the w/c in the proper place and sits on his cushion. Having the cushion on the ground and not in the w/c reduces the distance he has to lift himself.

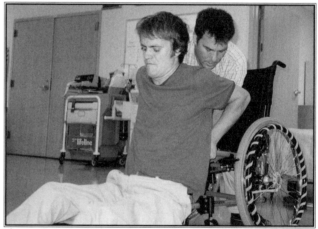

Figure 9-19D. With assistance, the patient lifts himself into the w/c.

Figure 9-19E. Patient puts a cushion under himself once he is in the w/c.

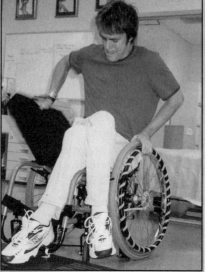

Figure 9-19F. Patient readjusts his sitting position.

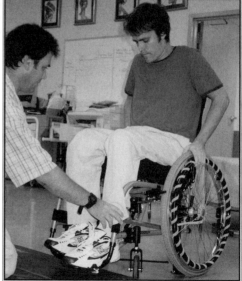

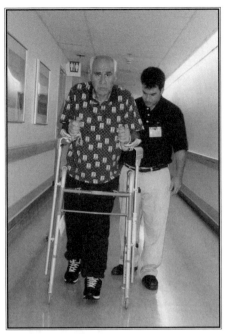

Figure 9-20. PTA walking with a patient with C6 tetraplegia, ASIA D. Bilateral arm troughs on the walker are needed due to weakness in the triceps and finger flexor muscles. Under his trousers, the patient is wearing bilateral polypropylene AFOs with a dorsiflexion assist and a dorsiflexion stop. Cosmesis with this type of AFO is excellent.

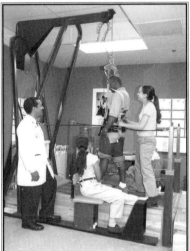

Figure 9-22. Physician consulting with staff about body-weight support treadmill training for a person with incomplete SCI. Training staff are positioned to assist in moving the legs and to control trunk rotation and weight shift. Note the black harness and overhead weight-support system.

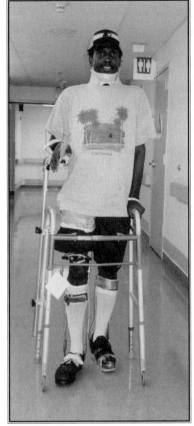

Figure 9-21. Patient with tetraplegia walking with trial orthoses. Use of these temporary orthoses, right KAFO and left AFO, allows ambulation before the patient's permanent orthoses are ordered and fabricated. The arm trough helps support the patient's right arm, which has weakness of the triceps muscle.

weakness that they are unable to navigate a 4% grade and no method of manual propulsion is efficient.[48]

Gait training is an important part of functional training for people who have sufficient motor recovery in their LEs, particularly those with incomplete injuries. People with SCI who ambulate may require LE orthosis to substitute for weak muscles.[49] An AFO can substitute for weak dorsiflexor muscles to prevent foot drop in swing and loading response. An AFO can also substitute for weak plantar flexor muscles by preventing unrestrained dorsiflexion in stance (Figure 9-20). A KAFO is used to substitute for weak quadriceps muscles (Figure 9-21). An erroneous, yet commonly held, belief of many clinicians is that use of a LE orthosis will prevent a muscle from contracting and, therefore, impede return of strength. This concept has not been supported in research of calf muscle

function in people with SCI,[50] so an AFO should be used when it improves patient function during gait or transfers. More extensive orthoses, such as a hip-knee-ankle-foot orthosis (HKAFO), are usually too cumbersome, although a reciprocating gait orthosis (RGO), which controls the hip, may be used to provide assistance in advancing the leg and, therefore, may be used by people with low cervical or thoracic injuries.

In recent years, body-weight support provided by an overhead unweighting system has been combined with walking on a treadmill or over ground to facilitate ambulation in people with incomplete SCI (Figure 9-22). Trainers or mechanical devices assist the patient in moving his or her legs in a normal gait pattern and speeds approaching those of normal walking are attained. No evidence currently exists that this intervention has carryover to walking over ground in people with complete injuries.

Although people with complete lesions are usually unable to rely on walking as their primary mode of mobility, they may use it as a form of exercise. The high energy cost of lifting the body with the arms, the slow velocity at which people in KAFOs or RGOs travel, and the demand on the shoulder musculature make this type of walking impractical. Another method of exercise ambulation, the ParaStep (Sigmedics, Fairborn, Ohio) uses electrical stimulation to activate the LE muscles. The energy cost per

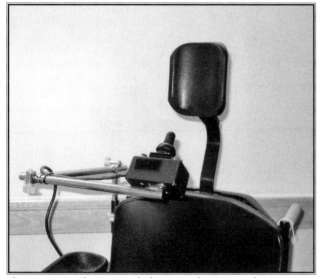

Figure 9-23. Chin control drive mechanism and positioning boom on power w/c.

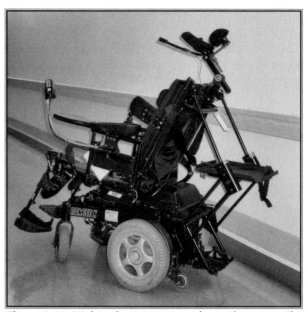

Figure 9-24. High-tech power w/c with ventilator tray. The cheek switch for operating the power recliner is attached to the headrest. Accessories include trunk supports and arm troughs.

meter traveled is similar for walking with KAFO's, RGO's, and ParaStep.™[51] ROM limitations, such as hip flexion, knee flexion, or ankle plantar flexion contractures, will interfere with the person's ability to walk. Plantar flexion contractures can usually be decreased by stretching in standing or using serial casts whereby sequential casts are applied to the ankle as the contracture is lessened. To stretch hip flexion contractures, the opposite hip must be flexed sufficiently to stabilize the pelvis. In supine, the hip being stretched hangs off the table in neutral abduction, with weights to help pull the leg down.

Provide Community Re-entry Activities

Visits into the community, with trips to movies, restaurants, amusement parks; introduction to w/c sports; and similar activities are coordinated by a multidisciplinary team.

Obtain Adaptive Equipment

The PT and OT are two team members responsible for selecting and prescribing most of the appropriate adaptive equipment. The PT may ask the PTA for input and suggestions, especially if the PTA has been practicing these functional activities with the patient and is more aware of the patient's status. Depending upon an individual facility's policies, the PTA may be responsible for ordering and obtaining some of the equipment once it has been selected by the team.

Wheelchair

Many people with SCI rely on a w/c for mobility. The most appropriate w/c for a given person depends on many factors, including the person's level of injury, age, UE strength, vocational or school plans,

living situation, resources, whether he or she has other medical problems, etc. People who are older, weaker, or have medical problems may require a power w/c, even with paraplegia or an incomplete injury. Patients with C1 to C4 injuries will require a power w/c with a head, chin (Figure 9-23), or sip and puff control to drive the chair. People who lack the ability to do pressure relief will need a w/c with power recline or tilt (Figure 9-24). Even people who walk limited distances may require a w/c for community mobility. Rigid ultra-lightweight manual w/cs (Figure 9-25) are often chosen over folding ones by people who are more active. w/c components, such as back height, wheel and caster size, tire type, armrests, "bucket" (the amount the seat back is lowered compared to the front), wheel camber (the amount the wheels flare away from the chair at the floor), and footplates can be customized for each patient's needs. The energy cost of propulsion of this type of chair is lower than in heavier regular-weight chairs.[52] Specialized hand rims, such as plastic covered or with projections, allow better contact with the push surface when hand function is limited, such as in the person with C6 to C8 tetraplegia (Figure 9-26). People who will rely on a w/c for mobility must learn enough about w/c maintenance and upkeep to prolong the life of the chair and assure that it will remain in good working condition.

Adaptive Equipment

Adaptive equipment includes a cushion, tub bench, raised toilet seat, and equipment that facilitates

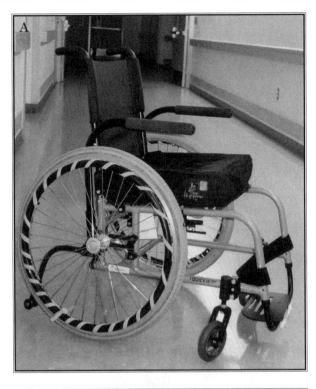

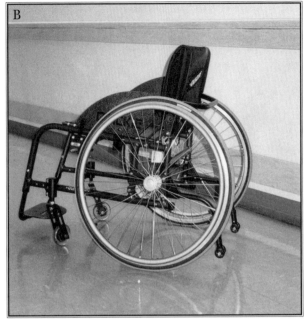

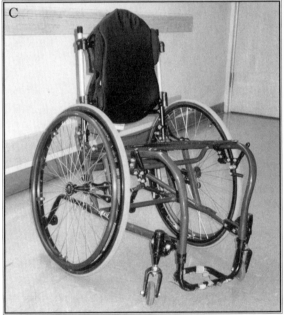

Figure 9-25. Examples of rigid ultralight w/cs. All w/cs have an adjustable axle plate, which allows the location of the wheels to be moved forward or backward relative to the seat. All have anti-tip tubes to keep the w/c from tipping over backwards. (A) High back and arm rests. Tubing is to permit greater contact on the pushrims during propulsion. (B) Low seat back, no arm rests, and small caster wheels. (C) An adjustable rigid back has been substituted for the back upholstery. This provides additional support and can improve sitting posture in patients with cervical or high thoracic-level injuries.

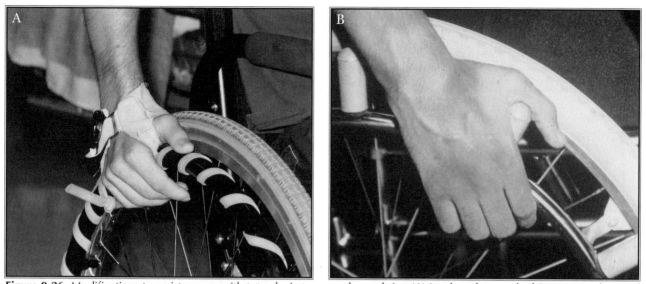

Figure 9-26. Modifications to assist person with tetraplegia to grasp the pushrim. (A) Leather glove and tubing wrapped around the handrim. Plastic coated handrims could be ordered on the patient's permanent w/c. (B) Vertical projections. These can also angle out at 45 degrees. Projections may increase the width of the w/c and make passage through doorways more difficult.

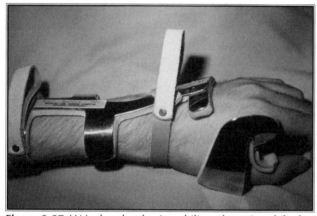

Figure 9-27. Wrist-hand orthosis stabilizes the wrist while the patient performs functional activities. Implements, such as a utensil or pen, can be inserted into the palm.

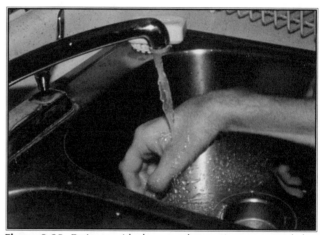

Figure 9-28. Patients with decreased sensations are at risk for being burned. Caution must be taken to avoid spilling hot liquids on arms or legs or using water that is too hot.

function, such as a reacher, UE orthosis (Figure 9-27), or gloves. A cushion, which helps to better redistribute pressure and provide sitting support, may be foam, gel, air-filled, or a combination. Anecdotal reports indicate that standing devices are helpful in reducing bladder problems, but clinical trials do not exist and third party payers may not consider this piece of equipment medically necessary.

Prevent Pressure Sores

Pressure sores, also called bedsores or pressure ulcers, are damage to the skin and or underlying tissues caused by excessive pressure or shear over bony prominences. Pressure on blood vessels limits the flow of blood and its oxygen supply to the tissues, just as the water supply is diminished when a garden hose is twisted or stepped on. Subsequently, the tissues supplied by these blood vessels die, and ulceration occurs. Pressure sores are common over any bony prominence, with some locations being more vulnerable than others, depending on the position the person assumes. For example, the sacrum is at most risk when the person is in supine or in a sitting position in bed, the heels are most vulnerable in supine, and ischial tuberosities in sitting.[53] When pressure is relieved, the blood supply returns and tissues are spared. Typically, people with SCI are at risk for pressure sores because they lack protective sensation and have a limited ability to move. Other factors that may cause pressure sores are thick, rough clothing (eg, decorative seams or rivets on jeans), lumpy or folded sheets, cushion covers, or clothing; moisture, especially due to bladder accidents; heat; burns (Figure 9-28); ill-fitting

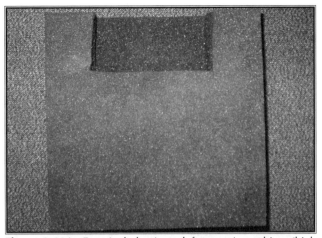

Figure 9-29A. Four-inch laminated foam w/c cushion (high density over extra high density) with ischial cutout. The cutout goes three-quarters of the way through the height of the cushion, thereby maintaining integrity of the cushion while eliminating pressure under the ischial tuberosities.

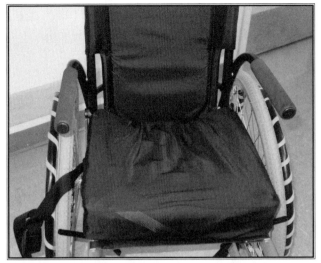

Figure 9-29B. Gel w/c cushion over a contoured foam base. Redistribution of sitting pressure is achieved with this cushion. The gel is primarily in the area of the ischial tuberosities.

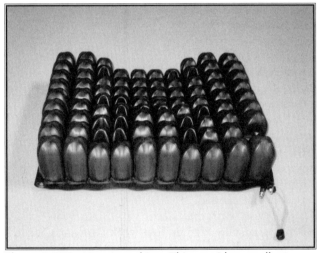

Figure 9-29C. Air w/c cushion. This provides excellent pressure redistribution for persons who have bony deformities of the pelvis. This cushion has lower bubbles over the area of the ischial tuberosities to aid with pressure relief. Cushion pressure must be checked every few days to prevent changes that could result in pressure sores.

RAISED

Reposition to
Alleviate
Ischial
Skin
Embarrassment and
Destruction

Figure 9-30. This easy-to-remember acronym, "RAISED," describes lifting body weight off the ischial tuberosities for pressure relief. (Adapted from *Methods of Ischial Pressure Relief for Patients with Spinal Injury*. Downey, Calif: Physical Therapy Department. Rancho Los Amigos Medical Center; 1980.)

---

clothing; poor nutrition; injuries due to carelessness with insensate skin; and orthopedic deformities (eg, scoliosis and pelvic obliquity).[53]

The two most important methods for preventing pressure sores are use of special pressure-relieving cushions (Figures 9-29 A to 9-29C) and mattresses and periodic relief of pressure over the bony prominences. To help people remember to do pressure relief, the acronym "RAISED" was coined[54] (Figure 9-30). This term conveys the process of lifting pressure off the ischii when sitting, which may be easier for the patient to remember than "pressure relief."

Studies of the optimum frequency of pressure relief are limited. In general, people with paraplegia or those who can use their arms for pressure relief are instructed to do their pressure relief for 15 seconds every 15 min. Other recommended time frames are 30 seconds of pressure relief every 30 min or 1 min of pressure relief every hour.[52] Further research is required to determine whether these time frames are sufficient to allow recovery of blood oxygen to resting levels.[55]

While in the sitting position, pressure can be relieved by lifting the buttocks from the seat, a depression pressure relief (Figure 9-31); leaning forward enough to raise the ischial tuberosities off the seat (Figure 9-32); or leaning side-to-side. In people with a power w/c equipped with a recliner or tilt system, pressure relief is accomplished by lying down or tilting backwards at least 65 degrees.[55]

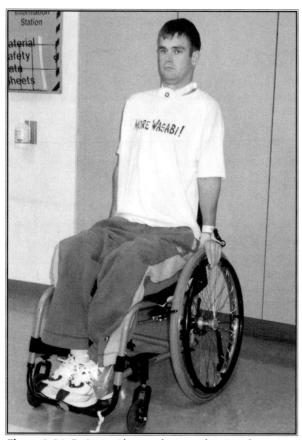

Figure 9-31. Patient with tetraplegia performing depression pressure relief.

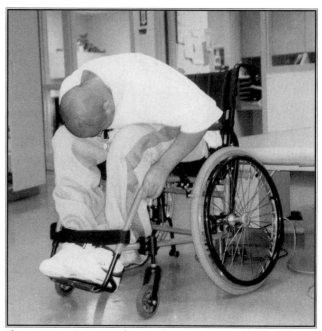

Figure 9-32. Patient with tetraplegia performing forward pressure relief.

Special equipment, such as a mattress, can help relieve pressure over bony prominences or redistribute pressures over larger and less bony areas. Just as in sitting, pressure relief is required in addition to any pressure redistribution provided by the mattress. Pressure relief is provided by turning the person in bed every 2 hours; using a pressure-changing mattress; or having the person lie prone or semi-prone. In the prone or semi-prone position, pillows are used to bridge bony areas, including the pelvis and knees. People who are able to lie in one of these positions can sleep for longer periods without turning, because pressure on prominent bony areas is minimized. The person is able to rest better, and the amount of nursing or attendant care required is decreased.

Pressure mapping with computerized pressure-sensing devices is a form of assessment performed by the PT to provide additional information about sitting pressures. Pressure can be measured on various pieces of adaptive equipment, such as mattresses or cushions, and the effectiveness of modified equipment or positions that relieve pressure can be compared. Both the PT and PTA can use the resulting pressure map as an education tool. The best screening for areas of excess pressure in sitting is by palpation of the bony prominences with the PT or PTA's hands. When areas of excess pressure are identified, the cushion or sitting position can be altered to minimize pressures.

Pressure sores take a toll on the person with SCI and society – physically, socially, and monetarily. To prevent sores or to identify them before they become severe, people with SCI are taught to inspect their skin morning and evening using a long-handled mirror and assistance, if needed.

Pressure sores may occur very quickly (ie, within 30 min) and may take up to a week for even a Stage I sore to heal. If a pressure sore does occur (Table 9-4), complete relief of pressure by staying off the sore is optimal to allow healing. The person who has a pressure sore may need to avoid or severely limit sitting.[53] If pressure sores progress to Stage III or IV, surgery may be required.[56]

Educate the Person With Spinal Cord Injury and Family

The person with SCI, family members, and hired attendant personnel must learn how to assist the person with SCI at home. People with SCI who are unable to care for themselves must learn how to direct others to provide their care. Many rehabilitation programs have classes for patients with SCI where a variety of subjects are covered. These may include presentations about the nature of SCI and how it affects the body, research on spinal cord regeneration, sexual function, adaptive vehicles, w/c maintenance, dealing with w/c vendors, hiring an attendant, and other topics that will assist the patient once he or she leaves the hospital.

Table 9-4
Classification of Pressure Sores

Stage I:	Nonblanchable erythema of intact skin (USPHS). In persons with dark skin, discoloration of the skin, warmth, edema, induration, or hardness may also be indicators.
Stage II:	Partial thickness skin loss involving the dermis, epidermis, or both.
Stage III:	Full thickness skin loss involving damage to or necrosis of subcutaneous tissue that may extend down to, but not through, underlying fascia. The ulcer is a deep crater, with or without undermining adjacent tissue.
Stage IV:	Full thickness skin loss with extensive destruction, tissue necrosis, or damage to muscle, bone, or supporting structures such as tendon or joint capsule.
***Non-Stagable:**	Sore is covered with eschar so that one is unable to determine the condition of the tissue below.

Note: Once a sore has been staged, it remains at that stage. For example, a Stage II sore becomes a healing Stage II (not a Stage III).

---

*Used at Rancho Los Amigos National Rehabilitation Center, Downey, Calif.
Adapted from Treatment of Pressure Ulcers. Clinical Practice Guideline #15 (AHCPR Publication #95-0652). Rockville, Md: U.S. Department of Health and Human Services; 1994.*

Evaluate the Home for Accessibility

A visit to the person's home may be recommended to assure that architectural barriers are minimized, make recommendations for mobility into and within the home, and maximize functional independence by making recommendations for furniture placement and bedroom and bathroom setup. When the PTA has worked directly with the patient in functional training, he or she can contribute to the problem-solving process during a home visit.

Discharge From the Rehabilitation Program and Reintegration Into the Community

Most people with SCI are discharged home, although people with more severe injuries or fewer resources may require discharge to an assisted living situation, such as a board-and-care, skilled nursing, or sub-acute facility. People with tetraplegia, and some with paraplegia, will require assistance from family members, friends, or a paid caregiver. Some communities have support groups to help people with SCI and their families continue to cope with the changes in their lives. A period of time is required for the person with SCI to adapt physically and emotionally to his or her new lifestyle, but successful social and vocational reintegration is an achievable goal. During the time following discharge from rehabilitation, the person may take advantage of vocational training to determine how the work environment and tasks can be modified to physical limitations that are present and how adaptive equipment can be utilized. People who have a valid driver's license may learn to drive with hand controls. Some medical centers have gyms that people with spinal injury can access, or they may be able to modify exercise methods to use a commercial gym. Medical follow-up is required to monitor bladder function and overall health and to assure that late complications are minimized. Each individual with SCI deserves to have a fulfilling and meaningful life and can achieve one with support and assistance.

CHAPTER QUESTIONS

I. John, age 22, sustained a C6 level SCI, ASIA A, in a motor vehicle accident 2 months ago. He was a student at a local community college studying computer science.

1. What muscles remain innervated?
2. Will he be able to continue using his computer?
3. What kind of adaptive equipment will be required to use the computer?
4. The PT has identified sliding board transfers as a goal for the patient. What activities or interventions would you want to initiate before attempting transfers?
5. What kind of w/c will he probably need, given his vocational goals?

II. A patient is on the tilt table having his hamstrings stretched to gain ROM for a straight leg raise. His injury level is T2. He starts sweating and complaining of a headache.

1. What do you suspect has occurred?
2. What should you do first?
3. If his BP is elevated, what should you do?

III. You are working with a patient with a SCI at L1 level, ASIA C, which he sustained 2 months ago. You know that the doctor has talked to the patient about recovery and the level of his injury. The patient now has Poor minus (P-) to Poor (P) strength in the hip flexor and quadriceps muscles and Trace (Tr) in his dorsiflexor, hamstring, and hip abductor muscles.

1. Is it important to continue to strengthen the muscles in his LEs?

2. Can he get stronger?

3. Would he still benefit from exercise if it were 13 months post injury? Why?

IV. You are asked to work with a patient who has T6 paraplegia and is sitting on a gel cushion. Yesterday was his first day sitting, and he had no problems with dizziness. The PT asks you to implement an education program on pressure relief and prevention of pressure sores.

1. What points would you want to cover with this patient?

V. You are running a class on power w/c mobility for patients with C2 to C5 tetraplegia.

1. What activities would be important for these people to learn in order to be able to function in the community?

2. What additional activities would be important if it were a class for patients using manual w/cs?

VI. You are working with a patient with T7 paraplegia.

1. What functional activities would you work on in preparation for a car transfer?

CASE STUDY

Social History. The patient, Randy, is a 26 year old male who is married and has two children, ages 3 and 5. The patient sustained a T9 complete SCI (ASIA A) when he fell off a roof while assisting in a family project to reroof his cousin's house. Use of alcohol was not implicated in his fall. He has worked for 8 years assembling parts for an electronics company. He lives in a one-story home, which he rents and which has three steps to enter. There is no rail. The bathroom is rather small and has a tub. His wife is a homemaker and takes care of the home and the children. He does the yard work on weekends. He has a large extended family and many friends from work. They are putting on a fund-raiser for him and visit him frequently in the hospital.

Medical History. At the time of his fall, he sustained no other injuries except for some bruises on his arms. The thoracic spine fracture was diagnosed by x-ray, and no surgery was required. He was placed in a thoraco-lumbo-sacral orthosis (TLSO) for 6 weeks. When the TLSO was discontinued, the physician cleared him for all functional activities, with no limitations. He had no pre-existing medical problems.

Rehabilitation Center. Randy was then referred to an inpatient rehabilitation center. Upon admission to the rehabilitation center, he was screened for the presence of deep venous thrombosis; none was found. Each of the team members evaluated the patient; the physician wrote medical orders for care and established the neurological level of injury as T9, ASIA A. Critical components of the rehabilitation program, including bowel, bladder, and skin care; increasing the patient's time out of bed; and initiating self-care and mobility, were implemented immediately while plans were made for the entire rehabilitation stay.

Physical Therapist Evaluation: The PT evaluated the patient and found the following:

Strength:

UEs = Normal (N)

LEs = Zero (0)

Trunk = Intercostals intact; abdominals absent except for those innervated by T8

Sensation (sharp or dull, light touch, proprioception):

UEs = Normal (N)

LEs = Absent

Trunk = Normal through T8; absent below

ROM:

Within functional limits, except for straight leg raise (SLR), which was 60 degrees bilaterally.

Functional capabilities. Previously, the patient had been independent in all functional activities. At the time of evaluation, he required moderate assistance for rolling in bed and coming to sit using the hospital bed rails, maximum assistance of one person for all transfers, and was independent for w/c propulsion on level terrain for short distances.

When the PT initially got the patient out of bed into a w/c as part of his initial evaluation, the patient experienced some dizziness, which resolved within the treatment session.

Arterial BP - 118/78.

HR - 70.

VC - 60% of normal.

Mild spasticity in the plantar flexor and adductor muscles, bilaterally and not interfering with function.

Patient Goals. The patient wants to be able to take care of himself, return to work, and take care of his family. He also wants to be able to walk again.

Discharge Goals. Physical therapy discharge goals are: independence in depression transfers to all surfaces, except the floor, for which he will require moderate assistance; independence in bed mobility and achieving the prone position in bed; independence in all w/c skills except stairs; and independence in knowledge of all aspects of his care. Specific information that physical therapy is responsible for teaching includes basic w/c maintenance, care of the cushion, performance of self-ROM, and sitting pressure relief. Other disciplines have established goals of independence in bowel and bladder care, skin management, independence in bathing and self-care.

Physical Therapy Program. The PT has not identified a respiratory program for this patient. Randy's VC is already 60% of normal and his inspiratory muscles are intact. Based on research[38] and experience, the PT anticipates that Randy's VC will return to previous levels by participating in the transfer training, w/c propulsion, and UE strengthening activities that are a part of his rehabilitation program.

The PT has identified the following program for Randy:

UE strengthening exercises. Although Randy's UE muscles test as N, he will need "supernormal" muscles to substitute for his LEs. The goals for strengthening the UEs will be accomplished by putting Randy in an UE exercise class designed specifically for patients with SCI.

Transfer training and functional activities. The PTA will be responsible for these activities. The PTA will progress Randy through transfers to and from the bed, mat, toilet, car, shower or tub, floor, and other surfaces, as needed and usually in that approximate order. The PT will also identify when Randy is ready to perform depression transfers. He may have a transition period when he is still using the sliding board for some transfers, such as the car, but is doing a depression transfer to other surfaces, such as the bed.

Randy is accustomed to being proactive in his work and solving problems that occur at work and home. Because of this attitude, he is always trying to figure out how to do his transfers more easily and to set up the environment to his advantage. This kind of behavior is critical in self-sufficiency and in solving problems that will arise after discharge and should be fostered. During the rehabilitation process, Randy is asked to make decisions about his care, to help determine the course of his program, and to prioritize goals.

The PTA will also work on functional activities, including sitting, rolling, coming to sit, scooting, and w/c skills. There is overlap in functional activities and transfer training. For example, sitting balance is critical for scooting, moving in bed, doing w/c activities, and for doing transfers. When the patient can get into the prone or semi-prone position with pillows protecting bony prominences, he can reduce the amount of turning that he must do at night and can, therefore, reduce the amount of assistance required. Proning for 1 to 2 hours is initiated during physical therapy treatment and is then carried over by nursing and Randy himself.

Randy has tight hamstring muscles. The PT has asked the PTA to oversee the stretching on the hamstring stretch apparatus and to assess the patient's progress daily.

Patient education about various aspects of his care. In addition to the education provided by the different health care disciplines involved in the patient's care, many rehabilitation centers provide classes for patient education on topics including how the body works after SCI, status of research in SCI, community resources, how to interact with w/c vendors, sexuality, and other topics. In addition, education of the family is important. This patient's wife will be a great resource to him and needs to be educated about all aspects of his care. Because Randy's wife will be an important support, she is included in training, including transfer training before he leaves the hospital.

The PT will consult with the patient about a w/c. All patients with complete injuries benefit from an ultralight w/c.[52] A variety of ultralight w/cs are available, each with specific features. Factors, such as whether Randy will transport the w/c in a car, whether he will return to work, and what his insurance will allow, will be considered. If possible, Randy should try a variety of ultralight w/cs before making a decision. The PTA will work with Randy on the basics of w/c maintenance, such as how to fix a flat tire and how to adjust the wheel camber, casters, and brakes.

The PTA will train the patient on w/c skills and teach the patient how to get the w/c in and out of the car.

Evaluation of the home environment. The PT and PTA should also discuss with Randy his home layout and coordinate with other disciplines for equipment Randy will need, such as a raised toilet seat, bath bench, and grab bars. They will also discuss the need for a home visit. Even though Randy can skillfully and independently perform his transfers and has good problem-solving skills, he has identified the small size of the bathroom as a potential problem. Based on this potential barrier, the PT or the PTA will make an on-site visit, typically with the OT, to come up with the best solution to bathroom access. From the beginning of Randy's stay, other equipment needs, such as a ramp, were discussed so that everything would be available at the time of discharge. Randy's father and brother made a ramp according to specification given them by the PTA. Near the end of his rehabilitation stay, Randy is scheduled for a day pass on Sunday and an overnight pass the next weekend so that he has an opportunity to test his skills away from the hospital and at home. Any problems that are identified can be dealt with while he has easy access to the hospital resources.

Questions

1. What muscle groups should be emphasized?

2. What kind of transfers will the PTA begin with?

3. What activities will be compromised by his lack of 90 to 110 degrees SLR?

4. When would the PTA stop stretching to gain SLR?

5. Would you expect to need to be concerned about autonomic dysreflexia with this patient?

6. What specific education would be covered by physical therapy?

7. What would this patient need to know about his cushion, pressure relief, skin care, and LE ROM?

8. What w/c skills would the PTA work on with this patient?

Suggested author answers are available at www.slackbooks.com/neuroquestions.

Final Results

Randy underwent a four-week rehabilitation program.

During the first week, the physician discussed the prognosis of his injury. He indicated that while it is impossible to know with certainty what the outcome would be, most people with his kind of injury did not have recovery of muscles or the ability to walk. Randy was sad about what the doctor had said, but ready to move forward with learning how to take care of himself. During the second week, a meeting was held during which the team discussed questions the family had about Randy's discharge. The psychologist met with Randy to help him deal with the injury and plan for the future.

By the end of the second week, Randy was dressing himself, doing his self-care, learning tub and toilet transfers, doing a depression transfer to the bed and mat, and doing his own self-IC. Nursing was working with him on morning skin inspection and extending the time between catherizations, so he would not have to do IC so often at night. He was also attending daily multi-disciplinary classes. His SLR was still limited, but modifications were made by all disciplines in activities he performed in the long sitting position.

By the third week, he was transferring to the toilet with assistance for his bowel program, transferring with assistance and a tub bench to a tub for showering, transferring to the car using a sliding board, and proning half the night. During this week, he had a small setback when he developed a bladder infection. He was lethargic, had a fever, was sweating, and missed a day of therapy. A few days of treatment with antibiotics cleared the infection, and he was able to return to therapy even before the infection completely resolved. Despite the infection, he was able to go on an overnight visit and identify problems that were resolved on the home visit the next week. His SLR reached 100 degrees.

By the end of the fourth week, Randy was ready to go home—able to perform most of his care independently. He and his wife had learned a great deal about take care of him and were able to identify resources for when problems arose. He had achieved all the goals that the PT established for him. In addition, Randy had accomplished most of the goals he had set for himself. He was not able to walk, although he was looking forward to trying to walk with orthoses and crutches in the future. He was not ready to return to work yet, but he has a job waiting for him that can be performed, with slight modifications, from a w/c. His fellow-workers are looking forward to his return. He has a great support network in his family and friends, and this will be important to his life. His life has changed, and some aspects will never be the same. He and his wife (and the children) are adapting to his injury and the life-style changes it will bring. He will still need to be followed for potential medical problems and will need to continue to have emotional and psychological help as he adapts to his changed life.

Resources for people with SCI and individuals interested in SCI issues:

ORGANIZATIONS

Christopher Reeve Paralysis Foundation
A foundation committed to funding research to develop cures and treatment for paralysis due to SCI. Also provides grants for quality of life for people living with disabilities.
500 Morris Avenue
Springfield, NJ 07081
(800) 225-0292
www.apacure.com

American Spinal Injury Association
An organization for physicians and other health care professionals specializing in care of patients with spinal cord injury.
2020 Peachtree Road NW
Atlanta, GA 30309-1402
(404) 355-9772
www.asia-spinalinjury.org

National Spinal Cord Injury Association (NSCIA)
Provides information on a variety of topics related to SCI and an on-line newsletter.
6701 Democracy Blvd., Suite 300-9
Bethesda, MD 20817
(800) 962-9629, 301-214-4006
www.spinalcord.org

National Spinal Cord Injury Statistical Center (NSCISC)
Spinal Cord Injury Network. Provides information about research projects and statistics about SCI.
1717 6th Avenue South, Room 544
Birmingham, AL 35233-733
(205) 934-3320; FAX (205) 934-2709
www.spinalcord.uab.edu

OTHER WEBSITES

www.ninds.nih.gov/disorders/sci/sci.htm
A site of the National Institute of Neurological Disorders and Stroke, National Institute of Health, which supports biomedical research on disorders of the brain and nervous system.

REFERENCES

1. Atkinson PP, Atkinson JLD. Spinal shock. *Mayo Clin Pro.* 1996;71:384-389.

2. National Spinal Cord Injury Statistical Center. Birmingham, Ala: Accessed January 2004.

3. Kolakowsky-Hayner SA, Gourley EV 3rd, Kreutzer JS, et al. Pre-injury substance abuse among people with brain injury and people with spinal cord injury. *Brain Inj.* 1999;13:571-581.

4. Marino RJ, Barros T, Biering-Sorenson F, et al. International standards for neurological classification of spinal cord injury. *J Spinal Cord Med.* 2003;26(Suppl 1):550-556.

5. International standards for neurological classification of spinal cord injury. Chicago, Ill: American Spinal Injury Association; 2002.

6. Dittunno JF, Little JW, Tessler A, et al. Spinal shock revisited: a four-phase model. *Spinal Cord.* 2004;42:383-395.

7. Merriam WF, Taylor TKF, Ruff J, McPhail MJ. A reappraisal of acute traumatic central cord syndrome. *J Bone Jt Surg.* 1986;68-B:708-713.

8. Baydur A, Adkins RH, Milic-Emili J. Lung mechanics in individuals with spinal cord injury; effects of injury level and posture. *J Appl Physiol.* 2001;90:405-411.

9. Short DJ, Silver JR, Lehr RP. Electromyographic study of sternocleidomastoid and scalene muscles in tetraplegic subjects during respiration. *Int Disabil Stud*. 1991;13:46-49.

10. Bach JR. Mechanical insufflation-exsufflation. Comparison of peak expiratory flows with manually assisted and unassisted coughing techniques. *Chest*. 1993;104:1553-1562.

11. Alvarez S, Peterson M, Lunsford BR. Respiratory treatment of the adult patient with spinal cord injury. *Phys Ther*. 1981;12:1737-1745.

12. Jackson AB, Groomes TE. Incidence of respiratory complications following spinal cord injury. *Arch Phys Med Rehabil*. 1994;75:270-275.

13. Neurogenic bowel management in adults with spinal cord injury. *Consortium for Spinal Cord Medicine*. Washington, DC: Paralyzed Veterans of America; 1998:11.

14. Benevento BT, Sipski ML. Neurogenic bladder, neurogenic bowel, and sexual dysfunction in people with spinal cord injury. *Phys Ther*. 2002;82:601-612.

15. Comarr AE. Autonomic dysreflexia (hyperreflexia). *J Am Paraplegia Soc*. 1984;7(3):53-57.

16. Acute management of autonomic dysreflexia: adults with spinal cord injury presenting to health-care facilities. Consortium for spinal cord medicine. *J Spinal Cord Med*. 1997;20(3):284-307.

17. Naftchi NE, Richardson JS. Autonomic dysreflexia: pharmacological management of hypertensive crises in spinal cord injured patients. *J Spin Cord Med*. 1997;20(3):355-360.

18. Kubler-Ross E. *On Death and Dying*. New York, NY: Macmillan Publishing; 1969.

19. Siddall PJ, Loeser JD. Pain following spinal cord injury. *Spinal Cord*. 2001;39:63-73.

20. Burchiel KJ, Hsu FPK. Pain and spasticity after spinal cord injury: mechanisms and treatment. *Spine*. 2001;26(245):S146-S160.

21. Gellman H, Sie I, Waters RL. Late complications of the weight-bearing upper extremity in the paraplegia patient. *Clin Orthop Related Res*. 1998;233:132-135.

22. Subbarao JV, Klopfstein J, Turpin R. Prevalence and impact of wrist and shoulder pain in patients with spinal cord injury. *J Spinal Cord Med*. 1995;18:9-13.

23. Curtis KA, Drysdale GA, Lanza RD. Shoulder pain in wheelchair users with tetraplegia and paraplegia. *Arch Phys Med Rehabil*. 1999;80:453-457.

24. Davidoff G, Morris J, Elliot. Rath E, Bleiberg J. Closed head injury in spinal cord injured. patients: retrospective study of loss of consciousness and post-traumatic amnesia. *Arch Phys Med Rehabil*. 1985;66:41-43.

25. Garland DE. A clinical perspective on common forms of acquired heterotopic ossification. *Clin Orthop*. 1991;263:13-29.

26. Banovac K. The effect of etidronate on late development of heterotopic ossification after spinal cord injury. *J Spinal ord Med*. 2000;23(1):40-44.

27. Garland DE, Stewart CA, Adkins RH, et al. Osteoporosis after spinal cord injury. *J of Orthop Res*. 1992;10:371-378.

28. Thompson L, Yakura J. Aging related functional changes in people with spinal cord injury. *Top Spinal Cord Rehabil*. 2001;6:69-82.

29. Bauman WA, Adkins RH, Spungen AM, et al. The effect of residual neurological deficit on serum lipoproteins in individuals with chronic spinal cord injury. *Spinal Cord*. 1998;36(1):13-17.

30. Pollard ME, Apple DF. Factors associated with improved neurologic outcomes in patients with incomplete tetraplegia. *Spine*. 2003;28(1):33-39.

31. Roth EJ, Lawler MH, Yarkony GM. Traumatic central cord syndrome: clinical features and functional outcomes. *Arch Phys Med Rehabil*. 1990;71:18-23.

32. Pointillart V, Petitjean ME, Wiart L, et al. Pharmacological therapy of spinal cord injury during acute phase. *Spinal Cord*. 2000;38:71-76.

33. Waters RL, Adkins R, Yakura J, Sie I. Functional and neurologic recovery following acute SCI. *J of Spinal Cord Med*. 1998;21:195-199.

34. Waters RL, Adkins RH, Yakura JS, et al. Motor and sensory recovery following incomplete tetraplegia. *Arch Phys Med Rehabil*. 1994;75:311.

35. Mulroy SJ, Gronley JK, Newsam CJ, et al. Electromyographic activity of shoulder muscles during wheelchair propulsion by paraplegic people. *Arch Phys Med Rehabil*. 1996;77:187-193.

36. Powers CM, Newsam CJ, Gronley JK, et al. Isometric shoulder torque in subjects with spinal cord injury. *Arch Phys Med Rehabil*. 1994;75:761-765.

37. Gronley JK, Newsam CJ, Mulroy SJ, et al. Electromyographic and kinematic analysis of the shoulder during four activities of daily living in men with C6 tetraplegia. *J Rehab Res*. 2000;37(4):423-432.

38. Silva AC, Neder JA, Chiurciu MV, et al. Effect of aerobic training on ventilatory muscle endurance of spinal cord injured men. *Spinal Cord*. 1998;36:240-245.

39. Gilgoff IS, Barras DN, Adkins HV. Neck breathing: a form of voluntary respiration for the spine-injured ventilator-dependent quadriplegic child. *Pediatr*. 1988;82;741-745.

40. Warren VC. Glossopharyngeal and neck accessory muscle breathing in a young adult with C2 complete tetraplegia resulting in ventilatory dependency. *Phys Ther*. 2002;82:590-600.

41. Derrickson J, Ciesla N, Simpson N, et al. A comparison of two breathing programs for patients with quadriplegia. *Phys Ther.* 1992;72:763-769.

42. Liaw MY, Lin MC, Cheng PT, et al. Resistive inspiratory muscle training: its effectiveness in patients with acute complete cervical cord injury. *Arch Phys Med Rehabil.* 2000;81:752-762.

43. Lin KH, Chuang CC, Wu HD, et al. Abdominal weight and inspiratory resistance: their immediate effects on inspiratory muscle functions during maximal voluntary breathing in chronic tetraplegic patients. *Arch Phys Med Rehabil.* 1999;80:741-745.

44. Lerman RM, Weiss MS. Progressive resistive exercise in weaning high quadriplegics from the ventilator. *Paraplegia.* 1987;25:130-135.

45. Linn WS, Spungen AM, Gong H Jr, et al. Forced vital capacity in two large outpatient populations with chronic spinal cord injury. *Spinal Cord.* 2001;39:263-268.

46. Outcomes following traumatic spinal cord injury: clinical practice guidelines for health-care professionals. *Consortium for Spinal Cord Medicine.* Washington, DC: Paralyzed veterans of America; 1999:9, 10-20.

47. Somers MF. *Spinal Cord Injury: Functional Rehabilitation.* Norwalk, Conn: Appleton and Lange; 1992.

48. Newsam CJ, Mulroy SJ, Gronley JK, et al. Temporal-spatial characteristics of wheelchair propulsion. *Am J Phys Med.* 1996;75(4):292-299.

49. Waters RL, Miller L. A physiologic rationale for orthotic prescription in paraplegia. *Clin Prosth Orthot.* 1987;11:66-73.

50. Beekman CE, Miller-Porter L, Schoneberger M. Energy cost of propulsion in standard and ultra-light wheelchairs in people with spinal cord injuries. *Phys Ther.* 1999;79:146-158.

51. Waters RL, Mulroy S. The energy expenditure of normal and pathologic gait. *Gait and Posture.* 1999;9:207-231.

52. Beekman C, Perry J, Boyd L, et al. The effects of a dorsiflexion-stopped ankle-foot orthosis on walking in individuals with incomplete spinal cord injury. *Top Spinal Cord Inj Rehabil.* 2000;4(4):54-62.

53. *Treatment of Pressure Ulcers. Clinical Practice Guideline #15 (AHCPR Publication #95-0652).* Rockville, Md: U.S. Department of Health and Human Services; 1994.

54. Methods of ischial pressure relief for patients with spinal injury. Downey, Calif: Physical Therapy Department, Rancho Los Amigos Medical Center; 1980.

55. Coggrave MJ, Rose LS. A specialist seating assessment clinic: changing pressure relief practice. *Spinal Cord.* 2003;41:692-695.

56. Rubayi S, Pompan D, Garland D, et al. Proximal femoral resection and musculocutaneous flap for the treatment of pressure ulcers in spinal cord injury patients. *Ann Plast Surg.* 1991;27:132-138.

Chapter

10

CLIENTS WITH TRAUMATIC BRAIN INJURY

Dennis Klima, PT, MS, GCS, NCS

KEY WORDS

coma
contre-coup injury
coup injury
diffuse axonal shearing
Glasgow Coma Scale
persistent vegetative state
Rancho Los Amigos Levels of Cognitive Function
traumatic brain injury

CHAPTER OBJECTIVES

- Describe major causes of TBI.

- Discuss mechanisms of injury and medical complications associated with TBI.

- Describe the major categories of the Glasgow Coma Scale.

- Outline the major levels and associated cognitive behavior included in the Rancho Los Amigos Levels of Cognitive Function.

- Describe key components of the PT's examination for patients recovering from a TBI.

- Identify common cognitive, musculoskeletal, and neuromuscular impairments seen in this special patient population.

- List physical therapy management precautions for individuals with TBI.

- Describe major interventions performed for those musculoskeletal and neuromuscular impairments noted in the PT's examination.

- Discuss techniques for integrating both cognitive and functional training strategies to advance the patient towards those established goals.

- Describe key activities associated with patient discharge planning, home programs, equipment procurement, and community integration.

INTRODUCTION

Management of clients with TBI presents a major challenge for all health care professionals working with this special patient population. Over 1 million people sustain a TBI each year in the United States; moreover, 80,000 to 90,000 individuals will have a lifelong disability secondary to the injury.[1]

A *traumatic brain injury* (TBI) may be defined as "an insult to the brain, not of degenerative or congenital nature but caused by an external physical force, that may produce a diminished or altered state of consciousness and which results in an impairment of cognitive or physical functioning."[2] TBI accounts for one-third of all injury-related deaths in the United States, though 70% to 90% of all treated injuries are only classified as mild.[1,3]

Major causes of head injury include motor vehicle and recreational vehicle accidents as well as firearm-related injuries. Males sustain nearly twice as many injuries as females, and individuals between the ages of 15 and 24 or over 75 years of age demonstrate the greatest risk for a TBI.[4] Motor vehicle crashes are the leading cause of head injury in minorities, though violence and pedestrian vehicle trauma account for greater incidences of injury than in nonminority populations.[5] No significant differences exist, however, in functional recovery patterns between minority and nonminority groups.[5] For individuals 65 or older, the leading cause of TBI is a fall-related episode.[6]

Head injury sequelae can be devastating and affect virtually every component of the quality of life: self care, home management, work responsibilities, and leisure activities.[7] Poor recovery outcomes can eventually lead to long-term institutional placement if caregiving demands exceed available resources in the home environment. Public awareness has increasingly focused on injury prevention through vigilance with fall-prevention strategies for older individuals and increased helmet use during recreational sports and cycling activities. Local and national brain injury associations serve as strong advocacy catalysts for both children and adults recovering from a TBI.

THEORETICAL FRAMEWORK: ROLE OF THE PHYSICAL THERAPIST ASSISTANT

The theoretical framework outlining interventions performed by the PTA was discussed in Chapter 1 (see Figure 1-1). Neurologic interventions with this special patient population require a level of expertise beyond entry-level practice. PTAs working with these clients have gained experience through mentoring, continuing education, and shadowing activities in the clinical arena. Clinical expertise and additional responsibilities may have also developed through a career ladder progression in the rehabilitation setting.[8] PTs and PTAs with expertise in neurologic patient management serve as powerful expert mentors in facilitating clinical expertise among novice clinicians and students.[9] It should be noted that PTs and PTAs may initially elect to approach patient management through a team effort to enhance the PTA's intervention skills with patients with TBI. The seasoned PTA may then be delegated select interventions with more complicated patients where patient and situational considerations are less stable and predictable.[10] For example, functional activities with the agitated patient dictate immediate modification of intervention strategies given potential outbursts of hostility or inappropriate behavior. Effective delegation strategies are enhanced by ongoing communication with the supervising PT to optimize interventions performed by the PTA in the trajectory of care.

MEDICAL AND RECOVERY ISSUES

Mechanisms of Injury

The initial site of impact following a traumatic insult to the brain is known as the *coup injury*. Because of the rebound effect, which occurs in the cranium following the initial impact, a *contre-coup injury* will often occur (Figure 10-1). The term *diffuse axonal shearing* refers to the neuronal damage associated with traumatic rotational acceleration of the brain during unrestricted movement.[11] Extensive brain tissue deformation occurs through shearing forces and inertial loading incurred during the injury. Head injuries generally fall into two categories: open and closed. The skull and meninges remain intact following a closed head injury, whereas open injuries cause fracture and rupture of these protective structures. *Contusions* refer to more localized hemorrhages that occur at the site of injury and are commonly seen in the frontal and temporal regions of the brain.

Injuries sustained within the cranial vault may also be accompanied by concomitant edema, which adversely increases intracranial pressure (ICP). Normal ICP levels of between 0 to 15 mm Hg can substantially escalate to near fatal levels. In addition, cerebral perfusion pressure may be impaired following a sustained head injury and neural oxygen supply becomes inadequate.[12] Additional secondary damage results from tissue hypoxemia or infection, with infection more commonly arising when open penetration to the skull occurs during the injury.

Complications

Unfortunately, TBI rarely occurs in isolation without other orthopedic or internal organ trauma. Skull fractures may be present and are classified by the specific type of fracture line or location. Common fractures include linear, depressed, and basilar skull fractures; additionally, each type of fracture is usually associated with unique characteristics. For example, depressed skull fractures often occur following a blow to the skull, whereas basilar skull fractures are associated with a high incidence of meningitis.[13] In addition to these complications, patients can also experience multiple facial fractures and scalp lacerations. Facial fracture severity is outlined in the LeFort classification system. Extremity fractures and internal organ damage further create potential life-threatening complications, which lengthen recovery periods. Common areas of injury include pelvic, femoral, and humeral fractures. The presence of heterotopic ossificans, a condition

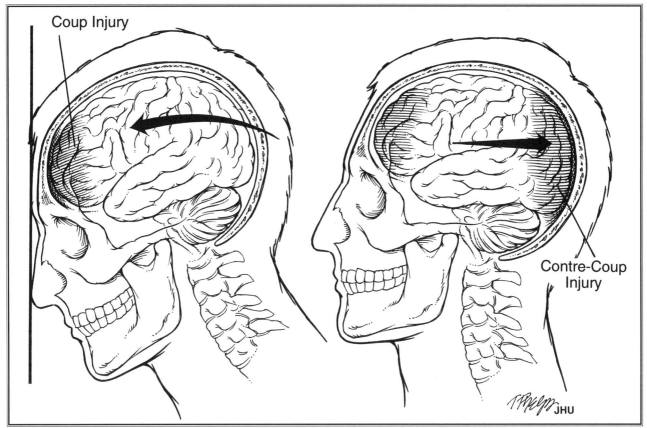

Figure 10-1. Mechanisms of injury: coup and contre-coup injuries. (Drawings by Tim Phelps.)

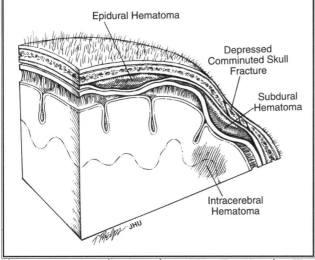

Figure 10-2. Complications from TBI. (Drawing by Tim Phelps.)

characterized by the formation of ectopic bone in patients following SCI and TBI, may cause further joint motion restrictions.[14]

Another complicating factor to recovery is the presence of a hematoma after the head injury (Figure 10-2). Subdural hematomas refer to rupture of the cerebral bridging vein complex with resultant bleeding into the subdural space. Fluctuating periods of lucency characterize this type of bleeding episode.[15] An epidural, or extradural hematoma, is usually caused by a tear in the middle meningeal artery. Patients sustaining these types of hematomas can experience varying degrees of altered consciousness, headaches, or other signs and symptoms specific to the areas of the lesion.[15] Intracerebral hematomas are located deeper within the brain and accompany more severe traumatic injuries and basilar skull fractures. Extensive hematoma formation may require surgical evacuation though a craniotomy procedure. These massive hematomas can potentially cause a hemispheric midline shift because of the size of the space-occupying lesion. Patients sustaining severe injuries undergo radical craniotomy procedures with burr hole drilling and resultant removal of portions of the skull. Subsequent cranioplasty procedures with bone grafting are later performed to ensure neural tissue protection.

Seizures present further medical complications following a TBI and may vary from mild in nature to those of the tonic-clonic variety. Seizures can occur immediately following the injury or can develop later in the course of recovery. Recent evidence suggests that the development of late post-traumatic seizures is linked to more extensive brain damage.[16] Patients are placed on prophylactic anticonvulsant medications (eg, Dilantin [Parke-Davis, Morris Planes, NJ]) following a head injury to manage the recurrent seizure activity. Health care professionals who work with patients recovering from a TBI should be versed in emergency procedures for those patients having post-traumatic seizure episodes to ensure patient safety during a seizure event. Patients should be protected during the episode and the type and duration of behavior should be well documented.

Recurrent, spontaneous seizure activity necessitates medication management. Common medications utilized for seizure management include Dilantin, Tegretol (Novartis, Basel, Switzerland), and Phenobarbitol. Pertinent adverse effects of seizure medications should also be recognized in the rehabilitation setting. Targeting specifically the motor cortex, Dilantin inhibits abnormal electrical discharge activity in the brain.[17] Major side effects include ataxia, nervousness, and confusion. Phenobarbitol and Tegretol may both induce drowsiness as a potential side effect and patients should be monitored for problematic oversedation while in therapy.[17] Zonisamide, a more recent medication introduced in the US, demonstrates less adverse cognitive side effects though may induce distal UE dyskinesias.[18]

Intensive Care Unit Management

Following TBI, appropriate medical intervention must immediately address both direct injuries and secondary complications. Multi-trauma patients are often transported to local or regional trauma centers. Severe injuries necessitate intubation and the need for multiple intravenous lines. An ICP monitor may be placed to record ongoing pressure changes and gradients. Osmotic diuretics such as Mannitol (Baxter, Deerfield, Ill) are utilized to decrease adverse ICP. Damage to the abdominal or thoracic cavities can warrant chest tube placement, and those patients requiring extensive ventricular or fluid monitoring may have a specialized pulmonary artery monitor, the Swan-Ganz catheter (Baxter, Deerfield, Ill), inserted.

In the very acute stage of medical intervention, patients will be evaluated using the *Glasgow Coma Scale* and resultant scores will categorize the severity of the injury. The instrument assesses three domains of function in individuals following head injury: motor performance, eye opening, and verbal response (Table 10-1).[19] The scale is comprised of 15 points, and injury severity is depicted through summation of the points from each of the three sections. Glasgow Scale scores from 13 to 15 designate mild injury, 9 to 12 moderate injury, and 3 to 8 reflect severe TBI.[11,20] Patients with mild brain injury generally demonstrate less severe of loss of consciousness (<20 to 30 min) and

Table 10-1 *Glasgow Coma Scale*			
Eyes	Open:	Spontaneously	4
		To verbal command	3
		To pain	2
	No response		1
Best motor response	To verbal stimulus:	Obeys command	6
	To painful stimulus:	Localizes pain	5
		Flexion-withdrawal	4
		Flexion-abnormal (decorticate rigidity)	3
		Extension (decerebrate rigidity)	2
		No response	1
Best verbal response	Oriented and converses		5
	Disoriented and converses		4
	Inappropriate words		3
	Incomprehensible sounds		2
	No response		1
Total Range		3 to 15	

Adapted from Teasdale G, Jennett B. Assessment of coma and impaired consciousness: a practical scale. Lancet. 1974;2:81-84.

post-traumatic amnesia (<24 hours).[21] Manifestations of moderate and severe brain injury are more pronounced and are often linked to brainstem injury. Factors associated with poorer outcomes include associated secondary injuries, persistent coma, and lingering post-traumatic amnesia.[22] The rehabilitation team members should be aware of the initial Glasgow score and ensuing complications at the time of injury to modify any examination or intervention activities.

Classification of Levels of Recovery

Recovery from a TBI depends upon a multitude of factors related to the extent of the injury, associated medical complications, and the patient's premorbid status. The *Rancho Los Amigos Levels of Cognitive Function* are often utilized to categorize patients following TBI and to describe behavioral patterns in the sequence of recovery (Table 10-2).[23] Comprised of 8 levels, this scale illustrates a recovery continuum which begins with the patient's initial unresponsive status and then tracks cognitive improvement to the final behavioral category.[24] The initial three levels reflect the patient's minimally responsive phase. Level I denotes no response, whereas Level II reflects an observed generalized response to a designated stimulus.[23,24] Such generalized responses often are characterized by gross body movements or an increase in vital signs. Patients in the Level III begin demonstrating more specific elicited response patterns, such as a hand squeeze or visual tracking, in response to a verbal stimulus. It should be noted that patients

---

Table 10-2

Rancho Los Amigos
Levels of Cognitive Function

I. No response
II. Generalized response
III. Localized response
IV. Confused-agitated
V. Confused-inappropriate
VI. Confused-appropriate
VII. Automatic-appropriate
VIII. Purposeful-appropriate

Adapted from Malkmus D. Integrating cognitive strategies into the physical therapy setting. Phys Ther. *1983;63:1952-1959.*

---

with massive injuries and severe brain damage could permanently remain within these initial classification levels. Level IV of the Rancho scale describes behavior related to the agitated patient. At this level, the patient is unable to integrate the multitude of sensory experiences in the immediate environment. The patient's gross attention to the environment is very limited. Periods of aggression may arise when periods of overstimulation occur, and the patient becomes distracted very easily.[23,24]

Levels V through VIII demonstrate gradual resolution of cognitive deficits toward behavior that is both purposeful and appropriate. In Level V, agitated behavior wanes, though the patient continues to demonstrate substantial deficits in language, memory, and praxis. The patient remains highly distractible, shows difficulty focusing on a specific task, and demonstrates inappropriate behavior. Confused appropriate behavior is designated in the sixth level, and the patient begins demonstrating increased goal-directed behavior with the ability to follow simple commands.[23,24] In the remaining two Rancho levels (VII-Automatic/ Appropriate and VIII-Purposeful/Appropriate), the patient becomes increasingly oriented and demonstrates improved learning capacity. In addition, responses become more automatic in nature. Judgment may continue to remain impaired in the final levels. The patient, for example, may have difficulty performing appropriate activities during emergencies at home.

Following the acute rehabilitation phase, patients will be discharged to receive further rehabilitation at a rehabilitation center, sub-acute facility, or nursing home. Patients may even return home if sufficient care and monitoring can be provided by the caregiver. Inpatient settings may initially be preferred to offer more intense therapy on a daily basis. Rehabilitation

centers, however, often have specific policies that dictate minimum Rancho levels for admission, and placement may be difficult for patients at lower functional levels.[25]

PHYSICAL THERAPY MANAGEMENT

Examination

The PT will perform an examination before the initiation of select intervention activities by the PTA. Given the patient's potential altered mental status, pertinent social history and home environment information may have to be obtained through family members or other caregivers. In performing a detailed systems review and examination, the therapist will ascertain the degree to which the patient's injury has affected the overall baseline cognitive and functional status. Target tests and measures will further assess the extent of impairments and functional limitations.

The PTA should be clearly aware of those alterations in arousal, mentation, and cognitive status, which may be encountered when dealing with patients with TBI. Examination findings may indicate varied levels of arousal impairment consistent with coma or *persistent vegetative state*. The term *coma* refers to a lack of responsiveness to verbal stimuli, variable responses to other forms of stimuli, and an absent sleep-wake cycle.[15] Persistent vegetative state denotes similar patterns of unresponsive behavior, though tends to reflect a condition of longer duration. Severe disturbances in cognition, arousal, and communication may impede standard testing procedures. For instance, patients are often able to only follow simple one-word commands, and examination strategies must be augmented. Key components of the cognitive examination area include orientation, level of consciousness, and memory. Confusion and disorientation may be considerable, and residual lethargy and sluggishness are often associated with delirium following head injury.[26] Furthermore, the patient may exhibit a concomitant period of post-traumatic amnesia and display persistent memory deficits during the recovery period.

Additional neurologic testing will include assessment of select cranial nerves, sensation, and coordination. Patients with cerebellar deficits should be screened for extremity deficits such as dysmetria and dysdiadochokinesia; moreover, central ataxia patterns may be noted in sitting posture or gait activities. Neurologic tests may uncover important findings, which have implications for interventions by the PTA. For example, sensory disturbances may call for therapeutic handling adaptations, and cranial nerve deficits require intervention adjustments because of conditions such as hemianopsia.

A detailed musculoskeletal examination will yield findings related to muscle tone, strength, and joint ROM. Abnormalities in tone may be found in any one or all extremities. Patients with more severe injuries may demonstrate postural patterns consistent with decorticate or decerebrate rigidity. Patients with decerebrate rigidity display strong extension posturing in all four extremities. Patients with decorticate rigidity demonstrate grossly flexed UEs with a similar LE extension positioning. The PT may elect to quantify tonal disturbances through the Modified Ashworth Scale. In this scale, muscle tone is described through varying resistance felt throughout the available ROM.[27] Given the potential for joint contractures and limitations due to abnormal posturing or heterotopic ossificans, joint integrity must be thoroughly assessed. Detailed goniometric measurements will underscore pertinent ROM limitations. When cognitive deficits impede formal testing procedures, examination of muscle performance may be completed through motor pattern analysis demonstrated in both gravity-eliminated and antigravity planes. Patients at higher functional levels may be candidates for more traditional strength-testing techniques.

Examination of the integument involves a systematic skin inspection to detect any possible skin irritation, rashes, or pressure ulcer areas. Patients who have begun posturing extremities are particularly at risk. The therapist must examine those areas that are particularly vulnerable for pressure sore development. These include the ischial tuberosities, greater trochanters, and sacrum. Patients who are bed-confined should be inspected for less common areas of skin compromise such as the spine of the scapula or olecranon process. Protection devices may be indicated when the patient is unable to volitionally change positions in bed.

For higher-level patients, examination activities will continue with assessment of all areas of functional mobility. Bed mobility activities, including bridging, rolling and supine to sit transitions, will be observed for level of assistance required and qualitative performance strategies. Static and dynamic balance will be assessed to investigate postural control in both sitting and standing. Common balance instruments utilized to identify fall risk in the elderly have been extrapolated to quantify balance performance in individuals with head injury and include the Performance Oriented Mobility Assessment[28] and the Berg Balance Test.[29] These tools have not been thoroughly validated in the population of patients with TBI; however, the PT may elect to utilize these instruments with geriatric patients who have sustained a head injury because of a fall.

Careful examination of the patient's gait and locomotion status will allow such important findings as pertinent gait deviations, required level of

---

Table 10-3

Practice Patterns Associated With Adult Head Injury

Pattern 5D Impaired motor function and sensory integrity associated with nonprogressive disorders of the CNS acquired in adolescence or adulthood.

Pattern 5I Impaired arousal, ROM, and motor control associated with coma, near coma, or vegetative state.

---

assistance, and muscle substitution patterns. Lastly, aerobic capacity and functional endurance will be measured through vital sign response to activity, perceived exertion, or other standardized measures of aerobic capacity. These baseline measures are particularly important for patients recovering from TBI because of reported diminished exercise capacity and fitness levels.[30]

Evaluation, Diagnosis, and Prognosis

Following the examination, the PT will formulate a summation of findings in the evaluation and establish both a diagnosis and prognosis. Diagnoses may be related to impaired mobility, motor function, or sensory integrity secondary to the TBI. Parameters of management for patients with TBI are delineated in the *Guide to Physical Therapist Practice*, Second Edition.[7] Two key practice patterns address management of the adult patient with head injury and include related practice content such as the expected range of number of visits; factors impacting the duration of care; and applicable tests, measures, and interventions (Table 10-3). Prognostication for patients with TBI is based upon characteristics of the injury, comorbidity conditions, and previous level of function. The PT's clinical decision-making process regarding the patient's prognosis will also be based on current evidence to support those short- and long-term goals established. For example, the therapist must consider that patients with decreased awareness of their limitations following head injury tend to set less realistic goals.[31] In addition, brain injury severity, LE hypertonicity, and concomitant LE injuries are factors which have been shown to predict ambulation potential in children and adolescents following a TBI.[32] Complications, such as heterotopic ossificans, have been associated with poorer functional outcomes following TBI.[14]

Interventions

Initiating interventions within the PT's plan of care requires careful analysis of those mitigating

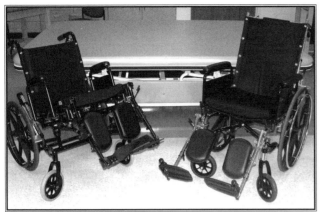

Figure 10-3. The tilt-in-space and recliner wheelchairs are often utilized for patients with special seating needs.

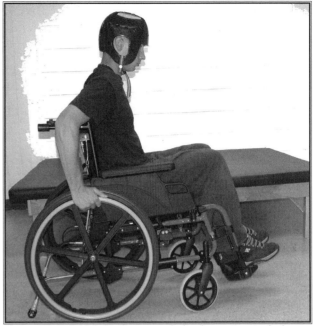

Figure 10-4. Initial short-term goals for the patient include performing w/c parts management independently and propelling to and from therapy sessions.

impairments and functional limitations identified in the initial examination. Moreover, the PTA must carefully review the results of the PT's tests and measures in order to target effective interventions aligned with those established goals within the plan of care. ROM goniometric measurements and muscle test grades will corroborate specific areas to be addressed. Furthermore, attention to upper motor neuron deficits will effectively allow the assistant to incorporate therapeutic exercise strategies to improve the patient's motor control. Patients recovering from a TBI may demonstrate varying levels of hemiplegia in accordance with the severity of the insult. Motor performance may progress through Brunnstrom's recovery sequence, and active dissociation should be recognized to track and facilitate recovery patterns.[33] For example, the PTA must note progress through increased complexity of extremity movement combinations, as compared to abnormal synergy patterns. Finally, functional mobility activities are implemented to address major deficits in bed and w/c mobility, transfers, balance, and gait performance. Along with the PT evaluation, the PTA should look at the occupational therapy and speech and language pathology (SLP) evaluations and progress notes for additional information pertinent to the patient's plan of care. These evaluations will provide information related to perceptual, communication, and cognitive impairments that may be present, which affect performance of essential ADLs.

SPECIFIC INTERVENTIONS FOR IMPAIRMENTS AND FUNCTIONAL LIMITATIONS

Seating Considerations

All aspects of the patient's condition should be carefully considered when creating an initial seating system for the patient. The PTA may work in conjunction with the supervising PT in making adaptive changes to the w/c for optimum positioning and seating alignment. Patients lacking postural control may benefit from a tilt-in-space w/c with attached head positioning.[34] A recliner w/c may be utilized for a patient with orthopedic fixation devices and associated fractures (Figure 10-3). A patient with residual hemiparesis deficits may find a hemiheight w/c effective for propulsion maneuvers given the reduced seat to floor height. When adapting any seating system for the patient's needs, it becomes important to recognize the advantages and disadvantages of any change that is proposed. For example, the addition of desk style armrests to a w/c may be beneficial for approaching any table surface, though may impede a patient's ability to perform a sit to stand maneuver if UE assistance is required.

For the patient initially utilizing a w/c, appropriate time should be allotted for instruction in propulsion maneuvers and parts management. Patients should be taught brake-locking maneuvers, leg rest management, and general propulsion strategies for level surface and turn negotiation. Important points of safety should be reinforced when cognitive deficits exist and judgment is impaired. Frequently, an initial short-term goal for the patient will be to independently propel between the physical therapy department and the rehab gym for scheduled sessions (Figure 10-4).

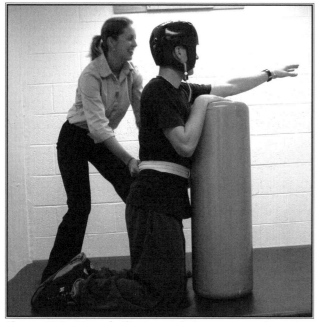

Figure 10-5. Neurofacilitation techniques are performed to enhance optimum motor performance when upper motor neuron deficits are present.

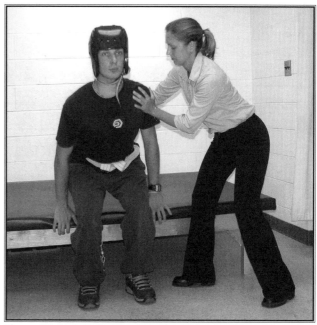

Figure 10-6. Activities such as the sit-to-stand transition allow patients to perform exercise programs within the context of a task.

Therapeutic Exercise

The PTA may be delegated selected activities involving the application of various therapeutic exercise programs for impaired joint integrity or muscle performance.[7] Given the prevailing weakness that develops from either the injury itself or the adverse effects of bed rest, patients may exhibit considerable deficits in muscle performance. The assistant should be cautious in scrutinizing examination findings to discern specific muscle grades of tested muscles or the ratings of muscle tone to effectively position and stabilize affected areas. Appropriate therapeutic exercise programs and mobility activities should be implemented based upon these test findings. For example, in an analysis of patients with a TBI, Duong et al[35] found that those patients having less than three-fifths LE strength on admission required greater assistance with transfers and locomotion. Passive ROM and active assisted strategies may be indicated for flaccid limbs, and the PTA may be required to don and doff various splints, braces, or other orthoses to effectively position an extremity.[36] Splints should not be used in place of comprehensive stretching programs but, rather, as an adjunct to treatment.[37] Aggressive passive ROM regimens are necessary to maintain joint integrity when hypertonicity results in prolonged flexed or extended posturing of extremities. In a study of 105 patients diagnosed with moderate or severe TBI, it was noted that a major predisposing factor to ankle contracture development included dystonia in both the inversion and plantarflexion musculature.[38]

Depending on the resultant impairments from a TBI, neurofacilitation techniques may be required to enhance optimum motor performance with upper motor neuron deficits (Figure 10-5). Active dissociation patterns can be utilized in conjunction with functional activities to promote active use of hemiparetic extremities.[39] In addition, strategies employing techniques such as weight bearing can facilitate stabilization in flaccid extremities. PTAs may elect to have patients perform bilateral extremity patterns for activation of weakened muscle groups.[40] Use of air splints may be beneficial to position an extremity during an activity. Current interventions involving constraint-induced therapy in stroke rehabilitation have also proven to be beneficial in individuals recovering from a TBI.[41] This procedure involves restraining the patient's unaffected UE in an effort to promote increased functional use of the hemiparetic extremity.

The effective clinician should be innovative in adapting therapeutic regimens around prevailing cognitive deficits. Patients may benefit more from exercise activities within the context of a task rather than conventional cardinal plane performance (Figure 10-6). Patients sustaining additional extremity or spinal fractures may require additional adjustment of therapeutic exercise programs based upon the location and severity of the fracture. Caution should be used when handling any extremity with a cast or external fixator apparatus.

Functional Mobility Training

Functional training interventions are germane to the patient's rehabilitative success. It is within this domain that PTAs can effectively and strategically progress the patient towards both the short- and long-term mobility goals established by the supervising PT. In accordance with both cognitive and mentation recovery, appropriate mobility maneuvers will guide patients in achieving optimum functional independence. Patients at lower functional or cognitive levels require extensive practical training in transfer techniques and bed mobility sequences.[42] Patients with severely impaired coordination, dense hemiparesis, or orthopedic trauma may initially require a dependent transfer strategy in an effort to maneuver from surface to surface. Patients sustaining TBI with associated fractures or other complications particularly present a challenge. Extensive fractures and orthopedic complications necessitate modified transfer strategies secondary to weight-bearing restrictions on multiple extremities. Furthermore, fixation devices such as Halo vests alter balance responses[43] and normal postural transitions such as supine to sit. Devices, such as sliding boards and UE fracture platform devices, are beneficial to perform the transfers and bed mobility tasks.

The PTA should guide the patient toward independence in all bed mobility skills including bridging, rolling, and supine to sit. Sit-to-stand transitions may be especially difficult during recovery.[44] Patients having hemiparetic extremities should be taught strategies to utilize and facilitate use of these limbs. Activities such as bridging merge functional tasks with active dissociation patterns. Adjuncts to treatment such as physioballs and bolsters may prove helpful in securing patient positioning.

Interventions for Balance Impairments

Patients recovering from TBI may demonstrate balance impairments related to their injury. Balance interventions are aimed at maintaining the body's COM within the LOS given environmental factors and the individual's own biomechanics.[45] The regulation of balance reflects contributions by the vestibular, somatosensory, and visual systems to effectively maintain postural control. The interaction of these systems illustrates a systems approach to motor control and represents an integrated, multi-system network among various structures within the CNS to modulate balance responses. This more current model better displays the dynamic nature of the CNS compared to previous hierarchal paradigms.

The initial examination by the PT should clarify the extent of the balance impairment and the degree to which functional sitting and standing require attention. The PTA should recognize key components, as well as score interpretation, of common balance instruments. The Performance Oriented Mobility Assessment,[28] also known as the Tinetti instrument, was formulated to assess balance and gait disturbances in the geriatric population. The instrument contains 28 available points and utilizes a simple ordinal scale. The Berg Balance Scale is a simple battery utilized to assess an individual's balance control during a series of tasks, which are graded on a four-point scale. Fifty-six available points are possible from performance on the 14 skill categories.[29] Subjects must perform a variety of tasks, which include a transfer, picking up an object from the floor, and alternately touching a step stool with each foot. A score below 45 is strongly predictive of assistive device use in the community-dwelling elderly.[46] Scores from the therapist's initial examination may point to those target interventions that are needed in the rehabilitation program. For example, patients having difficulty with the sit to stand maneuver on a standardized balance instrument may require preliminary activities, such as strengthening activities or arising from varied surfaces, to successfully master the activity. Additional research validating these instruments in stroke and TBI patient populations is needed.

It should be noted that patients demonstrating balance improvements from rehab programs might not have concomitant gait progress.[47] Moreover, medical complications from the patient's acute care hospitalization impact balance performance. In a recent multicenter analysis of factors associated with balance deficits among patients recovering from TBI, it was found that the incidence of medical complications (eg, respiratory complications and urinary tract infections) were strongly related to sitting balance impairment.[48]

Balance impairments can be caused or further exacerbated by existing muscle weakness. The presence of abductor weakness may result in a compensated abnormal trunk-lean in unilateral stance towards the affected side.[49] This compensation strategy becomes especially treacherous if the patient has a decreased UE protective response because of hemiplegia or processing latency. Simple light-touch contact with a cane or other assistive device may prove beneficial in improving postural control by enhancing hip abductor activation.[50]

Balance training should also reflect activities with attention to designated strategies utilized to maintain postural control. The sequential ankle, hip, and stepping strategies may be interrupted due to motor control problems or abnormal coactivation. In addition, flexibility limitations at the hip and ankle may further impede strategy activation. Recent evidence in the application of Tai Ch'i techniques suggests that this intervention approach has demonstrated efficacy in improving standing balance with individuals who had sustained a severe head injury.[51] Patients with severe balance impairments or vestibular dysfunction require more advanced interventions by the PT. Unfortunately, persistent dizziness following TBI has been shown to be a major barrier to reemployment among patients desiring to return to work following their injury.[52]

Gait and Locomotion Training

Gait interventions are major constituents in the functional mobility program of the patient. It is essential that both qualitative and quantitative parameters of gait performance be addressed. Patients should not be advanced with gait training activities without the appropriate muscle activity or assistive device to support a limb or advance the LEs in gait. Patients who often achieve independent functional ambulation within 3 months of their head injury include those who are younger, less severely injured, and have a better functional ambulation profile before the onset of rehabilitation.[53]

Gait quality for the patient with head injury becomes a major priority in rehabilitation training. PTAs should link gait deviation causality to those concomitant impairments. For example, tightness in the gastrocnemius muscle may be linked to a genu recurvatum tendency in stance phase. Likewise, residual weakness in the ankle dorsiflexors may induce a steppage or circumducted swing pattern.[49] Because of the duality in roles of the dorsiflexor muscles in both stance and swing phases, an abrupt slap may be observed during the loading response. Persistence of gait deviations should be communicated to the supervising PT to assess the patient for possible orthotic candidacy.

Patients with resultant spastic hemiplegia in the LE may have additional gait deviations. Particular problematic gait issues include the adductor or scissoring gait, the stiff knee, and the equinovarus foot.[54] Specific interventions should be employed to address gait quality. Stretching techniques can be performed to elongate spastic muscle groups. Aggressive stretching is indicated following select chemodenervation procedures, such as BoTox (Allergan, Irvine, Calif) injections or phenol nerve blocks, to improve gait quality.[54] In addition, the PTA may assist the PT with serial casting procedures. This technique involves a cast application for a period of days to maintain a static stretch force across a designated joint.[55]

Correction strategies during gait and locomotion training are implemented to normalize gait quality and to improve quantitative parameters such as speed, distance, and BOS. Independence in ambulation for short distances may take 6 months or longer for those individuals recovering from severe injuries.[42] Selection of the appropriate gait device may be problematic

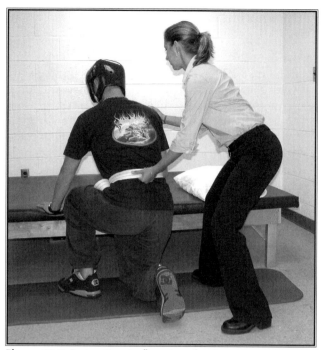

Figure 10-7. Instruction in floor transfers is an integral part of those interventions for higher-level patients.

when extensive cognitive deficits persist. Patients often exhibit difficulty with sequencing and placement of the cane, crutches, or walker. Patients at higher functional levels should be trained on all surfaces and should perform activities on inclines, curbs, and uneven surfaces. Instruction in floor transfers is also an integral part of the management plan for the patient who is at risk for falls (Figure 10-7). Often, slight gait deviations are persistent following a TBI, and patients attempt to maximize safety through a slower walking pattern and increased guardedness.[56] Recent application of gait treadmill unweighting techniques to patients with TBI has been employed, though limited evidence exists to support the intervention's effectiveness with this population.[57]

SPECIAL CONSIDERATIONS FOR THE PATIENT WITH BRAIN INJURY

Coma Emergence

Patients with from severe TBIs may require extensive medical management on the intensive care unit. Following medical stabilization, patients will be discharged to those facilities where coma emergence programs may be implemented. The PT may track progress through a standardized coma emergence rating form. Three commonly utilized instruments include the JFK–Revised instrument, the Coma Near Coma

Scale, and the Western Neuro Sensory Stimulation Profile.[58] These tools assist in quantifying designated responses to standardized sensory stimuli. Patients reaching maximum scores on these instruments may then have more advanced goals and intervention plans established. The Western Neuro Sensory Stimulation Profile[59] is especially beneficial for monitoring patients who demonstrate slow recovery progress. Patients emerging from minimally responsive states may be progressively mobilized using tilt table or standing frames activities. Patients begin with a sitting schedule to gradually increase sitting time. Vital signs should be carefully monitored for orthostatic changes and adverse physiologic responses to positional changes. Patients can demonstrate abnormal fluctuations in BP and diaphoresis. PTAs often work in tandem with supervising PTs in coma emergence programs given the complexity of the multiple medical issues and ongoing need for re-examination. In addition, patients often require two people for lifts, positioning, serial casting, and standing activities.

The Agitated Patient

Perhaps one of the most challenging issues for all rehabilitation team members is management of the agitated patient. Significant agitation can contribute to the patient's length of stay, hinder functional independence, and ultimately, hinder impending discharge to home.[60] PTs and PTAs must be attentive to the multitude of sensory experiences that are communicated to the patient during this stage because of potential adverse responses from the patient. Patients often become anxious and aggressive when they cannot process the immediate sensory information within their environment. Moreover, patients may overreact in the presence of relatively minor requests or tasks.

The PTA must effectively strategize interventions to deliver appropriate sensory experiences. Sessions should be structured properly to prevent sensory overload.[23] Often, quiet areas are helpful in reducing distractions, and reducing voice volume may be more calming. Treatment sessions may have to be modified to multiple shorter sessions. "Time-out" periods can be implemented when undesired behavior is unable to be redirected. Caution must be taken with both verbal and manual cues during mobility maneuvers because agitated patients may demonstrate periods of tactile defensive behavior.

Integration of Cognitive and Neuromuscular Interventions

The ultimate challenge in head trauma rehabilitation is to integrate both cognitive and functional training strategies to effectively guide the patient towards those target goals established and to maximize independence. The added cognitive dimension within therapeutic interventions adds a level complexity that necessitates skills of the experienced PTA. Cognitive impairments following a TBI may be substantial. Sleep disorders arising after the injury can also interfere with treatment sessions.[61] Patients may demonstrate slower processing and require increased time to optimize task performance.[62] Diminished attention span is also apparent, and patients require ongoing redirection to the designated task. Simple strategies such as reducing background distraction noise can be helpful. The PTA must consider that learning often occurs at a considerably diminished rate in the rehabilitation activity. Appropriate time allotment and cue sequence must be constructed within a treatment session to facilitate skill attainment. The effective PTA will recognize processing latencies when teaching motor tasks and allow appropriate time for problem solving. Finally, physical therapy clinicians must be reminded that the issue of impaired judgment is still evident even in the latter stages of the Rancho scale. Cognitive and motor recovery rates do not necessarily occur in synchrony, and while independent in mobility skills, the patient with poor judgment creates a potentially dangerous situation if left unsupervised in the clinic or home environment.

Cognitive and functional interventions are frequently fused in a variety of ways. The PTA can perform gait interventions while requiring that the patient perform the necessary speed changes required during an emergency, such as exiting a building during a fire drill. Reinforcing safety strategies taught during previous sessions will assist the patient in identifying critical components of a desired task. PTAs should employ critical problem-solving strategies to maximize patients' ability to prepare for home or community situations. Such activities might include performing safety maneuvers with rail support in dim lighting during stairs negotiation or practicing dialing 911. Patients' cognitive recovery can be monitored through a cognitive log.[63] This is a simple bedside tool that is utilized to track progress in such measures as memory, language, attention, and reasoning. Progress achieved and patient outcomes may also be monitored through such assessment measures such as the Functional Independence Measure (FIM) tool. This outcomes measure has demonstrated validity with patients recovering from a TBI.[64]

Precautions

Functional mobility programs and interventions for patients with TBI require attention to several key issues. Patients who are agitated should be monitored closely and should never be left alone if 24-hour direct supervision is required. Furthermore, rehabilitation professionals should make sure assistance is immediately available within the treatment area if a sudden occurrence of agitation should occur. Functional activities in enclosed areas (eg, stairwells) dictate additional personnel nearby. Policies should be in place for a silent "show of force" pending significant outbursts of aggressive behavior. For example, multiple staff may be required to rush to a patient's room to diffuse a hostile behavioral event. PTAs must be cognizant of policies implemented to protect patients who have been victims of family abuse or assault; moreover, alias names are utilized as part of the facility's procedures to maintain patient protection and confidentiality.

Management of patients at lower levels of function also mandates precautionary measures. Patients who have undergone craniotomy procedures may require helmet utilization. Patients are regularly required to wear a helmet when out of bed. When patients are mobilized without the helmet, care should be taken not to put excess pressure over the affected area. Rehabilitation team members must also demonstrate competency with management of catheters, oxygen canisters, and tube-feeding lines during treatment sessions.

DISCHARGE PLANNING AND COMMUNITY REENTRY

Equipment Procurement and Family Training

The PTA is involved in all aspects of discharge planning following the designated course of rehabilitation. Appropriate ordering of durable medical equipment will be required at the time of discharge, and the PTA will participate in the ordering of required assistive device and ambulation needs. If a w/c is required, appropriate features should be ordered to sufficiently address the needs of the patient. For example, appropriate seat width and depth should accommodate the patient's size, and front-rigging features should provide for necessary LE support and orthopedic considerations.[34] Elevating leg rests may also be required for individuals with LE fractures or circulatory impairments.

An important component of the discharge disposition includes family training activities for those patients being discharged who require care and assistance at home. The PTA will effectively train the caregiver in mobility strategies that are linked to those functional needs of the patient. These activities may include transfer techniques, ambulation guarding, w/c management skills, and supervision of home exercise programs. Family training programs should also address car transfers and stairs and curb negotiation.

Table 10-4

Key Questions Addressed During the Home Visit

1. Will the patient be able to enter and exit the living environment safely?
2. What environmental barriers are present?
3. Are any grab bars or additional devices needed in the bathroom?
4. If a w/c is to be used, will it be able to clear the doorways?
5. Where are steps encountered in the home?
6. Are rails available in stairways? If so, right or left?
7. Are safety devices present such as smoke alarms or telephone access?
8. Will the patient be able to navigate around furniture in all rooms?

In conjunction with recommendations by the supervising PT, the PTA may suggest the need for continued therapy interventions. Patients may require a course of outpatient or home therapy in an effort to continue work toward the long-term goals established for the patient in the plan of care. Patients who are at higher functional levels may benefit from a community re-entry program to transition into previous employment and societal roles.

Home Assessment

Before discharge, the PTA or supervising PT may elect to do a home visit to assess the patient's home environment and identify potential environment barriers. The setting should be thoroughly inspected for possible safety issues that may arise when the patient returns home. Scrutiny of doorway widths, inclines, and floor surfaces is especially important for the client who will be returning home in a w/c. In addition, the PTA should analyze major entrance and exit passageways to the home. In some rehabilitation settings, patients may be allowed to return home for a scheduled visit before discharge for a trial run of mobility skills acquired. Often, rehabilitation team members perform a joint home assessment to address multiple areas of potential patient needs (Table 10-4). The PTA serves as an important conduit to the supervising PT for identification of issues related to the discharge disposition and recommendations.

Home Programs

Fabrication of an individualized home program following discharge from an inpatient rehabilitation stay requires careful attention to all components of the patient's functional status. Exercise interventions should target weakened muscle groups and incorporate functional activities; moreover, the exercises should be sufficient in quantity to address pertinent needs yet not overwhelming in number. Home programs should provide for ambulation activity with the caregiver, where possible. It is crucial that the program extend beyond a simple instructional sheet. Performance logs will help assure adherence, especially when caregiver supervision is not optimum. Written instructions should be clear, with large print, and should contain key terms familiar to both the patient and caregiver.[65]

Use of medical jargon or unknown terms becomes detrimental to the teaching process. Diagrams are often useful, especially when the PTA wants to accentuate important performance strategies or points of emphasis in the program. Effective home programs consider those residual cognitive deficits that may still be pervasive at the time of discharge. Caregivers supervising home programs should receive appropriate instructions regarding strategies to facilitate optimum performance in lieu of any attention or processing deficits.

Community Integration

Patients who are recovering from a TBI often begin community reentry activities during the inpatient rehabilitation stay. The rehabilitation team members may accompany patients, for example, on a community outing (eg, to the mall) or a recreation activity. Patients who display behavior consistent with the final Rancho stages, Levels VII and VIII, are particularly appropriate for such activities, and the PTA will be able to observe such phenomena as abstract reasoning processes and social interactions. Gait and locomotion progress within the environmental context can also be analyzed during community outings.

Patients may also continue community reentry activities with adult day programs designed for this special patient population. These programs assist patients in transitioning to employment initiatives and provide important psychosocial support. Important activities aimed at optimizing problem-solving skills are addressed because of those residual cognitive deficits which still exist.[66] Factors associated with a good quality of life following head injury include inveterate community and social support.[67] Key factors impeding patients' successful return to employment include significant cognitive impairment and low education levels.[68] Day programs can also provide resource assistance for those patients who experience depression, which is one of the most common secondary conditions associated with TBI.[69]

CONCLUSION

Rehabilitation of individuals with TBI offers the PTA the unique opportunity to interlock principles of functional training with key cognitive strategies to improve the overall quality of life for their clients. Carefully planned intervention programs range from basic therapeutic exercise to community reentry activities. Interventions by the PTA are pivotal components of both the Nagi Disablement and Patient/Client Management Models as they relate to management of patients with TBI. More recent models of enablement, such as the ICIDH-2 (WHO-2) framework, emphasize additional themes of activity and participation in having patients assume previous societal and employment roles.[70] The approach to individuals with complex impairments and functional limitations should be one of partnership between the PTA and supervising PT. The effective PT/PTA team will successfully assemble appropriate intervention and reexamination activities, in conjunction with ongoing communication, to optimize functional and neurobehavioral outcomes for the patient.

CHAPTER QUESTIONS

1. What are some of the medical complications that occur following TBI?

2. What are some types of strategies that can be utilized in gait training for a patient with cognitive impairment who also has a LE weight-bearing restriction?

3. What are various safety precautions that must be maintained when treating a patient whose behavior is consistent with Rancho Level IV?

4. What is meant by the terms coup and contrecoup injury?

5. What are important intervention considerations for the patient with post-traumatic seizures who is taking Dilantin?

Suggested author answers are available at www.slackbooks.com/neuroquestions.

CASE STUDY

The patient, Leszek, is a 19-year-old Polish student who was an unrestrained passenger in a motor vehicle accident. He suffered a right frontal cerebral contusion with diffuse axonal shearing. He also sustained a mild subdural hematoma in the right frontal lobe pole. The initial Glasgow Coma Scale score was 12 in the emergency room. His acute care admission was significant for episodes of post-traumatic seizures, which lengthened his stay considerably. Following medical stabilization, he was transferred to a rehabilitation setting where an initial examination was performed by the PT. The patient's cognitive status is consistent with Rancho Level VI.

On admission, the PT performed the examination. Findings include the following:

History and Systems Review: Information was obtained from the patient's family due to the patient's memory deficits. Leszek's parents are Polish immigrants, and they moved to this country 16 years ago. Leszek is a student at the university and is majoring in accounting. He works as a waiter at a local restaurant on weekends. His past medical history is significant for asthma, and he has had no major surgeries. He enjoys dancing and playing soccer. They characterize Leszek as a "quick learner." He lives with his family in a two-story home. There are eight steps between floors. The family has a pet dog, Borek, who is in good health. The patient has one sister, who will be getting married in 1 month. The patient's current medications include Dilantin and Albuterol.

Tests and Measures:

Orientation: Oriented to name only.

Arousal/Mentation: Lethargic; Slow in initiating activity.

Short-Term Memory: Poor: unable to remember three objects

Cranial Nerves: Intact I-XII

Sensation: Intact to light touch and proprioception in all extremities.

ROM/Joint Integrity: No UE limitations noted passively. LE passive ROM is significant for a lack of full hip extension on the right by 5 degrees and a lack of 10 degrees on the left. Knee and ankle joints demonstrate no limitations. No significant muscle tone abnormalities detected.

Strength:
UE: 4/5 in major shoulder and elbow muscle groups. 5/5 wrist and hand musculature
LE: Proximal weakness: 3+/5 hip abductors and extensors; 4/5 hip rotators, flexors; 4/5 quadriceps/hamstrings; 5/5 ankle/foot musculature

Reflexes: 2+: Biceps, Triceps, Brachioradialis; 1+ Quadriceps; 2+ Gastrocnemius

Coordination: Mild right UE dysmetria noted in the finger to nose test.

Balance: Maintains static unsupported sitting >3 min. Patient loses balances when reaching outside BOS. Unable to stand unsupported; demonstrates a (+) Romberg.

Bed Mobility: Moderate assistance for supine to sit; minimal assistance for bridging; minimal assistance for rolling; moderate assistance for sit to stand.

Gait and Locomotion: Patient ambulates 10 feet with a rolling walker with moderate assistance. He demonstrates decreased step and stride lengths; displays strong tendency to shuffle feet in gait. (+) Trendelenburg noted bilaterally.

W/c Mobility: Supervision required for parts management. Propels 20 feet with minimal assistance and extensive cues for turns and direction changes.

Aerobic Capacity: Resting heart rate – 64 bpm. Following amb – 88 bpm. No shortness of breath observed following ambulation.

Oxygen Saturation:
Resting-95%, Postambulation-92%

Lungs: Clear to auscultation other than mild congestion heard in upper airways.

Goals

Long-term (3 weeks)

1. Supervision with household ambulation with assistive device.

2 Walks (distances up to 75 feet) with verbalized safety precautions.

3. Independent transfers and bed mobility.

4. Supervision with stairs negotiation with right rail and correct step sequencing.

5. Supervision with home exercise program.

6. Hip strength: 4/5 bilaterally and ROM: 15 degrees passive hip extension.

7. Durable medical equipment procurement.

8. Completion of family training activities.

9. Dancing with supervision with family members in preparation for upcoming wedding.

Short-term (1 week)

1. Ambulation 40 feet with minimal assistance with rolling walker.

2. Transfers with minimal assistance and minimal cues for safety.

3. Rolling and bridging with supervision and minimal cues; Sit to stand with minimal assistance.

4. Hip extension PROM increase by 5 degrees.

5. W/c propulsion to and from PT sessions with supervision.

6. Independent w/c parts management.

Evaluation, Prognosis, and Diagnosis

The PT noted that Leszek demonstrates excellent rehabilitation potential because of his current functional profile, age, and minimal restrictions by comorbidity conditions. The prognosis for improving his overall functional mobility status is good, though impaired cognition may impede immediate involvement with previous community and work-related activities. The PT's diagnosis conveys impaired motor function associated with the TBI along with related balance impairments and functional limitations in transfers, bed mobility, and gait.

Plan of Care

The patient will receive physical therapy for 1 hour daily for gait training, therapeutic exercise, balance activities, and transfers. Appropriate DME procurement and family training activities will be included. The patient's estimated length of stay is 3 weeks.

Interventions

Following the initial examination, the PTA began seeing the patient daily. Leszek was also followed by occupational therapy and speech therapy. A w/c and temporary seating system was prepared. Leszek performed a daily regiment of functional training involving those activities included in the plan. Therapeutic exercises included performance of extremity Theraband activities, w/c push-ups, sit to stand repetitions, and pelvic lifts. Passive stretching of the hip joint was also included. Gait training focused on increasing distance while decreasing the overall level of assistance required. Consistent with Rancho Level IV, he followed simple directions well though displayed difficulty learning new tasks. The PTA utilized repetition and visual cues to enhance the learning process; for example, the w/c brakes were covered with colored tape to serve as a reminder to lock the brakes before a transfer. In addition, the PTA learned some key Polish terms to emphasize particular skill components. Signs were also placed in the patient's room to indicate times for scheduled activities, and the patient maintained a daily log of activities performed in physical therapy. In each PT session, the patient would verbalize those key safety strategies involved in the performance of the particular skill. Leszek began transporting himself independently to therapy sessions.

The patient steadily progressed through his therapy regimen and incrementally achieved designated goals. Leszek's cognition also improved, along with his speed of processing in mobility maneuvers. The PTA was soon able to utilize a straight cane with contact guarding in ambulation activities. As his balance progressed, the PTA had the family bring in his soccer ball to perform more challenging dynamic activities. Moreover, the ball represented a past activity that he enjoyed and could now revisit in therapy. The PTA progressed the patient with more advanced activities, such as floor transfers and uneven surface ambulation. He scored a 48 on the Berg Balance Test during the therapist's reexamination, and the patient began working on tasks involved with the instrument's most demanding categories. The PTA challenged his judgment with various emergency maneuvers such as running to dial 911. In the final week of therapy, he was able to perform a quick polka step in preparation for his sister's upcoming wedding. Discharge planning activities included a family training session and ordering of required equipment. Leszek still required a temporary w/c for longer community ambulation distances. A foam cushion and straight cane were also ordered. His parents demonstrated safe and effective guarding in gait, stairs negotiation, and car transfer techniques. A full home exercise program was formulated and reviewed with Leszek and his parents. A course of outpatient therapy was recommended. Two weeks following discharge, the PTA received a photo in the mail of Leszek dancing at the wedding.

PT and PTA Collaboration

Throughout the intervention regimen, both the supervising PT and PTA discussed the patient's progress toward the established goals. On one occasion, the therapist was asked to examine a developing skin rash on the patient's distal UEs. In addition, the PTA communicated to the therapist that Leszek's gait had been noticeably less steady over the past few days. Following the assessment, the physician was notified and it was determined that the rash was due to an adverse side effect of the patient's Dilantin.

REFERENCES

1. Thurman DJ, Alverson C, Dunn KA, Guerrero J, Sniezek JE. Traumatic brain injury in the United States: a public health perspective. *J Head Trauma Rehabil.* 1999;14:602-615.

2. Brain Injury Association of America. Causes of brain injury. Available at: http://www.biausa. org/Pages/causes_of_brain_injury.html. Accessed November 1, 2004.

3. Cassidy JD, Carroll LJ, Peloso PM, Borg J, Von Holst H, Holm L, Kraus J, Coronado VG. Incidence, risk factors, and prevention of mild traumatic brain injury: result of the WHO collaborating center task force on mild traumatic brain injury. *J Rehab Med.* 2004;43:28-60.

4. Centers for Disease Control and Prevention. Traumatic brain injury. Available at: http://www. cdc.gov/doc.do/id/0900f3ec800081d7. Accessed May 27, 2004.

5. Burnett DM, Kolakowsky-Hayner SA, Slater D, Stringer A, Bushnik T, Zafonte, R, Cifu DX. Ethnographic analysis of traumatic brain injury patients in the National Model Systems Database. *Arch Phys Med Rehabil.* 2003;84:263-267.

6. Brain Injury Association of America. CDC report shows prevalence of brain injury. Available at: http://www.biausa.org/Pages/cdc_report.html. Accessed July 20, 2004.

7. *Guide to Physical Therapist Practice.* 2nd ed. Alexandria, Va: American Physical Therapy Association; 2001.

8. Carpenter CA. The physical therapist assistant. In: Pagliarulo, MA, ed. *Introduction to Physical Therapy.* 2nd ed. St. Louis, Mo: Mosby; 2001:47-71.

9. Jenson GM, Gwyer J, Shepard KF, Hack LM. Expert practice in physical therapy. *Phys Ther.* 2000;80:28-43.

10. Watts NT. Task analysis and division of responsibility in physical therapy. *Phys Ther.* 1971;51:23-30.

11. Smith DH, Meaney DF, Shull WH. Diffuse axonal injury in head trauma. *J Head Trauma Rehabil.* 2003;18:307-316.

12. Murdock KR. Physical therapy in the neurologic intensive care unit. *Neurol Rep.* 1992;16:17-21.

13. Murdock KR, Klein P. Physical therapy intervention for acute head injury. *Phys Ther Prac.* 1994;3:19-36.

14. Johns JS, Cifu DX, Keyser-Marcus L, Jolles PR, Fratkin MJ. Impact of clinically significant heterotopic ossificans on functional outcome after traumatic brain injury. *J Head Trauma Rehabil.* 1999;14(3):269-276.

15. Paz JC, West MP, eds. *Acute Care Handbook for Physical Therapists.* 2nd ed. Boston, Mass: Butterworth-Heinemann; 2002.

16. Englander J, Bushnik, Duong TT, Cifu DX, Zafonte R, Wright J, Hughes R, Bergman W. Analyzing risk factors for late posttraumatic seizures: a prospective, multicenter investigation. *Arch Phys Med Rehabil.* 2003;85:365-373.

17. Keltner NL, Folks DG. *Psychotropic Drugs.* Philadelphia, PA: Mosby; 2002.

18. Hoch MB, Daly L. Anticonvulsants. *J Head Trauma Rehabil.* 2003;18:383-386.

19. Teasdale G, Jennett B. Assessment of coma and impaired consciousness: a practical scale. *Lancet.* 1974;2:81-84.

20. Graham DI. Pathophysiological aspects of injury and mechanisms of recovery. In: Rosenthal M, Griffith ER, Kreutzer JS, Pentland B, eds. *Rehabilitation of the Adult and Child with Head Injury.* 3rd ed. Philadelphia, Pa: FA Davis; 1999:42-52.

21. Kay T, Harrington DE, Adams R, et al. Definition of mild traumatic brain injury. *J Head Trauma Rehabil.* 1993;8:86-87.

22. Evans RW. Predicting outcome following traumatic brain injury. *Neurol Rep.* 1998;22:144-148.

23. Malkmus D. Integrating cognitive strategies into the physical therapy setting. *Phys Ther.* 1983;63:1952-1959.

24. Hagen C, Malkmus D, Durham P. Levels of cognitive functioning. In: *Rehabilitation of the Head Injured Adult: Comprehensive Physical Management.* Downey, Calif: Professional Staff Association of Rancho Los Amigos Hospital; 1979.

25. Gray DS, Burnham RS. Preliminary outcome analysis of a long-term rehabilitation program for severe acquired brain injury. *Arch Phys Med Rehabil.* 2000;81:1447-1456.

26. Nakase-Thompson R, Scherer M, Yablon SA, Nick TG, Trzepacz PT. Acute confusion following traumatic brain injury. *Brain Inj.* 2004;18:131-142.

27. Bohannon RW, Smith MB. Interrater reliability of a modified Ashworth scale of muscle spasticity. *Phys Ther.* 1987;67:53-54.

28. Tinetti, M. Performance-oriented assessment of mobility programs in elderly patients. *J Am Ger Soc.* 1986;34:119-126.

29. Berg K Measuring balance in the elderly: validation of an instrument. *Can J Public Health.* 1992;83:S9-11.

30. Bhambhani Y, Rowland G, Farag M. Reliability of peak cardiorespiratory responses in patients with moderate to severe traumatic brain injury. *Arch Phys Med Rehabil.* 2003;84:1629-1636.

31. Fischer S, Gauggel S, Trexler LE. Awareness of activity limitations, goal setting and rehabilitation outcomes in patients with brain injuries. *Brain Inj.* 2004;18:547-562.

32. Dumas HM, Haley SM, Ludlow LH, Carey TM. Recovery of ambulation during inpatient rehabilitation: physical therapist prognosis for children and adolescents with traumatic brain injury. *Phys Ther.* 2004;84:232-242.

33. Sawner K, LaVigne J. *Brunnstrom's Movement Therapy in Hemiplegia.* 2nd ed. Philadelphia, Pa: JB Lippincott; 1992.

34. Bergen AF. The prescriptive wheelchair: an orthotic device. In: O'Sullivan SB, Schmitz TJ, eds. *Physical Rehabilitation: Assessment and Treatment.* 4th ed. Philadelphia, Pa: FA Davis; 2001:1061-1091.

35. Duong TT, Englander J, Wright J, Cifu DX, Greenwald BD, Brown AW. Relationship between strength, balance, and swallowing deficits and outcome after traumatic brain injury: a multicenter analysis. *Arch Phys Med Rehabil.* 2004;85:1291-1297.

36. Blanton S, Grissom SP, Riolo L. Use of a static adjustable orthosis following tibial nerve block to a residual plantarflexion contracture in an individual with brain injury. *Phys Ther.* 2002;82(11):1087-1097.

37. Lannin NA, Horsley SA, Herbert R, McCluskey A, Cusick A. Splinting the hand in the functional position after brain impairment: a randomized, controlled trial. *Arch Phys Med Rehabil.* 2003;84:297-302.

38. Singer BJ, Jegasothy GM, Singer KP, Allison GT, Dunne JW. Incidence of ankle contracture after moderate to severe acquired brain injury. *Arch Phys Med Rehabil.* 2004;85:1465-1469.

39. Platz T, Winter T, Muller N, Pinkowski C, Eickhof C, Mauritz KH. Arm ability training for stroke and traumatic brain injury patients with mild arm paresis: a single-blind, randomized, controlled trial. *Arch Phys Med Rehabil.* 2002;82:961-968.

40. Mudie MH, Matyas TA. Can simultaneous bilateral movement involve the undamaged hemisphere in reconstruction of neural networks damaged by stroke? *Disabil Rehabil.* 2000;22(1-2):23-37.

41. Karman N, Maryles J, Baker RW, Simpser E, Berger-Gross P. Constraint-induced movement therapy for hemiplegic children with acquired brain injuries. *J Head Trauma Rehabil.* 2003;18(3):259-267.

42. Watson MJ, Hitchcock R. Recovery of walking late after a severe traumatic brain injury. *Physiotherapy.* 2004;90:103-107.

43. Richardson JK, Marr Ross AD, Riley B, Rhodes RL. Halo vest effect on balance. *Arch Phys Med Rehabil.* 2000;81:255-257.

44. Zablotny CM, Nawoczenski DA, Yu B. Comparison between successful and failed sit-to-stand trials of a patient after traumatic brain injury. *Arch Phys Med Rehabil.* 2003;84:1721-1725.

45. Shumway-Cook A, Woolacott MA. Normal postural control. In: Shumway-Cook A, Woolacott MA, eds. *Motor Control: Theory and Applications.* 2nd ed. Philadelphia, Pa: Lippincott Williams and Williams; 2001:163-191.

46. Bogle Thorbahn LD, Newton RA. Use of the Berg balance test to predict falls in elderly persons. *Phys Ther.* 1996;76:576-585.

47. Wade LD, Canning CG, Fowler V, Felmingham L, Baguley IJ. Changes in postural sway and performance of functional tasks after traumatic brain injury. *Arch Phys Med Rehabil.* 1997;78:1107-1111.

48. Greenwald BD, Cifu DX, Marwitz JH, Enders LJ, Brown AW, Englander JS, Zafonte RD. Factors associated with balance deficits on admission to rehabilitation after traumatic brain injury: a multicenter analysis. *J Head Trauma Rehabil.* 2001;16(3):238-252.

49. Lippert LL. *Clinical Kinesiology for the Physical Therapist Assistant.* Philadelphia, Pa: FA Davis; 2000.

50. Jeka JJ. Light touch contact as a balance aid. *Phys Ther.* 1997;77:476-487.

51. Shapira MY, Chelouche M, Yanai R, Kaner R, Szold A. Tai Chi Chuan practice as a tool for rehabilitation of severe head trauma: three case reports. *Arch Phys Med Rehabil.* 2001;82:1283-1285.

52. Chamelian L, Feinstein A. Outcome after mild to moderate traumatic brain injury: the role of dizziness. *Arch Phys Med Rehabil.* 2004;85:1662-1666.

53. White DK, Katz DI, Alexander MP, Klein RB. Recovery of ambulation after traumatic brain injury. *Arch Phys Med and Rehabil.* 2004;85:865-869.

54. Esquenazi A. Evaluation and management of spastic gait in patients with traumatic brain injury. *J Head Trauma Rehabil.* 2004;19(2):109-118.

55. Singer BJ, Jegasothy GM, Singer KP, Allison GT. Evaluation of serial casting to correct equinovarus deformity of the ankle after acquired brain injury in adults. *Arch Phys Med Rehabil.* 2003;84:483-491.

56. McFadyen BJ, Swaine B, Dumas D, Durand A. Residual effects of a traumatic brain injury on locomotor capacity: a first study of spatiotemporal patterns during unobstructed and obstructed walking. *J Head Trauma Rehabil.* 2003;18:512-525.

57. Seif-Naraghi AH, Herman RM. A novel method for locomotion training. *J Head Trauma Rehabil.* 1999;14(2):146-162.

58. Duff D. Review article: altered states of consciousness, theories of recovery, and assessment following a severe traumatic brain injury. *Axone.* 2001;23(1):18-23.

59. Ansell BJ, Keenan JE. The Western neuro sensory stimulation profile: a tool for assessing slow-to-recover head-injured patients. *Arch Phys Med Rehabil.* 1989;70(2):104-108.

60. Bogner JA, Corrigan JD, Fugate L, Mysiw WJ, Clinchot D. Role of agitation in prediction of outcomes after traumatic brain injury. *Am J Phys Med Rehabil.* 2001;80(9):636-644.

61. Castriotta RJ, Lai JL. Sleep disorders associated with traumatic brain injury. *Arch Phys Med Rehabil.* 2001;82:1403-1406.

62. Rios M, Perianez J, Munoz-Cespedes JM. Attentional control and slowness of information processing after sever traumatic brain injury. *Brain Inj.* 2004;18:257-272.

63. Alderson AL, Novack TA. Reliable serial measurement of cognitive processes in rehabillitation: the cognitive log. *Arch Phys Med Rehabil.* 2003;84:668-672.

64. Corrigan JD, Smith-Knapp K, Granger CV. Validity of the Functional Independence Measure for persons with traumatic brain injury. *Arch Phys Med Rehabil.* 1997;78:828-834.

65. Mostrum E, Shepard KF. Teaching and learning about patient education. In: Shepard KF, Jenson GM, eds. *Handbook of Teaching for Physical Therapists.* 2nd ed. Boston, Mass: Butterworth Heinemann; 2002:287-319.

66. Rath JF, Hennesy JJ, Diller L. Social problem solving and community integration in postacute rehabilitation outpatients with traumatic brain injury. *Rehabil Psychol.* 2004;48(3):137-144.

67. Kalpakjian CZ, Lam CS, Toussaint LL, Merbitz NK. Describing quality of life and psychosocial outcomes after traumatic brain injury. *Arch Phys Med Rehabil.* 2004;83:255-265.

68. Franulic A, Carbonell GC, Pinto P, Sepulveda I. Psychosocial adjustment and employment outcome two, five, and ten years after TBI. *Brain Inj.* 2004;18:119-129.

69. Gordon WA. Community integration of people with traumatic brain injury: introduction. *Arch Phys Med Rehabil.* 2004;85:S1-S2.

70. The international classification of function, disability, and health. *Disability Date Breifing.* Canberra, Australia: Austr Inst Health Welfare; 2002;20:1-5.

Chapter

11

CLIENTS WITH STROKE

Jim Smith, PT, MA

Becky McKnight, PT, MS

KEY WORDS

affective disorder
anosognosia
aphasia
apraxia
body-weight support during gait training
constraint-induced movement therapy
cerebrovascular accident (CVA)
dysphagia
dysphasia
hemiparesis
hemorrhagic stroke
homonymous hemianopia
ischemic stroke
lacunar infarction
learned nonuse
pusher syndrome
shoulder pain after stroke
stroke
transient ischemic attack (TIA)
unilateral neglect

CHAPTER OBJECTIVES

- Describe the types of cerebrovascular accidents.
- Describe the impairments and functional limitations that typically accompany stroke, and identify strategies that a PTA may use to

accommodate for these during the provision of physical therapy interventions.

- Identify the data collection techniques that a PTA may employ to determine a patient's progress within the PT's plan of care.
- Describe strategies for effective physical therapy interventions, including patient- or client-related communication and instruction and procedural interventions that may be included within a PT's plan of care for a patient who has had a stroke.

INTRODUCTION

Cerebrovascular disease refers to any disorder involving the blood supply to the brain. When cerebrovascular disease results in the death of brain tissue, a *stroke*, also called a *cerebrovascular accident* (CVA), occurs. Diverse symptoms can develop depending on the location and size of the brain injury. Stroke is, unfortunately, common: in the United States, about 750,000 strokes occur each year, making it the most common neurological disorder and the leading cause of disability among adults.[1,2] Physical therapy interventions are usually indicated for the impairments and functional limitations that follow a stroke. Appropriately applied physical therapy interventions can diminish disability related to stroke symptoms.

Types of Stroke

There are two broad categories for stroke: ischemic and hemorrhagic. *Ischemic stroke*, which is more common, involves loss of the blood supply to part of the brain. This develops because of a blockage of one or more arteries that supply blood to the brain. The obstruction can occur from pathologic changes that gradually occlude the blood vessel, such as atherosclerosis; or from an embolus that blocks a blood vessel. There are two additional categories of ischemic stroke: *lacunar infarction* and *transient ischemic attack* (TIA). A *hemorrhagic stroke*, also referred to as intracranial hemorrhage, occurs when a blood vessel in the brain ruptures, resulting in blood flooding into the surrounding tissues.

Ischemic Stroke

Ischemia involving the brain is a great concern because of the high-energy demands of brain tissue. There is no mechanism to store metabolic reserves in the brain, so adequate blood supply is required to provide all of the glucose, oxygen, and nutrients used by these tissues. When a blood vessel becomes blocked, the blood supply is interrupted distal to the blockage. In the area of complete or near complete interruption of blood supply ischemic necrosis, the death of the tissue occurs within a couple minutes. This cell damage is irreversible. Surrounding the area of necrosis is an area where the blood supply is diminished but not completely interrupted. The tissues in this area will have diminished functioning during the time of ischemia but can return to normal function if blood supply is restored quickly. If, however, blood supply is not restored within a short period of time, the necrotic area will expand, resulting in greater tissue death and greater disability. Because of this, immediate medical attention is imperative.[1]

Lacunar Infarction

Lacunar infarcts are small strokes deep inside the brain that are named for their crescent-shaped appearance. They are common in the putamen, the basal ganglia, the thalamus, and the internal capsule. As with all strokes, the symptoms associated with lacunar infarctions vary depending upon the exact structures that are involved. Although these involve a small area, the effects can be quite dramatic since the areas involved can serve a variety of functions.[1]

Transient Ischemic Attack

TIAs are caused by a temporary interruption in blood supply to the brain and result in sudden onset of impairments or functional limitations, such as extremity weakness, sensory deficits, and difficulties with functional mobility. TIA symptoms vary in duration, but most are resolved within 1 hour and within 24 hours, there is a full recovery from all symptoms. TIAs often precede a stroke and require medical attention even though the symptoms do resolve.[1]

Hemorrhagic Stroke

The major effects of a hemorrhagic stroke are damage from the lost circulation and damage from the leaked blood itself. The blood that leaks into the brain tissue has volume (that is, it takes up space), but the skull cannot accommodate the increase in volume. This results in compression of brain tissue, which results in direct injury to neurons. It may also cause compression of adjacent blood vessels, resulting in those vessels narrowing or closing down. While this effect is greatest in the area of the bleeding, the enclosed nature of the skull may result in an elevated intracranial pressure throughout the brain, requiring special medical management. Another effect of the leaked blood is irritation of the adjacent tissues. The chemical composition of the blood is noxious to brain tissue, causing further damage.[1]

CONFOUNDING PROBLEMS

When caring for an individual who has had a CVA, the major emphasis will be on the impairments and functional limitations that are results of the stroke. However, most individuals who are recovering from a stroke have preexisting medical problems that cannot be ignored. These medical problems can directly impact the patient's ability to participate and progress with physical therapy interventions.

Common cardiovascular diseases found in patients recovering from a stroke include hypertension, coronary artery disease with a history of a heart attack or of a coronary artery bypass surgery (CABG), and peripheral vascular disease (PVD). The PTA will need to monitor the cardiovascular status of these individuals during therapeutic activities. If the individual has a history of a heart attack or CABG, it is important to know when these occurred so that the appropriate precautions related to exercise intensity can be followed. For example, a patient who recently underwent a CABG and subsequently had a CVA will have precautions related to the amount of pressure that can be put through the UEs during functional activities. This will lead to the need for alternative strategies for sit-to-stand transfers because the patient cannot push through the hands on the chair.

Common musculoskeletal conditions that may be encountered include arthritis, joint replacement, amputation, osteoporosis, pathologic fractures (hip, wrist, back), back pain, and rotator cuff injury and repair. Again, impairments and limitations related to these conditions can impact the patient's progress during recovery after a CVA. For example, a patient who has had a trans-femoral amputation of the left leg and who now demonstrates hemiparesis of the right side may require a one-arm drive w/c for functional mobility. Precautions related to preexisting conditions must be taken into consideration during provision of interventions (eg, weight-bearing restrictions or total joint precautions).

Other common conditions that are encountered in this patient population are diabetes and chronic obstructive pulmonary disease (COPD). When working with individuals with diabetes, it is important for the PTA to be able to recognize symptoms of hypoglycemia so that appropriate action can be taken. A patient with a diagnosis of COPD may need oxygen supplementation during therapeutic activities. The PTA will need to monitor the patient's response to exercise by noting the respiratory rate and monitoring oxygen saturation. The patient may need verbal cues for appropriate breathing strategies during the physical therapy session. These patients may be limited in their endurance for therapy, and the session may need to be divided to allow the patient to rest in between different activities.

When beginning to work with a patient who is recovering from a CVA, the PTA must not only consider the limitations due to preexisting medical conditions but also should have an idea of the patient's prior level of functioning as reported in the PT's initial evaluation. Each patient is unique regardless of the diagnostic label(s). Many individuals with multiple medical conditions continue to be active and are reportedly "healthy," while other patients have a sedentary lifestyle with obesity and generalized weakness due to inactivity but may not have any diagnosed medical conditions. Therefore, an understanding of the patient's prior level of function will help to shape the expectations for therapeutic intervention. In addition, knowledge of the patient's prior functional activity will provide insight into the patient's perception of exercise or activity and can guide the PTA in determining how to best approach the patient to ensure optimal participation in therapy.

Psychosocial issues that can impact the provision of physical therapy must also be recognized. The patient's cultural background and belief system related to disability and medical intervention must be considered. For example, a social and cultural background that views disability as a personal weakness that must be hidden can result in differing responses. One patient may be motivated to overcome the disability to be able to reenter his or her previous social role whereas another individual may become depressed and lose interest in participation with therapy. Regardless of the belief system or response, it is the responsibility of all health care providers to be sensitive to these issues and to work within the patient's belief system to ensure optimal recovery. Family and social support can often make the difference in a patient being able to return home or needing alternate discharge arrangements. The PTA should review the initial evaluation to gain insight into the social support that is available to the patient and note the prognosis for discharge environment. A patient with mild limitations in functional mobility may not be able to return to independent living, but if a spouse or other family member is available, this could mean the difference between the individual returning home or needing to move into an assisted living facility. Care must be taken to determine the abilities and the willingness of the family to provide the needed assistance. Patients who have a CVA are often elderly and many times their spouses are not in good health; it may be dangerous to the patient as well as the spouse if the patient were to return home.

ROLE OF THE PHYSICAL THERAPIST ASSISTANT

Although symptoms from a stroke can vary widely depending upon the size and location of the brain injury, recovery from a stroke often follows a predictable pattern. When a patient is medically stable and the stroke symptoms appear to be following the predictable prognosis, the PT may choose to direct the PTA to provide selected physical therapy interventions. To be prepared to assist with these interventions, it is important that the PTA has a basic understanding of common impairments and functional limitations as well as contemporary intervention strategies that can be utilized to address them.

TYPICAL IMPAIRMENTS AND FUNCTIONAL LIMITATIONS

Following a stroke, the patient and her or his family will recognize and want to address the hemiparesis and accompanying functional limitations. However, because this is a form of brain injury, physical therapy intervention must address the broad spectrum of symptoms the patient displays. These may include impairments of cognition, communication, cardiopulmonary capacity, strength, coordination, sensation, and the functional limitations that accompany these impairments. Physical therapy interventions will directly address some of these common impairments, whereas other impairments will not be the focus of the intervention but must be taken into consideration since they can impact participation in physical therapy and the patient's progression toward anticipated goals. The PT may direct the PTA to provide interventions to directly address impairments including motor planning and apraxia, diminished cardiopulmonary capacity, impaired vestibular sensation, impaired strength or motor control, shoulder pain, and balance deficits. Impairments including cognitive impairments, visual perceptual deficits (unilateral neglect), anosognosia, affective disorders, communication disorders, dysphasia, impaired somatosensation, and impaired vision may not be directly addressed by physical therapy intervention. However, it is important that the PTA be able to recognize the impact these impairments can have on the patient's functional limitations and disabilities. Often, modification to the therapy intervention will need to occur to take into consideration these additional impairments. The PTA should consult with the PT and other members of the multi-disciplinary team to determine appropriate strategies to use in each case.

Impairments in Motor Planning and Apraxia

Praxis is the performance of intentional action(s) or skills. Apraxia, therefore, is an acquired impairment in the performance of purposeful movements. As defined by Shumway-Cook and Woollacott, *apraxia* "is a disorder of the execution of movement that cannot be attributed to weakness, to incoordination or sensory loss, or to poor language comprehension or inattention to commands."[3] It can develop after a stroke and appears to result from an inability to mentally formulate a plan of action for a motor task. The disruption in the formation or implementation of a plan may result in surprising functional limitations: the inability to comply with a request to lie down on a bed or comb one's hair, consistently putting clothes on inside-out, drinking from an empty cup, or attempting to cut one's food with a spoon.[3]

Symptoms among persons with apraxia vary greatly. Some of the types of apraxia that may be encountered in the clinic include the following:

- "**Ideational apraxia:** failure to conceive or formulate an action, either spontaneously or to command.

- **Ideomotor apraxia:** the patient may know and remember the planned action, but... he cannot execute it with either hand.

- **Kinetic limb apraxia:** clumsiness and maladroitness of a limb in the performance of a skilled act that cannot be accounted for by paresis, ataxia, or sensory loss.

- **Facial-oral apraxia:** patients are unable to carry out facial movements to command (lick the lips, blow out a match, etc)."[4]

- **Motor impersistence:** an inability to sustain a physical action; is usually identified when a patient cannot close the eyes, protrude the tongue, or raise the nonparetic arm on request and persist in the action for 20 seconds.[5]

One-third of patients with a first stroke will have symptoms of apraxia, and it is more common among those who have had a left hemisphere lesion.[6] Apraxia present at the time of hospital admission for a stroke indicates there will be a higher dependency on others to support the patient upon discharge. When providing interventions to a person with apraxia, the PTA should recognize the tasks that are impaired by apraxia and focus on the patient's learning of strategies for those tasks. For example, if a patient is impaired in the initiation of an activity, the emphasis should be placed on instruction, and if the problem is more one of performance errors, the emphasis should be placed on feedback to enhance error detection.[7]

Diminished Cardiopulmonary Capacity

Persons who have had a stroke have impaired fitness (ie, capacity to perform physical activity and work). This acquired activity intolerance is attributable to the following:

- Decreased cardiorespiratory fitness.

- The energy demands that accompany hemiparesis, sensory loss, and incoordination.

- Deficient motor planning and deconditioning from bedrest and inactivity.[2,8,9]

In addition, current clinical practices for inpatient rehabilitation appear to contribute to deconditioning because activity levels among individuals receiving rehabilitation services during the 14 days following a stroke are very low. Bernhardt et al found that among patients receiving inpatient rehabilitation, only 13% of an individual's day included participation in therapeutic activities that contribute to the recovery of mobility.[10] The cumulative effect is that the leading cause of mortality among individuals who survive a stroke is vascular disease affecting either the heart (eg, cardiovascular disease) or the brain (eg, stroke).[2]

This has implications for the physical therapy interventions applied following stroke. Gordon et al recommend that exercise programs should be directed at the following:

- Regaining the endurance to participate in activities as soon as possible.

- Aerobic training for the benefits of decreasing body fat and improving glucose regulation.

- Improving aerobic fitness to minimize the functional limitations and mortality that accompany stroke.[2]

To achieve these goals, the exercise program, as designed by the PT, may contain elements similar to a cardiac rehabilitation program. That is, the exercise will need to be of sufficient frequency and duration and of a type that the patient can do to achieve training benefits. To individualize and safely implement the exercises, the PTA must collect data about the patient's response during exercise interventions. The data collection should include data on cardiovascular (ie, heart rate, BP, and arrhythmia monitoring) and cardiopulmonary (ie, respiratory rate and oxygen saturation) responses and the patient's perceived exertion.

Impaired Vestibular Sensation

The vestibular system senses head movement and head position relative to gravity. This information is used to inform the movement system for the extremities and trunk and to improve visual acuity. When a stroke interrupts the transmission or interpretation of vestibular information, it may cause symptoms of *vertigo* (an illusion of motion), *nystagmus* (involuntary back-and-forth movements of the eye), *disequilibrium* (a sense of imbalance), *ataxia* (incoordination of movement that is not a result of weakness), or a combination of these symptoms. The symptoms of vertigo or disequilibrium may cause nausea, and medications may reduce the nausea sufficiently to allow the patient to participate in physical therapy interventions.

Impaired Strength or Motor Control

Eighty-nine percent of patients admitted to the hospital following a stroke have weakness.[11] The severity of the weakness or paralysis that develops following stroke varies according to the location of the damaged brain tissue. The weakness is more a representation of the locale (ie, structures) damaged than it is the size (ie, volume of brain area) of the stroke.

Hemiparesis is the term that describes weakness of either the right or left half of the body, and hemiplegia describes a similar unilateral weakness combined with loss of sensation(s). Historically, the weakness that develops following a stroke has been described as hemiparesis or hemiplegia that involves the contralateral side (ie, the extremities and trunk of the half of the body opposite the side of the brain injured from the stroke). However, the loss of strength also involves the extremities and trunk ipsilateral (same side) to the stroke, although to a lesser extent. Therefore, the terms *weaker side* and *stronger side* are recommended for accuracy when describing the pattern of weakness that follows a stroke. This pattern of weakness is important when performing physical

therapy interventions because exercise to improve strength should be directed at both sides of the body and not just to the weaker side.[12]

Less than 15% of persons who have a stroke will fully recover motor function, and the more severe the weakness, the poorer the prognosis. That is, the individuals who have the greatest weakness following a stroke are expected to have a slower recovery and will remain weaker than those with lesser strength deficits. In addition, the severity of post-stroke weakness is related to the severity of functional limitations for transfers, standing, ambulating, and stair climbing.[11]

Shoulder Pain After Stroke

The development of shoulder pain following a stroke can cause psychoemotional distress and limit function. This is a frequent complication, with the literature indicating that it affects 34% to 84% of persons who have had a stroke.[13] Several theories have been proposed to explain the pathology responsible for this disorder, and Turner-Stokes and Jackson summarized these as follows:

- Development of muscle imbalance from the competing symptoms of spasticity and flaccidity, resulting in malalignment of the glenohumeral joint.
- Development of adhesive capsulitis (ie, frozen shoulder) with inflammation of the joint capsule restricting flexibility.
- Joint subluxation with incongruity of the glenohumeral joint developing due to inadequate muscular support to compensate for the tractioning effect of gravity.
- Inflammation of extracapsular structures, such as irritation or tears of the rotator cuff muscles or tendons.
- Nerve damage from traction or entrapment of peripheral nerves.
- Development of complex regional pain syndrome (eg, reflex sympathetic dystrophy).[14]

These theories propose that the pain develops due to irritation or repetitive trauma to the tissues about the shoulder joint, indicating that a proactive approach designed to prevent the development of shoulder pain is the preferred intervention strategy. Unfortunately, strong evidence supporting a specific method does not exist. Protective strategies have included adherence to a static positioning program and the use of a sling or other supportive device for the involved UE. The support devices are used to combat gravity's tractioning pull on the glenohumeral joint. An arm sling will effectively support the limb; unfortunately, it also limits and discourages active use of that UE. Another option is a cuff support that encircles the proximal humerus

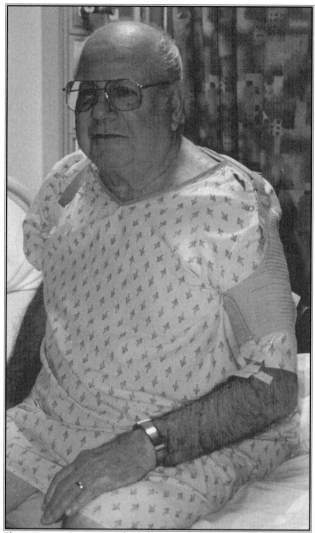

Figure 11-1. Patient with cuff supporting the shoulder of the hemiplegic upper limb.

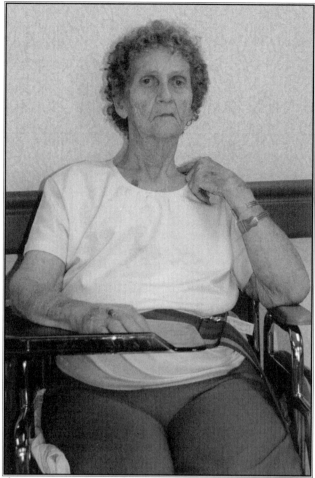

Figure 11-2. Patient utilizing arm support on wheelchair to support the weakened UE.

and is suspended from the upper trunk and opposite shoulder (Figure 11-1). Placement of an axillary roll or pad suspended under the involved limb has fallen out of favor because it does not adequately support the glenohumeral joint. Individuals in a chair can also support the arm in an arm trough attached to a lap tray or directly on the lap tray[14] (Figure 11-2).

Another protective strategy is preservation of flexibility about the shoulder joint. This can be achieved through passive ROM. However, care should be taken to inhibit (relax) the shoulder muscles, which may resist the movement due to spasticity or spasm.[14]

Neuromuscular electrical stimulation (NMES) is an electrotherapy intervention appropriate for the person with hemiparesis and can be applied as a component of physical therapy interventions to achieve contraction of the supraspinatus or posterior deltoid muscles. The goal of the NMES intervention is to preserve muscle strength in the flaccid or weakened

shoulder through peripheral stimulation. By doing so, the subluxation of the glenohumeral joint is reduced or prevented with benefits of decreased pain or increased mobility.[14]

Balance Deficits

The risk of falling is greater after stroke due to impaired balance. This is expected, as normal balance requires effective performance of the systems for sensation (visual, vestibular and somatosensation) and motor control (including the strength, coordination and rate of the person's response), and these abilities are often impaired following stroke. Therefore, a person who has had a stroke may require interventions to remediate impaired balance when sitting, standing, or walking.[15]

In addition to these balance disturbances, there is a subset of about 5% of persons who have had a stroke who demonstrate "pusher" behavior. As described by Roller, "*pusher syndrome* in patients post-stroke is characterized by leaning and active pushing toward the hemiplegic side with no compensation for instability"[16] while maintaining the head in a mostly upright position.[16] The person with this disorder will resist correction, and when a caregiver attempts to assist the person towards a neutral (upright) posture, the patient will complain that they are falling, and the pushing behavior will persist.

This "pusher" behavior develops because the brain injury from the stroke leaves the individual unable to sense and correctly interpret an upright posture (either in sitting and/or standing). This misinterpretation leads the individual to think he or she is upright when, in fact, he or she is leaning to the side. The individual may also have the sense of falling while being supported in the upright position by the PT or PTA. Therefore, the individual's response is to continue to lean, or push, away from the correct upright position.[17] Interventions performed by the PTA should include focusing the patient's attention on his or her available sensations, which may include his or her vision, vestibular sensation or proprioception, and awareness of the support surface. Interventions should augment this sensory feedback, such as using a mirror or training sitting balance on a firm (rather than soft) surface. Practice is a necessary strategy for improving the patient's ability to detect errors and then to develop corrective strategies.[16]

Cognitive Impairment

Cognitive abilities include the mental processes of comprehension, reasoning, and decision-making that guide our behaviors and actions. When a portion of the brain has been injured, there will be a disruption in the way that the brain receives, processes, interprets, or responds to information; the behaviors we observe following a stroke are a result of the disruption of these processes.[3] The cognitive impairments most frequently encountered while working with persons who have had a stroke are neglect, apraxia (discussed above), anosognosia, and communication disorders. These impairments are confusing to recognize and can present barriers to your patients' participation in physical therapy interventions, to their improvement, and to their attainment of goals. Therefore, when providing selected physical therapy interventions, a PTA should be able to recognize and respond appropriately to the behavioral expressions of these cognitive impairments.

Another contributor to cognitive performance in some individuals is an alteration in perception, which is the process of converting sensations into meaningful and understandable information. Because of the amount and types of sensory disturbances that may occur following a stroke, it is not surprising that these individuals have impaired cognition. When this type of impairment contributes to deterioration in cognitive performance, the PTA should work to augment sensory inputs (examples are provided below) and to educate the patient, family, and other caregivers about strategies to compensate for the sensory or perceptual deficit.

Unilateral Neglect

Unilateral neglect is a disorder that is important to recognize because of its frequency and its influence on the rehabilitation process. The symptoms of unilateral neglect are an inability to report, attend to, or recognize sight, sound, and/or touch opposite to the side of the brain affected by stroke.[18] It is also referred to as neglect, visuospatial neglect, hemispatial neglect or 'left' neglect.

Neglect is a frequently encountered impairment, with a reported incidence following stroke between 10% and 82%.[19] Neglect is classically associated with stroke involving the right half of the brain, causing neglect (inattention or unawareness) of the left environment or body; however, it may also be observed when a left hemisphere lesion causes a right neglect, although that form is more likely to resolve 4 to 8 weeks following the stroke.[19,20]

The PTA must be concerned with the functional impact from the symptoms that accompany the inability to attend to the left or right components of the patient's environment. The symptoms will present as deficiencies in the domains of memory (mental representation and recall), action-intention (motor performance), or attention (response to sensations).[19] Neglect involving memory is quite striking, as the patient may be impaired in their ability to describe aspects of their home based on the mental perspective from which they are recalling it. For example, a patient with a left unilateral neglect may not be able to recall the railing on his stairs if he is "picturing" the stairs from the perspective of the bottom of the stairs and the railing is on the left, but he will be able to recall the same railing if he changes his perspective to the top of the stairs (so that the railing will be on his right). When neglect involves motor intention, the patient will be impaired in his ability to act or plan movements involving the right or left half of the body. This will adversely affect function as seen by behaviors, such as not recognizing that food is on the left side of a plate and, subsequently, not eating that half of a meal; not dressing or applying makeup to half of the body; or not accounting for objects (eg, door frames) to one side and then walking into them, causing injury or falls. When the neglect involves attention, there may not be a response to stimuli that occur within a portion of the individual's environment. For example, a person with a neglect involving the left side of his environment may not respond to sounds, sights, and/or touch that originate from his left regardless of his integrity to those sensations. Another example is when an individual may not be able to identify when a car is approaching from the left side while the individual is crossing the street.

Neglect is associated with a poorer outcome following stroke because persons with neglect require longer programs of inpatient rehabilitation, achieve less recovery of functional abilities, and require greater assistance with daily activities.[19] Given the diverse intervention strategies in use, it is unlikely that the PTA will become trained in applying all of them. Therefore, when an unfamiliar technique is encountered, the PTA must request guidance from the PT. Pierce and Buxbaum comprehensively reviewed the interventions for unilateral neglect, which, briefly summarized, are categorized as interventional techniques directed at the following:

Achieving arousal through the following:

- Medications that stimulate excitatory neurotransmitters (such as dopamine).

- Feedback, either auditory or auditory and visual, that alerts the patient to her or his area of neglect.

Improving visual attention through interventions to increase visual tracking into the neglected visual field or through visuoperceptual training.

Improving hemi-spatial representation (eg, awareness) through interventions directed at the impaired side that include the following:

- Activation or movement of the hemiparetic limb(s).

- Constraint-induced therapy.

- Mental imagery training.

- Optical training with prism lenses to reorient the visual fields.

- Patching of one eye, or the modification of eyeglasses to block a hemi-field of vision for both eyes, to reorient visual attention.

- Caloric stimulation (placing cold water in the outer ear canal).

- Optokinetic stimulation via visual stimuli moving horizontally across the visual field.

- Vibratory stimulation to the posterior neck muscles.

- Trunk rotation (passive).[18]

All of these interventions have demonstrated some benefit in reducing the effects of unilateral neglect. However, when reviewed in total, the evidence on these interventions remains limited.[18]

Recognition of the conflicting evidence on the response to interventions for unilateral neglect is important for the PTA because this will result in the PT employing different strategies for interventions based on the patient's symptoms and the evolving evidence for this problem. Given the diverse intervention strategies, it is unlikely you will become trained in applying all of them, and when the PTA encounters an unfamiliar technique, she or he must request guidance from the PT. Also, PTAs need to identify when a patient is, or is not, responding to an intervention for unilateral neglect and communicate that information to the PT.

Anosognosia

Anosognosia is the denial of one's own neurological symptoms, such as weakness, functional limitation, and other deficits. Examples that have been observed following stroke include the denial of hemiparesis, visual loss, aphasia, movement disorder, and apraxia. This is typically observed by the PTA through the behaviors of persistent denial of the poststroke impairments, the minimizing of weakness, and indifference to the effects of the weakness (eg, blaming it on arthritis or fatigue or trauma to a limb). Common concurrent stroke symptoms are hemisensory disturbances, unilateral neglect, dressing or constructional apraxia, reduced intellectual functions, motor impersistence, and prosopagnosia (impaired recognition of familiar faces), although memory is usually spared. The incidence of anosognosia is greater than is recognized by most clinicians, as the literature indicates an occurrence of 28% to 85% among persons who have had a right hemisphere stroke and 0% to 17% among persons who have had a left hemisphere stroke. Even though this symptom usually resolves 12 to 22 weeks after the onset of a stroke, the presence of anosognosia is generally considered a poor prognostic indicator for functional recovery.[21,22] The authors are not aware of intervention strategies for those cases in which anosognosia symptoms persist. Fortunately, that occurs among less than 10% of persons with this symptom.

Communication Disorders

Dysphasia is an acquired impairment of communication, which may include expressive (speaking) ability, receptive (comprehension) ability, or both. *Aphasia* is the term more frequently used in the clinic for this disorder although that term more accurately refers to the complete loss of these communication abilities.

The brain's cortex contains two areas, Broca's and Wernicke's, which are primarily responsible for communication. Communication is a lateralized brain function, meaning that different components of communication are controlled predominantly on each side of the brain. In most people, spoken language is lateralized to the left hemisphere of the brain and nonverbal communication is lateralized to the right hemisphere (although this rule does not apply to about half of the people who are left handed). The communication impairments observed after a stroke vary depending on the location(s) affected by the stroke.

Following a stroke that involves Broca's area of the left cerebral cortex, a person will have troubles verbally expressing him- or herself. The impairment is with the process of motor programming for the production or the organization of spoken words. This may present as slow or nonfluent speech, poor articulation, or grammatically incorrect speech.

When a stroke affects Wernicke's area of the left cerebral cortex, an individual will be impaired with the receptive components of communication. The impairment is in the comprehension of language; therefore, these individuals may have difficulty following the PTA's spoken instructions. The person with this lesion will retain the ability to speak fluently, but the use of words is impaired, and the patient may demonstrate the use of meaningless words or phrases. In addition to the anticipated frustration that accompanies a disorder of communication, this type of lesion will also contribute to agitation and related emotional reactions.[23]

Nonverbal communication may be impaired following a stroke in the right hemisphere. If Broca's area is involved, the person will be impaired with expression, such as the use of emotional gestures, or with the intonation of speech. If Wernicke's area is involved, the individual will have trouble interpreting nonverbal signals (eg, facial expressions or gestures) from others. A lesion to this area will also cause a deficiency in comprehending spatial relationships (eg, distances).[24]

The PTA will encounter additional communication disorders, which may include the following:

- **Anomia:** naming and word-finding impairments.
- **Dysarthria:** impaired articulation during speech (from incoordination or weakness of the oral-facial muscles).
- **Dyslexia or alexia:** impaired reading (comprehension of written communication).
- **Dysgraphia or agraphia:** impaired ability to communicate through writing.
- **Paraphasia:** the inappropriate substitution of words when speaking.[25]

Communication impairments will adversely impact a patient's response to therapeutic interventions and his ability to function. Due to the complexity of these disorders, the PTA should consult with the PT, and possibly the speech language pathologist, to identify the communication strategy that is optimal for each individual.

Affective Disorders

Affect refers to mood or the emotional component of behaviors. It is expected that there will be emotional reactions among persons who have had a stroke, and these may include sadness, denial, passivity, agitation, mood swings, indifference, or the inability to control impulsive or socially inappropriate behaviors.[26] However, the location or type of injury from the stroke may contribute to severe or persistent affective changes that need to be managed within the context of the health care team. Due to the medical management options that may need to be employed, the PTA should consult with the PT when the following behaviors are encountered: *abulia* (extreme apathy), *anxiety*, *emotional lability* (rapid swings among emotional states), *pathological laughing and crying*, and *depression* (also called poststroke depression).

One challenge for some patients is demonstrating behaviors that are in keeping with the social and cultural expectations for a situation. Stroke may result in a loss of this ability, which is called a *loss of inhibitions* or *disinhibition*. When disinhibition occurs, a patient may act in a manner that would have been unacceptable to him or her before the stroke (eg, telling off-color jokes or physically grabbing at others). The PTA should address the inappropriate behavior when it occurs, because the action is not acceptable whether it is the patient's typical behavior or a symptom of stroke, and clarify the behavioral expectations. A patient with disinhibition may require a comprehensive behavioral shaping program, applied by all members of the health care team, to achieve an appropriate response to typical situations or improvements of behavior.

Dysphagia

Dysphagia is a disorder of swallowing that may result from incoordination or weakness of the oral, pharyngeal, laryngeal, or esophageal muscles. A patient with dysphagia may benefit from treatment to improve control or strength in these muscles. Until this is achieved, the patient may be on a restricted diet to prevent pulmonary aspiration. A common restriction related to dysphagia is the person is only allowed to drink fluids that have had a thickener added, which slows the swallowing process and makes it easier for the individual to swallow correctly. The PTA assisting a person at this stage of his rehabilitation must comply with the dietary restriction because a variation may result in aspiration, which can lead to complications (eg, pneumonia).

Impaired Somatosensation

The somatosensory system conveys information to the brain from the musculoskeletal system and the skin. When a portion of the brain responsible for processing or interpreting this information is affected by a stroke, the person will have an impairment of somatosensation. This will affect safety because the person will be delayed or unable to sense pain and withdraw from harm. It will also impair movement, coordination, and balance because somatosensation informs us about the position(s) and rate(s) of movement of our limbs and body. Without this information, we cannot move accurately, and this is one of the causes of ataxia (incoordination of movement that is not a result of weakness).

Another symptom that may develop is *learned non-use*, in which the absence of sensation from a limb contributes to the adaptive behavior of relying on the limb with intact sensation to assist with all functions while the limb with impaired somatosensation is not used to assist with functions. Interventions directed at improving somatosensation may include tactile stimulation, through electrical stimulation or stroking of the skin, or training for tactile perception, through recognition of objects, discrimination of textures, or recognition of positions.[27]

Impaired Vision

A stroke that interrupts the pathways for transmitting or interpreting visual information will cause an impairment of vision. *Homonymous hemianopia* is a commonly encountered visual impairment following stroke and results in defective or lost vision in the right or left half of the visual field. This visual field loss occurs in both eyes and should not be confused with unilateral neglect. Homonymous hemianopia is an impairment of visual sensation and unilateral neglect is an impairment of attention or awareness. These different disorders may present concurrently or alone.

Visual acuity may also be impaired following stroke with symptoms such as blurred vision or diplopia (double vision). These develop due to disruption in the ability to stabilize gaze (eg, maintain visual fixation on an object), which is a prerequisite for normal vision. One cause for gaze instability is disruption of the brainstem nuclei responsible for stabilization (which is mediated by the vestibulo-ocular and optokinetic reflexes) or from loss of vestibular or visual sensory input to these nuclei. Another cause is disruption of the movement system for the eyes and control of the muscles that move the eye or the brainstem locations that innervate these muscles, which can result in diplopia (double vision) or blurred vision.[25]

Functional Limitations

The severity of the functional limitations that follow a stroke vary according to the location of the damaged brain tissue and the presence of the previously described impairments. Functional limitations may affect the patient's ability to move him- or herself, change positions, or complete ADLs. As outlined in

the *Guide to Physical Therapist Practice*[28] (the *Guide*) the functional limitations may also include the following:

- Difficulty planning movements.
- Difficulty with manipulation skills.
- Frequent falls.
- Loss of balance during daily activities.
- Difficulty negotiating terrains.[28]

In summary, the clinical presentation of individuals following a stroke will be diverse and range from the individual requiring total assistance for all ADLs to those with no obvious impairments or functional limitations. In addition, the stroke may influence any of the brain's functions so that cognitive skills such as communication, praxis, or even the ability to stay awake may be impaired.

It is also important to note that the symptoms will vary over time for each patient. It is important to develop a good understanding of each patient's baseline functional abilities from the information in the PT's initial evaluation. The PTA's expectation is that the patient will demonstrate improvement in functional abilities in response to physical therapy interventions, and this will usually be observed as progress towards, or achievement of, the goals established in the PT's plan of care. The rate of improvement should be communicated to the PT. In some cases, the PTA may note a deterioration of functional abilities, and this also should be communicated to the PT. This is particularly important when there is a notable deterioration in function or cognitive ability or when the patient becomes more lethargic because the patient may be experiencing complications that require acute medical services.

EXAMINATION TOOLS, TESTS, AND MEASURES

The PT's examination will identify baseline measures of the patient's impairments and functional limitations. This data is evaluated by the PT and informs the prognosis and the development of the PT's plan of care. As physical therapy moves more into evidence-based practice, it is more common to see PTs incorporate standardized tests and measures during the initial examination and evaluation and subsequent evaluations. Some of these standardized tests and measures are referred to as outcome measurement or scales. Two excellent resources for these types of scales are Lewis and McNerney's *The Functional Toolbox*[29] and *The Functional Toolbox II*.[30] Upon review of the PT's evaluative note of a patient, the PTA will have an idea of what to expect the patient to look and behave like. The PTA will want to take note of the data collected and the tests and measures utilized by the PT in the evaluation in order to choose the appropriate techniques for data collection to monitor the patient's response to the interventions provided, as delegated by the PT.

Motor Control: Strength and Coordination

Strength is measured as a component of the PT's examination although the method of collecting this data varies depending on the patient's capabilities (eg, ability to follow instructions and severity of weakness). Strength measures may be taken through manual muscle testing, hand-held dynamometry, or through a record of functional capabilities (eg, the ability to transfer from sitting to standing). Historically, there has been debate about the role of measuring the strength of persons who have had a stroke or related upper motor neuron lesion (ie, damage to the brain accompanied by symptoms that include spasticity); however, the evidence has indicated that measurement of strength following stroke will provide reliable and valid data and that this is valuable information in determining prognosis.[31]

As identified in the section on Impaired Strength (page 175) following a stroke, it is common to have weakness that is greater in the extremities opposite from the side of the stroke (eg, following a right middle cerebral artery CVA the left arm and leg will exhibit more pronounced weakness than the right arm and leg). In a majority of individuals, the strength will improve over time although impairment of strength will persist.[11]

However, as the strength improves, another impairment that often becomes evident is the inability to isolate extremity movements. That is, when attempting to move a single joint, the other joints in that limb also move in a pattern identified as a synergy (refer to page 45). One of the goals of physical therapy interventions will be to reduce the tendency for movement in these patterns and improve the ability to isolate movements.

Coordination may also be affected following stroke, and when impaired, the symptoms for this may be described as follows:

- Dysdiadochokinesia, which is a deficiency in the ability to perform rapidly alternating movements (RAM).
- Dysmetria, in which the ability to control the distance, power, and speed of movement is impaired.
- Action tremor, which indicates that a tremor or shaking occurs during the performance of voluntary (intentional) movements.

- A general slowing of movements, with additional delays in the ability to initiate a movement and to terminate a movement.

Refer to Chapter 4 for testing procedures for coordination.

Flexibility

Passive ROM is usually measured to identify any preexisting impairments that need to be addressed (eg, arthritis). In addition, this baseline data is collected because of the risk for the development of stiffness in the muscles affected by stroke. That is, in addition to the resistance to stretch that accompanies spasticity, the muscles often develop a gradual loss of flexibility due to a reduction of elasticity.

Functional Limitations

Following a stroke, a patient may have limited capabilities with the functions of bed mobility, transferring from sitting to standing or standing to sitting, ambulating, stair climbing, and many other ADLs. Documentation of functional abilities may be done by a description of the patient's ability to perform the function, by timing the patient's performance of the function, or by physical therapy outcome measurement scales.

The description of the patient's functional abilities should be based on efficiently and accurately describing the patient's (and not the caregiver's) ability or contribution to performing the function. The descriptors from the Functional Independence Measure (FIM) are effective for this and were described in Chapter 4.

Timed measurement of a patient's performance of tasks also provides valuable clinical data. Examples include using a stopwatch to time the functions of transferring from sitting to standing and ambulation speed. Transfers can be timed for the time needed to stand up from a chair once, the time needed to stand up three consecutive repetitions, or the number of repeated transfers (from sitting to standing to sitting) that can be completed within 10 seconds. Measures, such as the 6-minute walk test, are designed to measure exercise capacity and may be used for some patients following stroke.[3] However, patients with much lower ambulation or exercise capacity will be better described through measures such as rate of ambulation. One technique is to determine the time it takes an ambulating patient to traverse 10 feet. This should be measured during a period of walking, as starting and stopping will alter the results. Gait speed can then be easily calculated as the distance divided by the duration. A patient who ambulates across 10 feet in 5 seconds has a gait speed of 2 feet per second, while the speed of a patient who requires 15 seconds is walking at 0.67 feet per second.

Another important distinction in the ability to ambulate is the patient's ability to accommodate to different environments. The surface that is being walked on can alter performance because of the appearance (eg, visual contrast), texture (eg, tile versus carpeting), or the presence of obstacles. Environmental complexity will alter performance because the presence of obstacles, local activity (eg, other people walking nearby), or other distractions in the area may impair performance. For example, a patient may be able to walk effectively in a quiet physical therapy department, but his performance may deteriorate when he walks in a busy hospital hallway. When this occurs, the difference should be recorded and reported to the PT.

Evaluation of data from standardized examination tools, such as the Barthel Index, the Fugl-Meyer Assessment of Sensorimotor Recovery After Stroke, the Rivermead ADL Scale or the National Institutes of Health Stroke Scale, falls outside of the scope of the PTA. However, within the context of providing physical therapy interventions, the PTA will collect data to determine the patient's response to the intervention(s) provided. When the evaluating PT has employed a standardized examination tool, the PTA may need to apply components of the measures from that tool. To do this accurately, the PTA should review the tool with the PT to identify the data collection technique(s) to be used within the plan of care and the correct performance of each technique for collecting this data.

Balance Measures

Patient examination and evaluation of data from balance impairment tests falls outside of the responsibilities of the PTA. However, within the context of providing physical therapy interventions, the PTA may need to collect data about balance to determine the patient's response to the intervention(s) provided. If the evaluating PT employed a balance measurement tool, the PTA may need to apply components of the tool. As described above, the PTA should communicate with the PT to ensure the correct performance of the technique. Examples of these measures include the following:

- Timed up and go.
- Berg Balance Scale.
- Functional Reach Test.
- Unipedal standing (timed for duration).

In general, the PTA will want to note the patient's balance reactions based upon position (sitting vs standing) and in relationship to a functional activity. Often, the patient will have increasing difficulty with balance as the demands of the task increase. This information should be noted, documented, and relayed to the PT. Chapter 4 provides additional information on assessing balance.

Endurance

Exercise capacity is impaired following stroke. Some of this impairment may result from the hemiparesis because the patient must accommodate for weakness. However, cardiorespiratory fitness is also affected. MacKay-Lyons and Makrides reported that within 1 month after the stroke, the capacity to exercise was reduced to 60% of the typical capacity of a healthy, sedentary person, a response that is equivalent to that for person recovering from a myocardial infarction.[9] The PT's examination will contain measures of the patient's response to exercise to determine the baseline and because the reduced capacity raises the potential for an adverse response during exercise.

The data collected will usually contain information about the amount of exercise and the patient's response to that level of activity. The PTA should note the amount of activity, such as whether the patient was able to transfer repeatedly, ambulate a specific distance, or ascend a flight of stairs. This information will aid the PTA when determining the exercises and activity expectations for the first intervention session with the patient. The PT's examination should also contain information about the patient's response to exercise. This is usually identified through measuring (at rest and with activity) the patient's heart rate, respiratory rate, BP, and/or oxygen saturation (pulse oximetry). The PTA should continue to collect this data during exercise interventions in order to provide exercises that are within the patient's cardiopulmonary capacity.

INTERVENTIONS

By definition in the *Guide to Physical Therapist Practice*,[28] physical therapy interventions include three components: (1) coordination, communication, and documentation, (2) patient- or client-related instruction, and (3) procedural interventions.[28] Each of these components of providing an intervention must be included in the PT's plan of care for an individual recovering from a stroke. The PTA will participate in each of these areas as directed by the PT.

Coordination of services is very important for individuals who have suffered a stroke due to the diverse symptoms that may be present. Most patients recovering from a stroke will be receiving care from other health care providers including a physiatrist, OT, speech language pathologist, nurse, neuropsychologist, and others. It is important that all disciplines coordinate the care provided to ensure the patient will have the time and the energy necessary for participation in all of the rehabilitation and treatment sessions. In some settings, multidisciplinary meetings will allow for coordination and communication between the different health care providers working with the patient. This will provide the PT and PTA with invaluable information regarding the patient's impairments that are not directly addressed by the physical therapy procedural interventions, information about the patient's strengths, and can provide strategies to manage these issues. Skilled communication includes the verbal interactions between the PT and PTA and appropriate documentation by the PTA that clearly delineates the interventions provided and the patient's response to those interventions.

Provision of patient- or client-related instruction should be a part of every physical therapy session as well as recording an indication of the patient's response to instruction. That record of the response to instruction typically includes a description of the individual's ability to follow directions or his or her comprehension of instruction as evidenced by the presence or absence of behavioral changes. As the patient learns more about his or her condition, including unique impairments and functional limitations, he or she will be better prepared to take control over his or her own care even if independent physical functioning is never achieved. Additionally, when caring for patients recovering from a stroke, it is common that the patient's family and caregivers will require education related to provision of care and support for the patient. In summary, education should be a priority within the interventions provided to the patient who has had a stroke.

The procedural interventions that can be utilized with patients who are recovering from a stroke are many and varied. The challenge is selecting and applying the optimal intervention(s) based on the individual patient's needs at that point in his or her course of rehabilitation. That problem-solving must be done within the context of the PT's plan of care and with consideration of the patient's impairments and functional limitations, medical status, the contributions of other members of the health care team, the goals and discharge plan, etc.

Strategies for Therapeutic Exercise Interventions

The plan of care designed by the PT will be unique to each patient receiving physical therapy following a stroke. Therefore, the PTA must be able to interpret that plan of care and apply it to the individual needs of each patient. This can be a daunting challenge because diverse therapeutic strategies and techniques have been advocated for promoting improvements in impairment, function, and disability following stroke. To guide the PTA in this process, the authors recommend the conceptual framework for therapeutic

interventions for neuromuscular disorders recently described by Fell.[32] Fell categorized interventions as those related to motor learning and practice, those related to characteristics of a movement or task, and as other parameters for interventions (which will be described shortly). This framework is summarized in Table 11-1 and will be useful for streamlining the problem-solving process when providing physical therapy interventions to persons who have had a stroke.

Another great challenge when providing physical therapy interventions to the patient who has had a stroke is the dynamic presentation of the symptoms of the stroke. The PTA should expect that changes in symptoms will occur and, therefore, rigorously collect data to inform the process of modifying the intervention(s) to the patient. Changes in response to physical therapy interventions for the symptoms from a stroke may be subtle and observed over several days or may be sufficient to require intervention progressions to occur repeatedly within a single physical therapy session with the patient.

Finally, the interventions must be implemented within the individualized context for each patient. For example, the patient's baseline level of wellness or premorbid pathology will influence the intervention activities. A patient who has osteoarthritic changes in the LEs may not be able to participate in the same exercises as one who does not, or a patient with a history of cardiovascular disease will need exercise interventions and monitoring specific to their aerobic exercise capacity and situation. Other examples include consideration of the patient's prognosis and needs unique to his or her discharge destination. That is, if the discharge plan anticipates performance of ADLs at some level of independence, the interventions should be designed to facilitate acquisition of that independence, but if the expectation is that the patient will require assistance, the interventions should be designed for family or caregiver instruction and practice for the acquisition of the necessary abilities.

Therapeutic Exercise Interventions for Aerobic Training

An overarching concern when implementing therapeutic exercise interventions is impaired exercise capacity. The American Heart Association has recommended that the major rehabilitation goals following a stroke are the prevention of inactivity and disuse, decreasing the risk of a recurrent stroke or cardiovascular disorder, and increasing aerobic fitness.[2] To achieve this, each patient should engage in physical exercise as soon as possible to enhance his or her general activity level. When the PTA is providing therapeutic exercise interventions, she or he must be very considerate of providing sufficient aerobic challenges,

Table 11-1
Progressing Therapeutic Intervention in Patients With Neuromuscular Disorders

Parameters Related to Motor Learning and Practice

- Variability in practice (eg, blocked practice — random practice).
- Practicing components of movement (eg, part-task training — whole-task training).
- Task attention (eg, minimal distractions — cognitive/attentional demands).
- Feedback (eg, extrinsic feedback [knowledge of performance, knowledge of results] — intrinsic feedback).
- Environmental progression (eg, simple — complex).

Parameters Related to Characteristics of a Movement or Task

- Amplitude or magnitude of movement (eg, small range — large range of movement, mass synergy — isolated movement).
- Velocity (eg, slow gait — fast gait).
- Amount of work (eg, increase the frequency, intensity, or duration of activity/exercise).
- Endurance (eg, increase the capacity to persevere at a task).
- Regional (eg, isolated movement — multijoint movement; proximal movements — distal movements).

Other Parameters

- Developmental sequence (eg, low — high COG, large — small BOS).
- Supportive device (eg, AFO or cane).
- Assistance given (eg, verbal cues for guidance — minimal cues; moderate assistance — minimal assistance).

Adapted from Fell DW. Progressing therapeutic intervention in patients with neuromuscular disorders: a framework to assist clinical decision making. Journal of Neurologic Physical Therapy. *2004;28:35-46.*

preferably through upright activities (eg, training for gait or stair climbing) while monitoring the patient's response to those exercises.[2] Sample activities are described in Table 11-2. The PT will be a resource for determining precautions and thresholds for aerobic training (eg, target and maximum heart rates and acceptable BP). Some patients may have inadequate capacity for planned exercise interventions, and in those situations, the PTA should consult with the PT for options, such as decreasing the exercise intensity or duration while increasing the frequency of exercise sessions.

Neuromuscular Electrical Stimulation Interventions

NMES can be effective at increasing movement strength or at decreasing spasticity, making it an appropriate physical therapy intervention for some people who have had a stroke. Intervention strategies with NMES vary depending on the impairment or functional limitation being targeted, and this intervention is usually a component or adjunct within a therapeutic exercise program. As discussed previously, NMES can be applied to the shoulder to reduce glenohumeral joint subluxation and the accompanying pain by stimulating the supraspinatus and posterior deltoid muscles.[33,34] Another NMES application has been directed at improving UE performance with functional tasks. This strategy requires stimulation to the weakened muscle groups that is performed concurrent with a task that requires those muscles. This application may improve patterns of movement that are weak following a stroke, such as impaired strength for wrist and finger extension.[35,36] There have been few reports on the role of NMES interventions to the LEs following stroke. It appears to improve the recruitment of muscles[37] and gait (during the stimulation),[38] but the persistence of functional benefits has not been established.

Activities for Therapeutic Exercise Interventions

One challenge when working with patients following a CVA is determining the types of postures or activities that will be used as the foundation for the practicing that is necessary to foster the reattainment of functional abilities. A frequently-used framework for determining therapeutic exercise interventions is a developmental progression. According to Fell this typically is biomechanically based and progressed

Table 11-2
Summary of Exercise Programming Recommendations for Stroke Survivors

Mode of Exercise	Major Goals	Intensity/Frequency/Duration
Aerobic • Large muscle activities (eg, walking, treadmill, stationary cycle, combined arm-leg ergometry, arm ergometry, seated stepper).	• Increase independence in ADLs. • Increase walking speed/efficiency. • Improve tolerance for prolonged physical activity. • Reduce risk of cardiovascular disease.	• 40% to 70% peak oxygen uptake; 40% to 70% heart rate reserve; 50% to 80% maximal heart rate; RPE 11 to 14 (6 to 20 scale). • 3 to 7 days per week (d/wk). • 20 to 60 min per session (or multiple 10-min sessions).
Strength • Circuit training. • Weight machines. • Free weights. • Isometric exercise.	• Increase independence in ADLs.	• 1 to 3 sets of 10 to 15 repetitions of 8 to 10 exercises involving the major muscle groups.
Flexibility • Stretching.	• Increase ROM of involved extremities • Prevent contractures	• 2-3 d/wk (before or after aerobic or strength training). • Hold each stretch for 10 to 30 seconds.
Neuromuscular • Coordination and balance activities.	• Improve level of safety during ADLs.	• 2 to 3 d/wk (consider performing on the same day as strength activities).

Adapted from the American Heart Association. Gordon NF, Gulanick M, Costa F, Fletcher G, Franklin BA, Roth AJ, Shephard T. Physical activity and exercise recommendations for stroke survivors. Circulation. 2004;109:2031-2041.

by elevating the COG and/or narrowing the BOS.[32] Examples of activities include exercises in prone or prone on elbows, rolling or crawling activities, exercise in quadruped or during creeping, exercise in kneeling or half-kneeling, and standing and ultimately walking activities.[32] For example, a patient who is limited in the ability to transition from a supine to a sitting posture should receive exercise interventions addressing that task with activities of a similar nature. Exercises lower on the developmental progression (eg, prone on elbows) will provide insufficient challenge to facilitate improvement, and exercises higher on the developmental progression (eg, standing) will reduce the likelihood of success during practice.

Another framework for determining therapeutic exercise interventions is to choose tasks necessary to the patient and design exercise interventions to advance ability for that task. This is an important consideration given the wide scope of activities that may be relevant to an individual within his or her discharge environment. These tasks may range from self-care (eg, getting up from the floor or putting on a coat) to recreation (eg, handling a fishing rod or walking on a beach), and therefore, potential tasks to be considered are too numerous to list. Instead, the PTA must be considerate of this and keep in mind the following when choosing postures or activities for exercise interventions: (1) the types of tasks and demands unique to each patient's needs upon discharge from physical therapy, (2) the patient's current functional ability, and (3) those postures or activities that represent a developmental progression that the patient should practice.

The authors recommend that the choice of activities for therapeutic exercise interventions be guided by the following considerations:

The activity is, or is similar to, a task that is necessary (relevant) to the patient.

Learning and improved function will be fostered when:

• The patient is capable of some successful performance of the activity.

• The activity is sufficiently challenging (difficult) for the patient during the practice sessions.

Note that the developmental progression is not a sequential progression or an advancement of activities that should be followed. Also, a patient may be able to skip some activities and should increase his or her practice with those activities that have the greatest relevance to physical therapy goals.[32]

Therapeutic Exercise Interventions for Motor Learning

One component of the therapeutic exercise interventions for a patient who has had a stroke is the fostering of a change in abilities through motor learning. The need for learning will vary with each individual and with the types of tasks the individual must perform. Examples include learning how to obtain movement from weakened limbs, learning how to use something new (eg, an assistive device), or learning new strategies for ambulating in crowded areas. To promote learning, the PTA must apply strategies that have proven effective for motor learning. The essential strategies for this are variability in practice, practicing components of movement, task attention, feedback, and environmental progression.[32] Each of these strategies are discussed in Chapter 3 and will be built upon here; in the clinic the PTA should consider these individually and collectively when providing interventions.

Practice Strategies

Practice is a well-recognized technique for improving performance. This applies whether the learner is a canoer learning a paddle stroke, a child just learning how to walk, or a person rehabilitating from a stroke who needs to learn how to move a limb. PTAs should recognize that each session of providing physical therapy interventions is the patient's opportunity for practice and that the practice is an essential component of improving the ability to move and to function. Therefore, each session should be designed for motor learning, and should include those strategies that will make the act of practicing the most successful for the patient. Skilled applications of motor learning and practice strategies should be applied to *all* therapeutic exercise interventions so that the patient can gain the optimal benefit from physical therapy.

When designing practice of a new movement or task, one common strategy is to have the patient repeat a single component of the action. For example, the PTA may choose to have the patient who has had a stroke repeatedly practice transferring from sitting to standing to sitting, or the PTA may have the patient practice walking on a flat, smooth surface. This type of practice, which relies on repeating the same component of a task under the same conditions, is called *blocked practice*. Blocked practice assists with the preliminary learning of the movements or components

of the task; therefore, it should be used in the early stages of learning. However, "it has been found that recall and transfer of motor skills, as well as learning, retention, and refinement of a skill, are best facilitated by random repetition over blocked repetition."[32] This means that varying the activities being practiced (ie, *random practice*) has the potential to improve the learning. For example, the PTA may have the patient practice transferring from sitting to and from standing from chairs of different heights, or the PTA may have the patient practice walking on irregular surfaces or on an obstacle course. An appropriate progression of the intervention would be to advance exercises from the consistency of blocked practice to the variability of random practice of a task.[32]

Another strategy to advance learning in the early stages of the acquisition of motor learning is *part practice* (or part-task training), in which the components or the movement(s) that constitute a task are practiced. Once these components have been practiced, the intervention should be progressed to *whole practice* (whole-task training) to foster motor learning. For example, a patient who has had a stroke may practice standing weight shifting, then progress to stepping forward and backward with the right leg, and then stepping with the left leg for part practice. This may later be progressed to ambulating, which represents the strategy of whole practice.[32]

Attention

The patient's initial motor learning will be greatest if he or she is able to pay close *attention* to the task or exercise that is being learned. Stroke is a brain injury, and as described earlier, there is a risk for symptoms of altered cognition or attention. Therefore, a PTA should use an environment with minimal distractions, and that may mean planning your interventions in a quiet room or during quieter periods in the therapy area (Figure 11-3). As learning advances, the PTA must also consider the anticipated outcome for the patient. If the patient is preparing for a discharge that will include distracting settings (eg, social gatherings, restaurants, or attending religious services), the individual will require the ability to manage complex demands on attention. Therefore, the interventions applied should prepare for those demands by progressing practice sessions towards complex environments (eg, walking in a busy hallway [Figure 11-4]) or by increasing cognitive demands (eg, holding a conversation while ambulating).[32]

Feedback

Feedback is any of the sensory information that a person uses for learning and improving their performance. *Intrinsic feedback* is the information that an individual gathers "on their own," such as the

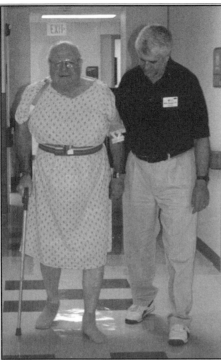

Figure 11-3. Gait training patient in an environment with minimal distractions.

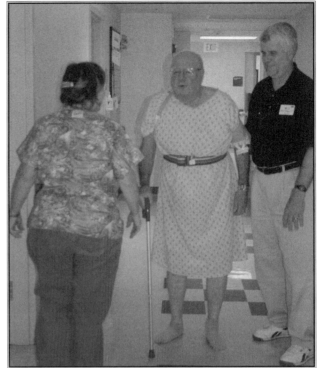

Figure 11-4. As the patient's attention to task improves, the environment should become more complex during the functional activity.

kinesthetic sensations of movement from the limbs. This type of feedback can be augmented by techniques such as using a mirror to allow a patient to observe his or her posture or how the posture changes as a result of his or her movements. *Extrinsic feedback* is when the physical therapy provider gives information to the patient to improve performance. Extrinsic feedback is characterized as *knowledge of performance*, which is information about the components or quality of movement(s), or *knowledge of results*, which is information about the outcome achieved from the movement(s). A PTA must use feedback as a tool to shape and improve his or her patient's motor performance and learning. To achieve this, Fell has advised that, as interventions are advances with a patient "regardless of the type and source of feedback, there should always be a progressive decrease in extrinsic feedback provided" in order to promote learning.[32] The PTA should also be considerate of the amount of feedback provided because excessive feedback will distract from the patient's ability to attend to the task at hand. The timing of feedback should also be considered. In many situations, the optimal time for feedback is delayed for a few seconds following the completion of the task, when feedback can be used to augment the patient's reflection and assessment of their performance of the task.[32]

Environmental Progression

The context that physical therapy interventions are provided in will influence the motor learning

based on the demands placed on the patient during the learning process. To better understand this, it is helpful to look at the taxonomy of tasks developed by Gentile presented in Table 11-3.[39] She has identified the following incremental demands, which are dependant on the type of task (described here as progressing from less to more complex):

- The person is stationary – the person is moving or being moved while performing the task (eg, riding in a w/c).
- The task remains consistent each time – the task varies with each performance.
- The person's posture is stable – the person is moving themselves during the task (eg, walking).
- The task does not require manipulation – the task requires manipulation (eg, buttoning a shirt).

As described by Gentile, these parameters can be combined (see Table 11-3) to identify the level of complexity of a task and, therefore, to categorize the types of demands that are imposed by different types of tasks or by different therapeutic exercise interventions.[39] While full analysis of this taxonomy exceeds the ability of the entry-level PTA, it is necessary for the PTA to apply these general concepts for progression of the interventions provided to a patient receiving physical

Table 11-3
Gentile's Taxonomy of Tasks

	Body Stability No Manipulation	Body Stability Manipulation	Body Transport No Manipulation	Body Transport Manipulation
Stationary No intertrial variability	Closed Consistent Motionless Body stability	Closed Consistent Motionless Body stability Manipulation	Closed Consistent Motionless Body transport	Closed Consistent Motionless Body transport Manipulation
Stationary Intertrial variability	Variable Motionless Body stability	Variable Motionless Body stability Manipulation	Variable Motionless Body transport	Variable Motionless Body transport Manipulation
Motion No intertrial variability	Consistent Motion Body stability	Consistent Motion Body stability Manipulation	Consistent Motion Body transport	Consistent Motion Body transport Manipulation
Motion Intertrial variability	Open Variable Motion Body stability	Open Variable Motion Body stability Manipulation	Open Variable Motion Body transport	Open Variable Motion Body transport Manipulation

Adapted from Gentile AM. Skill acquisition: action, movement, and neuromotor processes. In: Carr J, Shepherd R, Gordon J, et al, eds. Movement Science: Foundations for Physical Therapy in Rehabilitation. *1987:93.*

therapy interventions for stroke symptoms. This is best achieved by identifying, through the goals established by the PT, the types of environments and demands that the patient is likely to encounter. The exercise interventions must begin in the less demanding components described here and advanced according to the patient's response and success of performance. Advancement should follow these concepts to foster the patient's achievement of the PT's goals.

For example, a patient whose goal or anticipated outcome includes the expectation of ambulation in public areas (eg, restaurant or place of worship) will need to achieve the ability for body transport *and* be able to perform this when intertrial variability (ie, obstacles and other people also walking by) is occurring. If the earlier interventions are performed in a quiet physical therapy gym to foster attention for successful learning, it is expected that the patient will develop the ability to walk in a consistent (nonvariable) environment. However, the addition of variables, such as walking in a hallway in which other people are also walking so that the patient now has to respond to and avoid those people, results in a more complex task that places greater demands on the patient. If this is not practiced, it cannot be expected that the patient

will develop the necessary abilities to succeed with the task. Therefore, the therapeutic exercise interventions should be intentionally designed to advance the exercises to include this type of practice and, therefore, prepare the patient for the task and make the patient more likely to succeed when outside of the physical therapy environment.[32]

Factors Relating to the Movement or Task

The exercises employed should also be directed at advancing the ability to move a region of the body, including advancing the strength of the movement and the quality (skill) of the movement. For example, if a patient who has had a stroke has an impairment of weakness of the knee extensor muscles, which contribute to a functional limitation of requiring assistance to stand up from a chair, there are many exercise options that will promote strengthening of the knee extensor muscles. However, for the exercise to be therapeutic, the interventions should be designed so that the patient is exercising and practicing at the level that challenges that individual to improve performance for that movement or task. The following are examples of characteristics of a task or movement that should be advanced or progressed as the patient's improving performance allows:

- The amplitude (or amount) of movement that occurs (eg, progress from moving through a small range to large range of movement or progress from moving large regions of the body to isolated or fine movements).

- The velocity of the movement (eg, progress from training at a slow gait speed to a fast gait).

- The amount of work being performed (eg, increase the frequency, intensity, or duration of the exercise of the task that is being practiced).

- The patient's capacity for work (endurance) should be advanced (eg, increase the repetitions performed or the distance walked during gait training).

- Progression can be based on the region(s) of the body being addressed (eg, the challenge may be increased by training for proximal movements before distal movements or for the performance of isolated movement before multi-joint movements).[32]

Other Parameters

The ability to perform a task may be improved through the use of a supportive or adaptive device, allowing for practice and improved capability with that task. For example, a patient may use an ankle-foot orthosis to improve the ability to walk or a grab bar to provide additional support while rolling. Progression may be achieved by reducing the amount of support, the amount of reliance placed on the device, or by adjusting or adapting the device. For example, a patient may initially walk while supporting himself with parallel bars, followed by progression to a quad cane and then a straight cane.[32]

Another consideration during the provision of therapeutic exercise interventions is the amount or type of assistance provided by the PTA. This progression is commonly recognized for physical assistance, in which the PTA gradually and intentionally decreases the amount of support provided while the patient increases the amount of work she or he is able to perform. Progression can also be achieved by reducing other supports, such as the amount of verbal cues provided for guidance during task performance, with the progression being achieved by intentionally reducing the amount of cues provided to the patient.[32]

Additional Intervention Strategies in Stroke Rehabilitation

The last decade has seen an impressive growth in the evidence supporting some unique interventions to facilitate the recovery of functional abilities lost as a result of stroke. One of these interventions is partial *body-weight support during gait training*. This technique involves gait training on a treadmill or over land while the subject is suspended in a harness that supports the lower trunk and proximal LEs (Figures 11-5A and 11-5B). This harness supports a portion of the person's body weight so that he or she may practice the task of walking with a low risk for falling and with a reduction of gait deviation(s). This technique has achieved restoration of greater walking ability, as demonstrated by a significantly less reliance on assistance, greater walking speed, and greater walking endurance.[40,41]

This intervention typically involves walking on a treadmill while supported in the harness while two or three PTs and/or PTAs assist the patient to achieve the desired movement. Their manual assistance involves guidance with weight shifting, stance, and the swing and stance movements of the more involved LE. Progression of this intervention may be achieved by (1) decreasing the amount of assistance as the patient's skill improves, (2) providing less support through the harness (ie, increasing the weight-bearing demands on the patient's LEs), and/or (3) increasing the speed of walking on the treadmill.[40,41] Another option with body-weight support gait training that is showing promise is the use of a robotic device to provide movement and/or support of the LEs during the practice of walking.[40]

Recent research found that it was uncommon for individuals who have had a stroke to receive gait training interventions with a body-weight support device.[42] We believe that this intervention is infrequently chosen because it is relatively new, which has resulted in a lack of access to the equipment in many clinics, as well PTs' unfamiliarity with the intervention. However, we expect that this intervention will be used more frequently over the next decade.

Another strategy for rehabilitation of motor (movement) abilities following stroke is *constraint-induced movement therapy (CIMT)*. This intervention evolved from a fascinating series of investigations into *learned nonuse*, in which it was discovered in the lab of psychologist Edward Taub that a monkey relieved of sensation in an UE will cease to use that limb. The monkey has the *potential* to use the limb, but doing so is laborious. That level of effort is negative reinforcement, while use of the limb in which sensation is intact is easy and provides positive reinforcement. The combination reinforces the avoidance of using that limb, which Taub has identified as learned nonuse. Taub applied this understanding to the development of an intervention in which the limb that is not impaired is constrained by strapping it to the trunk, and the monkey is then required to use the impaired limb in order to feed itself and perform other essential functions. This results in

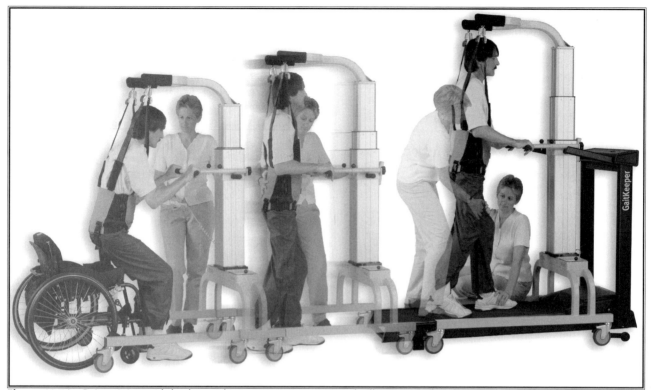

Figure 11-5A. Gait training with body weight support system on treadmill. (Reprinted with permission from Mobility Research, LLC; Tempe, Ariz. www.litegait.com.)

constraint-induced movement of the limb and a restoration of the ability to use it functionally.[43]

This technique has proven effective in the rehabilitation of movement ability of either the UE or the LE when the ability to move and use the limb is impaired following stroke. The intervention involves constraint of the less-involved extremity for 14 days, and during that period, the patient participates in training activities and tasks using the involved limb for 6 hours each weekday and for additional exercise periods on the weekends (Figure 11-6). This intervention is effective in increasing the amount and quality of movement in the involved limb and the use of the limb for functional tasks; the benefits from the intervention are sustained over time. The research on this protocol has been impressive in that it confirmed the efficacy of this intervention when massed practice (constraint of the less involved limb paired with approximately 70 hours of training activities) is provided to the patient.[43-45]

It appears that CIMT interventions are rarely employed outside of those clinics that specialize in this intervention.[42] The barriers to widespread use of this intervention may be related to the need for massed practice sessions, which encompass a full day of activities over 2 weeks.[44,45] This presents a problem for scheduling treatment sessions as well as achieving reimbursement by insurers. Fortunately, there is recent evidence that modifying the schedule also achieves

Figure 11-5B. Gait training with body weight support system on land. (Reprinted with permission from Mobility Research, LLC; Tempe, Ariz. www.litegait.com.)

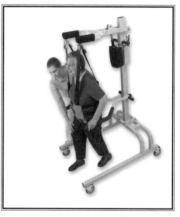

benefits because improved movement control and functional use of the limb has also been demonstrated following training sessions for 1 hour, 3 times a week over a 10-week period.[46]

CONCLUSION

The provision of interventions for patients with a CVA is based on the plan of care and considers the individual patient's goals, functional capabilities, and the discharge plan. Data collection is critical because the symptoms of the stroke may be changing between, and even within, the physical therapy sessions. While

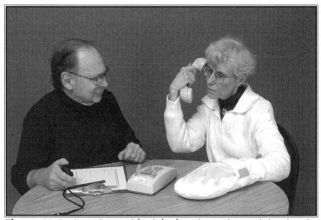

Figure 11-6. A patient with right hemiparesis participating in intensive repetitive task practice of a functional activity during constraint-induced therapy. (Used with permission from the Extremity Constraint Induced Therapy Evaluation (EXCITE) Trial, Steven Wolf, Principal Investigator.)

providing skilled interventions, the PTA must identify when changes occur and appropriately modify those interventions provided within the treatment plan established by the PT. Particular attention must be paid to the progression of interventions, such as therapeutic exercise or gait training techniques, so that the patient is challenged appropriately and advanced toward achieving optimal functional abilities.

During this process, it is important to recognize the potential for cognitive and communication deficits. Excellent strategies for modifying treatment to accommodate a cognitive impairment have been described by Shumway-Cook and Woollacott:

1. "Reduce confusion: make sure the task goal is clear to the patient.

2. Improve motivations: work on tasks that are relevant and important to the patient.

3. Encourage consistency of performance: be consistent with goals, and reinforce only those behaviors that are compatible with those goals.

4. Reduce confusion: use simple, clear, and concise instructions.

5. Seek a moderate level of arousal to optimize learning: moderate the sensory stimulation in the environment; agitated patients require decreased intensity of stimulation (soft voice, low lights, slow touch) to reduce arousal levels; stuporous patients require increased intensity of stimulation (use brisk, loud commands and fast movements, working in a vertical position).

6. Provide increased levels of supervision, especially during the early stages of retraining.

7. Recognize that progress may be slower when working with patients who have cognitive impairments.

8. Improve attention: accentuate perceptual cues that are essential to the task, and minimize the number of irrelevant stimuli in the environment.

9. Improve problem-solving ability: begin with relatively simple tasks, and gradually increase the complexity of the task-demands.

10. Encourage declarative as well as procedural learning: have a patient verbally and/or mentally rehearse sequences when performing a task."[3]

Finally, value the role of the patient, the patient's family, and the other caregivers in this process. The selected physical therapy interventions provided will only involve a small portion of the patient's day, but when others are encouraged to be involved in the process, a team effort is available to support the rehabilitation of the patient. This will extend and reinforce the activities and exercises necessary for the patient to achieve an optimal outcome from the process.

CHAPTER QUESTIONS

1. Explain the differences between ischemic stroke, hemorrhagic stroke, and TIA.

2. Describe how apraxia may limit a person's ability to perform functional tasks.

3. Identify the data that should be collected when providing interventions to a patient who has diminished cardiopulmonary capacity.

4. Define the following:
   a. vertigo
   b. disequilibrium
   c. ataxia
   d. hemiparesis
   e. unilateral neglect
   f. anosognosia
   g. aphasia
   h. dysphagia
   i. homonymous hemianopia
   j. learned nonuse.

5. Explain why shoulder pain is a concern following stroke, and describe strategies to prevent the development of shoulder pain.

6. Explain what pusher behavior is following stroke, and identify strategies to intervene to correct this behavior.

7. Identify the data collection techniques that a PTA may use to identify and document a patient's functional limitations, balance, and endurance when implementing the PT's plan of care for a patient who has had a stroke.

8. Describe strategies to enhance the effectiveness of patient-related communication and instruction with a patient who has had a stroke.

9. Describe therapeutic exercise interventions to enhance motor learning, the remediation of movement or function, and to increase aerobic capacity following stroke.

10. Identify the role of neuromuscular electrical stimulation (NMES), body-weight support during gait training and constraint-induced movement therapy (CIMT) as interventions for the patient who has had a stroke.

Case Studies

Case # 1

A 64-year-old gentleman was admitted to an acute rehab facility six days after having a CVA, which was diagnosed as a left internal capsule infarction. The patient displayed mild right extremity and trunk weakness. The patient also displayed diminished sensation throughout the right extremities. He demonstrated impaired balance and motor control and required minimal assistance for gait activities due to apraxia. The patient required constant verbal cues when ambulating and became easily distracted in cluttered environments or when other individuals walked past him. He had poor insight into his deficits and demonstrated impulsivity that placed him as a safety risk. The patient previously lived alone in a home with five steps to enter, and his goal was to return to that environment. The PT's plan of care called for therapeutic exercise to improve strength and motor control, gait training on level and uneven surfaces, and patient education.

Questions

1. List the impairments, functional limitations, and disabilities this patient demonstrates.

2. Within the plan of care, what activities could be used to address the right LE strength deficits? What parameters would be utilized (frequency, intensity, etc)?

3. This patient demonstrates safety issues during gait due to motor apraxia and anosognosia. How do you want to progress the environmental context in which this patient is practicing gait activities?

4. Discuss feedback strategies to utilize related to the patient's functional mobility deficits.

5. Utilizing the concepts of developmental sequencing, discuss other postures and activities you might choose to utilize with this patient to address the deficits of motor apraxia noted during gait.

6. What are you going to observe with this patient to determine if the intervention strategies being used are effective?

Case # 2

A 72-year-old female was on vacation with her sister when she had a left middle cerebral artery CVA. She was transported from her hotel room to the hospital via an ambulance. The patient displayed strength of 0/5 throughout the right UE. The patient had sufficient strength to initiate the movements of hip extension and adduction but demonstrated severe weakness and decreased tone throughout the right LE musculature. The patient required maximal assistance with all mobility, including rolling, supine to and from sit and sit to and from stand transitions, as well as transfers from bed to and from the w/c. When standing, she needed maximal assistance and a hemicane and was unable to support weight through her right leg. The patient's sitting balance was diminished, requiring minimal to moderate assistance to maintain an upright posture. The patient demonstrated mild pusher behavior and required frequent verbal cues to shift her weight to the left. The patient also demonstrated global aphasia. She did not attempt to speak and only communicated with head nods and shakes. The speech therapist's notes indicated the patient had only 50% accuracy with head nods and shakes. The patient was able to follow simple commands with physical and visual cues with 90% accuracy. Discharge plans are for the patient's son to come and assist with transporting the patient back to her hometown, where she will enter an acute rehabilitation unit. She will travel by commercial air. The son will need to be taught how to transfer the patient from a w/c into and out of a car and needs to practice a simulated transfer from a w/c into and out of an airplane seat.

Questions

1. List impairments, functional limitations, and disabilities this patient demonstrates.

2. Describe how this patient will need to be positioned when sitting in a w/c.

3. Discuss how you will approach this patient in relation to her aphasia.

4. Describe activities that can be utilized to help facilitate the patient's use of her right leg.

5. Discuss what parameters would be appropriate when addressing transitional movements (variability, components of movement, etc).

6. Detail the approach you will use when teaching the patient's son how to assist the patient in transfers.

Suggested author answers are available at www.slackbooks.com/neuroquestions.

REFERENCES

1. Fuller KS. Stroke. In: Goodman CV, Boissonnault WG, Fuller KS, eds. *Pathology: Implications for the PT.* 2nd ed. Philadelphia, Pa: Saunders; 2003:1054-1071.

2. Gordon NF, Gulanick M, Costa F, Fletcher G, Franklin BA, Roth AJ, Shephard T. Physical activity and exercise recommendations for stroke survivors. *Circulation.* 2004;109:2031-2041.

3. Shumway-Cook A, Woollacott MH. *Motor Control Theory and Practical Applications.* 2nd ed. Philadelphia, Pa: Lippincott Williams and Wilkins; 2001.

4. Adams RD, Victor M, Ropper AH. *Principles of Neurology.* 6th ed. New York, NY: McGraw-Hill; 1997:57.

5. Kertesz A, Nicholsom I, Cancelliere A, Kassa K, Black SE. Motor impersistence: a right-hemisphere syndrome. *Neurology.* 1985;35,662-666.

6. Donkervoort M, Dekker J, van den Ende E, Stehmann-Saris JC, Deelman BG. Prevalence of apraxia among patients with a first left hemisphere stroke in rehabilitation centers and nursing homes. *Clin Rehabil.* 2000;14(2):130-136.

7. Van Heugten CM, Dekker J, Deelman BG, Stehmann-Saris JC, Kinebanian A. Rehabilitation of stroke patients with apraxia: the role of additional cognitive and motor impairments. *Disability and Rehabilitation.* 2000;22(12):547-554.

8. Kelly JO, Kilbreath SL, Davis GM, Zeman B, Raymond J. Cardiorespiratory fitness and walking ability in subacute stroke patients. *Archives of Physical Medicine and Rehabilitation.* 2003;84:1780-1785.

9. Mackay-Lyons MJ, Makrides L. Exercise capacity early after stroke. *Archives of Physical Medicine and Rehabilitation.* 2002;83:1697-1702.

10. Bernhardt J, Dewey H, Thrift A, Donnan G. Inactive and alone: physical activity within the first 14 days of acute stroke unit care. *Stroke.* 2004;35(4):1005-1009.

11. Hendricks HT, van Limbeck J, Geurts AC, Zwarts MJ. Motor recovery after stroke: a systematic review of the literature. *Archives of Physical Medicine and Rehabilitation.* 2002;83:1629-1637.

12. Andrews AW, Bohannon RW. Distribution of muscle strength impairment following stroke. *Clinical Rehabilitation.* 2000;14:79-87.

13. Vuagnat H, Chantraine A. Shoulder pain in hemiplegia revisited: contribution of functional electrical stimulation and other therapies. *Journal of Rehabilitation Medicine.* 2003;35:49-56.

14. Turner-Stokes L, Jackson D. Shoulder pain after stroke: a review of the evidence base to inform the development of an integrated care pathway. *Clinical Rehabilitation.* 2002;16:276-298.

15. Murphy MA, Roberts-Warrior D. A review of motor performance measures and treatment interventions for patients with stroke. *Topics in Geriatric Rehabilitation.* 2003;19(1):3-42.

16. Roller ML. The 'pusher syndrome.' *Journal of Neurological Physical Therapy.* 2004;28(1):29-34.

17. Pérennou DA, Amblard B, Laassel EM, Benaim C, Hérisson C, Pélissier J. Understanding the pusher behavior of some stroke patients with spatial deficits: a pilot study. *Archives of Physical Medicine and Rehabilitation.* 2002;83:570-575.

18. Pierce SR, Buxbaum LJ. Treatments of unilateral neglect. *Archives of Physical Medicine and Rehabilitation.* 2002;83:256-268.

19. Swan L. Unilateral spatial neglect. *Physical Therapy.* 2001;81(9):1572-1580.

20. Stone SP, Wilson B, Wroot A, Halligan PW, Lange LS, Marshall JC, Greenwood RJ. The assessment of visuo-spatial neglect after acute stroke. *J Neurol Neurosurg Psychiatry.* 1991;54(4):345-350.

21. Maeshima S, Dohi N, Funahashi K, Nakai K, Itakura T, Komai N. Rehabilitation of patients with anosognosia for hemiplegia due to intracerebral hemorrhage. *Brain Injury.* 1997;11(9):691-697.

22. Pedersen PM, Jørgensen HS, Nakayama H, Raaschou HO, Olsen TS. Frequency, determinants, and consequences of anosognosia in acute stroke. *Journal of Neurological Rehabilitation*. 1996;10:243-250.

23. Ross ED. Acute agitation and other behaviors associated with Wernicke aphasia and their possible neurological basis. *Neuropsychiatry, Neuropsychology, and Behavioral Neurology*. 1993;6(1):9-18.

24. Lundy-Ekman L. *Neuroscience: Fundamentals for Rehabilitation*. Philadelphia, Pa: WB Saunders; 2002.

25. Waxman SA. *Correlative Neuroanatomy*. 23rd ed. Stamford, Conn: Appleton and Lange; 1996.

26. Ghika-Schmid F, Bogousslavsky J. Affective disorders following stroke. *Eur Neurol*. 1997;38(2):75-81.

27. Bohannon RW. Evaluation and treatment of sensory and perceptual impairments following stroke. *Topics in Geriatric Rehabilitation*. 2003;19(2):87-97.

28. *Guide to Physical Therapy Practice*. 2nd ed. Alexandria, Va: American Physical Therapy Association; 2001.

29. Lewis CB, McNerney T. *The Functional Toolbox: Clinical Measures of Functional Outcomes*. Washington, DC: LEARN Publications; 1994.

30. Lewis CB, McNerney T. *The Functional Toolbox II: Clinical Measures of Functional Outcomes*. Washington, DC: LEARN Publications; 1997.

31. Bohannon RW. Measurement, nature, and implications of skeletal muscle strength in patients with neurological disorders. *Clinical Biomechanics*. 1995;10(6):283-292.

32. Fell DW. Progressing therapeutic intervention in patients with neuromuscular disorders: a framework to assist clinical decision making. *Journal of Neurological Physical Therapy*. 2004;28(1):35-46.

33. Faghri PD, Rodgers MM, Glaser RM, Bors JG, Ho C, Akuthota P. The effects of functional electrical stimulation on shoulder subluxation, arm function recovery, and shoulder pain in hemiplegic stroke patients. *Archives of Physical Medicine and Rehabilitation*. 1994;75:73-79.

34. Price CI, Pandyan AD. Electrical stimulation for preventing and treating post-stroke shoulder pain: a systematic Cochrane review. *Clinical Rehabilitation*. 2001;15,:5-19.

35. Gritsenko V, Prochazka A. A functional electrical stimulation-assisted exercise therapy system for hemiplegic hand function. *Archives of Physical Medicine and Rehabilitation*. 2004;85:881-885.

36. Sullivan JE, Hedman LD. A home program of sensory and neuromuscular electrical stimulation with upper-limb task practice in a patient 5 years after a stroke. *Physical Therapy*. 2004;84:1045-1054.

37. Newsam CJ, Baker LL. Effect of an electric stimulation facilitation program on quadriceps motor unit recruitment after stroke. *Arch Phys Med Rehabil*. 2004;85(12):2040-2045.

38. Burridge JH, Taylor PN, Hagan SA, Wood DE, Swain ID. The effects of common peroneal stimulation on the effort and speed of walking: a randomized controlled trial with chronic hemiplegic patients. *Clinical Rehabilitation*. 1997;11(3):201-210.

39. Gentile AM. Skill acquisition: action, movement and neuromotor processes. In: Carr J, Shepherd R, Gordon J, et al, eds. *Movement Science: Foundations for Physical Therapy in Rehabilitation*. 1987:93.

40. Hesse S. Rehabilitation of gait after stroke: evaluation, principles of therapy, novel treatment approaches, and assistive devices. *Topics in Geriatric Rehabilitation*. 2003;19(2):109-126.

41. Visintin M, Barbeau H, Korner-Bitensky N, Mayo NE. A new approach to retrain gait in stroke patients through body weight support and treadmill stimulation. *Stroke*. 1998;29(6):1122-1128.

42. Jette DU, Warren RL, Wirtalla C. The relation between therapy intensity and outcomes of rehabilitation in skilled nursing facilities. *Arch Phys Med Rehabil*. 2005;86(3):373-379.

43. Taub E, Uswatte G, Pidikiti R. Constraint-induced movement therapy: a new family of techniques with broad application to physical rehabilitation--a clinical review. *Journal of Rehabilitation Research and Development*. 1999;36:237-251.

44. Blanton S, Wolf SL. An application of upper-extremity constraint-induced movement therapy in a patient with subacute stroke. *Physical Therapy*. 1999;79(9):847-853.

45. Kunkel A, Kopp B, Müller G, Villringer K, Villringer A, Taub E, Flor H. Constraint-induced movement therapy for motor recovery in chronic stroke patients. *Archives of Physical Medicine and Rehabilitation*. 1999;80:624-628.

46. Page SJ, Sisto S, Levine P, McGrath RR. Efficacy of modified constraint-induced movement therapy in chronic stroke: a single-blinded randomized controlled trial. *Archives of Physical Medicine and Rehabilitation*. 2004;85:14-18.

Chapter

12

CLIENTS WITH DEGENERATIVE DISEASES: PARKINSON'S DISEASE, MULTIPLE SCLEROSIS, AND AMYOTROPHIC LATERAL SCLEROSIS

Rolando T. Lazaro, PT, MS, DPT, GCS

KEY WORDS

amyotrophic lateral sclerosis
degenerative disease of the central nervous system
multiple sclerosis
Parkinson's disease
physical therapy examination
physical therapy intervention
therapeutic exercises

CHAPTER OBJECTIVES

- Discuss the signs and symptoms of Parkinson's disease (PD), multiple sclerosis (MS), and amyotrophic lateral sclerosis (ALS), and explain their implications to physical therapy examination and intervention.

- Discuss common intervention strategies for patients and clients with degenerative diseases of the CNS

- Identify some "clinical pearls" which can assist a PTA in treating patients with degenerative conditions of the CNS.

INTRODUCTION

Many of the patients and clients referred for physical therapy intervention have conditions that are caused by the degeneration of specific portions of the CNS, specifically those that involve or influence movement. The degeneration may be caused by the normal aging process, mediated by genetic abnormalities, or exacerbated or hastened by environmental factors. As movement specialists, PTs and PTAs play an important role in helping patients and clients with degenerative neuromuscular diseases achieve their highest functional capacity and optimum health and well being. A thorough understanding of the specific functions of the various structures of the CNS will allow the clinician to make inferences on potential movement disorders based on the structures involved. It will allow the PTA to determine what to expect assuming a typical presentation of the condition, and, consequently, to communicate to the PT possible changes in the patient's condition that do not follow the specific presentation for the disease. For example, if the PTA who is treating a patient with *Parkinson's disease (PD)* notices that this patient has developed paralysis in one side of the body, the PTA should communicate this finding to the PT because this is not consistent with a medical diagnosis of PD.

This chapter will focus on the three most common degenerative diseases: *PD, multiple sclerosis (MS)*, and *amyotrophic lateral sclerosis (ALS)*.

PARKINSON'S DISEASE

Parkinson's disease (PD) is a medical condition that results in a variety of movement disorders that impair an individual's ability to perform normal everyday tasks. In the US, 100 to 150 of every 100,000 people is affected by PD, with 1% of those over 60 years of age afflicted by the condition.[1]

A person with PD may exhibit one or more of the following motor impairments: bradykinesia (extreme slowness of movement), rigidity, resting (nonintentional) tremors, postural instability, and festinating gait.[2] Bradykinesia in PD is also associated with "on-off phenomenon," characterized by freezing episodes in which the person appears to be fixed or "stuck" in space, and is usually seen during a gross motor activity.[3] Other physical traits associated with PD include increased thoracic kyphosis and decreased lumbar lordosis, producing a stooped and flexed posture.[2] Each of these manifestations of PD impairs the gross motor function of all extremities, thus negatively impacting balance. Poor balance leads to falls, which, added to all the other aging problems, can create life-threatening results. One study, which used a questionnaire that reported on the frequency of falls in patients with PD, stated that more than one-third of these patients had fallen, and more than 10% fall at least once a week. Causes of these falls were attributed to postural instability, movement dysfunction, gait abnormalities, and difficulty with sitting and rising.[4] Poor balance also increases the risk of falling. Falls may occur due to the delayed motor responses when standing, walking, turning, and sitting without back support.[5] As normal individuals age, falls become an increasing problem. With age and a preexisting diagnosis of a disease such as PD, an individual may not only be at risk of falling, but the resulting problems following a fall may have greater consequences.

Because PD is a progressive degeneration of the basal ganglia, time brings on increasingly altered posture and increases in rigidity and bradykinesia, which lead to decreases in the ability to balance. Eventually, movement requires so much energy that the individual may become bed ridden with a fixed trunk and flexion contractures. In the advanced stages, inspiration is decreased, coughing is difficult, and bronchopneumonia may be one of the reasons for morbidity.[2]

Traditionally, drug therapy has been the primary intervention to delay the progression of impairments, functional limitations, and disabilities related to PD. The general effect of these PD medications is to replenish the brain's supply of dopamine, a neurotransmitter that is important in basal ganglia function. Common medications for PD include Sinemet (Merck and Company, Whitehouse Station, NJ), a Levadopa-Carbidopa combination. The "next generation" medications that have been approved include Permax (Eli Lilly and Company, Indianapolis, Ind) and Mirapex (Boehringer Ingelheim Pharmaceuticals, Ridgefield, Conn), which are dopamine agonists that bind to and stimulate cerebral dopamine receptors to improve motor performance.[6] While on these medications, patients may experience motor fluctuations causing unpredictable on-off episodes, which interfere with performance of ADLs and ambulation.

MULTIPLE SCLEROSIS

Multiple sclerosis (MS) is the most common neurologic condition affecting young adults. It is characterized by degeneration and subsequent loss of myelin scattered throughout the CNS, primarily in the white matter. In this condition, plaques of demyelination are accompanied by destruction and inflammation of oligodendroglia, which form part of the supporting structure of the CNS. Due to the degeneration of the myelin, neurotransmission is disrupted and will manifest as delayed or absent transmission of nerve impulses.[7]

Since demyelination can occur anywhere in the CNS, the resulting signs and symptoms and clinical manifestations will then vary based on the areas affected. These symptoms can develop slowly over days and weeks, or rapidly within hours. Common symptoms include fatigue, motor weakness, paresthesia, unsteady gait, double vision, tremor, and bladder and/or bowel problems. Fatigue is the most common MS symptom and is frequently misunderstood by family, friends, and employers because it is not a visible symptom. Some researchers and clinicians have noted that the fatigue experienced by patients with MS increases as the day progresses.[7]

In terms of the pattern of the disease, the classic presentation is characterized by periods of exacerbations (relapses) and remissions (partial or total disappearance of symptoms). As the disease progresses, the period of exacerbations becomes more frequent and longer, while the periods of remissions become more limited. Individuals afflicted with this disease then demonstrate progressive deterioration of function. Factors that have been associated with exacerbations include excessive fatigue, hot weather, rise in body temperature due to fever, trauma, and hot baths or showers.[7]

Over the last decade, treatment with disease-modifying agents has been developed. These agents have been found to reduce the frequency and severity of relapses, reduce the numbers of brain lesions as shown on MRI, and possibly reduce future disability. The medications are divided into two categories: (1) *immunomodulators*, which modify the immune system and include beta interferon 1a-intramuscular (Avonex [Biogen, Cambridge, Mass]), beta interferon 1a-subcutaneous (Rebif [Serono, Rockland, Mass]), beta interferon 1b (Betaseron [Berlex, Montville, NJ]), and glatiramer acetate (Copaxone [Teva Pharmaceuticals, Kansas City, Mo]); and (2) *immunosuppressants*, which shut down the immune system temporarily and include mitoxantrone (Novantrone [Serono, Rockland Mass]).[8]

AMYOTROPHIC LATERAL SCLEROSIS

Amyotrophic lateral sclerosis (ALS), also known as Lou Gehrig's disease, is the most common progressive neurodegenerative disease affecting adults. This disease involves the progressive degeneration of the motor neurons in the brain and the spinal cord. Progression of the disease is rapid, and death due to compromise of the respiratory system is noted within 2 to 5 years.[9]

Clinical symptoms include fasciculations (involuntary twitching of muscle fibers), muscle cramps, fatigue, weakness, and atrophy. There is a highly varied pattern of onset in ALS, with the most common pattern being LE onset, the second most common pattern being UE onset, followed by bulbar onset, and the least common pattern demonstrating symptoms in the distal musculature of the UEs and LEs. With each pattern of onset, the eventual progression of ALS is similar for most patients, with a spread of weakness to other muscle groups ultimately leading to complete paralysis. The cause of death is usually related to respiratory failure.[9]

There are several phases and stages that characterize the progression of ALS.[9]

Phase I

Phase I is termed *independent phase* and is characterized by the patient's ability to perform most everyday activities without any limitation. There are three stages under Phase I. In Stage 1, the patient exhibits mild weakness and complaints of "clumsiness." Stage 2 is characterized by more evident weakness affecting certain muscle groups. It is also in this stage that a noticeable decrease in the ability to perform ADLs appears. Stage 3 shows more severe selective weakness in the distal portions of the extremities. Respiration is also starting to be affected in this stage, as shown by increased fatigue and slight increase in breathing effort.

Phase II

Phase II is termed *partially independent*. As the name implies, the patient requires assistance in several ADLs in this phase. Phase II has two stages: Stages 4 and 5. In Stage 4, the patient is still able to perform most ADLs but tires easily. In terms of locomotion, the patient is mostly using a w/c at this point. Muscular weakness is evident, and tone abnormalities (spasticity) may be evident. More affectation in functional performance due to progression of the disease is evident in Stage 5, which is characterized by significant weakness of LEs and moderate to severe weakness of the UEs. Due to decreased mobility, the risk of skin breakdown is also evident in this stage.

Phase III

Phase III is termed the *dependent* phase of the disease. There is one stage under this phase, which is Stage 6. In this stage, the patient is bed bound and requires maximal assistance in ADLs. Respiratory function is severely compromised in this stage.

EXAMINATION AND EVALUATION: THE ROLE OF THE PHYSICAL THERAPIST ASSISTANT

The *physical therapy examination* of a patient with degenerative disease must be guided by several factors. First and foremost, it is important to identify from the patient's perspective the impact of the presenting signs and symptoms on his or her ability to function. It is important to determine, in terms of function, what the patient can and cannot do and then hypothesize the impairments that may be causing the identified functional limitations. The *Guide to Physical Therapist Practice*[10] (the *Guide*) is a helpful tool to guide the clinician in identifying the pertinent tests and measures that will provide the best representation of the patient's functional level. The PTA may be delegated portions of a reexamination (see Chapter 4), and it is of the utmost importance for the PTA to clearly communicate the results of the tests and measures to the PT.

As a PTA, it is important to identify the specific signs and symptoms associated with the condition, to monitor these signs and symptoms, and communicate to the supervising PT any significant changes in these signs, which may indicate the progression of symptoms, ineffectiveness of the prescribed physical therapy intervention, medication issues, or the possibility of other comorbidities. The rehabilitation team must be cognizant of other signs and symptoms that may necessitate referral to other medical practitioners. For example, symptoms of chest congestion, difficulty breathing, increased coughing, and mucus may be indicative of aspiration pneumonia and must be resolved expediently. This congestion may have been precipitated by decreased respiratory function (chest expansion, decreased inability to clear secretions, or ineffective cough) and is a fairly common complication in patients with degenerative disorders.

In looking at examination, it is important to identify the patient and family goals in making the determination regarding exercises and activities that will be implemented. Standardized functional tests often provide the clinician useful information regarding the impact of the disease progression on the patient's function. Serial testing of function allows the clinician to generate objective documentation of function; however, it should always follow a thoughtful interpretation of the results afforded by the PT. Examples of *general* functional tests that could be administered to patients with PD, MS, or ALS include the Performance Oriented Mobility Assessment (POMA),[11] Berg Balance Scale (BBS),[12] Functional Reach Test (FR)[13] or TUG.[14] These tests could give the clinician insights regarding the patient's level of function and risk of falls. Several disease-specific tests have also been developed: for PD, the United Parkinson's Disease Rating Scale (UPDRS),[15] and for MS, the Kurtzke Extended Disability Status Scale (EDSS).[16]

All the examination areas mentioned in Chapter 4 must be assessed in patients with degenerative diseases to provide the clinician with a clear picture of the patient's functional limitations, impairments, and disabilities.

INTERVENTION

Physical therapy intervention for patients with degenerative disorders should be based on the correction, remediation of, or compensation for the identified functional limitations and impairments. The *Guide*[10] identifies procedural interventions commonly used by PTs when treating patients with PD, MS, and ALS. All of the following interventions could be delegated to a PTA as long as the patient is stable and does not need ongoing (formal) assessment during the intervention period.

Aerobic and Endurance Conditioning and Reconditioning

The ability of the patient to have the cardiopulmonary capacity to be able to perform functional activities is central to optimal health and well being. Graded exercise must allow the patient to perform activities within the safe levels of cardiopulmonary functioning to allow the patient to tolerate increased activities. ADL training, gait, and locomotion activities can be incorporated to achieve this end. Aquatic exercise programs also allow the patient to perform these activities with less impact on the joints; however, increased workload due to increased hydrostatic pressure must be monitored accordingly. Examples of aerobic and endurance conditioning and reconditioning include the use of an upper body ergometer (UBE), LE pedal exerciser or an exercise bike, treadmill training, or walking using an appropriate assistive device, increasing distance as tolerated while making sure that vital signs are within safe limits. In terms of ADL training, the therapist can start with facilitation of simple ADL tasks (eg, maintaining sitting balance while the patient puts on socks and shoes) and then progress to those activities that require higher demands on the system in terms of postural control, coordination, endurance, and safety.

Balance, Coordination, and Agility Training

There must be an emphasis on decreasing the risk of falls to avoid the deconditioning effects of decreased activity and the medical complications following such an incident. Task-specific performance training could be employed to improve performance of everyday tasks, increase confidence in mobility activities, and improve quality of life. Vestibular training might be indicated to heighten the role of the vestibular system in balance tasks and compensate for loss in somatosensory and visual systems. Examples include standing weight-shifting activities with eyes open and eyes closed; standing or balancing on foam; tandem walking; braiding; Tai Ch'i; and maintaining balance while performing functional tasks like brushing teeth, getting something from the refrigerator or kitchen cabinets, or putting on socks and shoes. Balance exercises may be performed by incorporating them with ADLs, gait training, or endurance training. The therapist could start by having the patient sit upright, providing adequate support as necessary, instructing the patient to "sense" the upright position, improving stability in this position via compression (approximation through the shoulder will allow cocontraction and, therefore, stability), PNF rhythmic stabilization, and then strengthening the postural muscles using PNF or progressive resistance using manual and machine-generated resistance. Once the patient achieves relative stability in the static sitting position, the therapist can progress to working on dynamic sitting. To achieve this, the clinician could incorporate ADL training. For example, the clinician could ask the patient to reach for an object that is outside his or her BOS and then guide to make sure that the patient maintains balance. Performing isometric holds when the patient is in varying degrees of leaning will allow the patient to be stable in those increments of motion and achieve proprioceptive input in that position. The patient can then utilize the newly learned balance strategies in more ADLs (eg, putting on shoes and socks while sitting) or in recreational activities (eg, tossing a balloon, beanbag "basketball," or throwing darts). These same principles can be done while facilitating static and dynamic standing balance as well.

Flexibility Exercises

It is important for patients with degenerative diseases to maintain or improve their ROM and flexibility to allow for normal excursions of the body during functional tasks, thereby decreasing the risk of falls. Flexibility exercises also allow for easier transfers from one surface to another or easier performance of ADLs such as lower body hygiene and grooming. These exercises can also normalize tone, which is a major problem for patients with PD, MS, or ALS. As daily ROM is important, the patient must be taught how to perform self-assisted ROM activities and the family instructed on performing these activities. Examples include passive to active-assisted to active ROM of shoulder movements (flexion, abduction, and internal-external rotation), elbow (flexion and extension), forearm (pronation and supination), wrist and hand (flexion, extension, abduction, and adduction), hip (flexion, extension, abduction, and internal-external rotation), knee (flexion and extension), and ankle and foot (dorsiflexion, plantarflexion, inversion and eversion).

Relaxation

An often forgotten but nevertheless important component of a successful rehabilitation program for patients with degenerative disorders is relaxation training. Relaxation in the form of breathing exercises allows for increased oxygenation of the muscles and vital organs, thereby leading to increased performance and endurance, which may lead to improved swallowing and speech, while allowing chest expansion and improved posture in the process. Examples of activities include rhythmic breathing, progressive relaxation by contracting and relaxing muscle groups, and the use of imagery or music.

Neuromuscular Education or Reeducation

It is important to maintain the patient's ability to run normal functional motor programs to optimize functional performance. If this is impaired due to PD, MS, or ALS, the PTA could facilitate the performance of these functions using various neurological approaches that aim to allow for a window by which normal tone is achieved. These approaches facilitate the performance of normal movement while that window is open and consciously and consistently open and widen that window so the patient might eventually run an entire program sequence in the most efficient, effective, and functional manner possible. Examples of these neurological approaches include the use of Proprioceptive Neuromuscular Facilitation (PNF) or Neurodevelopmental Techniques (NDT) to strengthen muscle and facilitate functional mobility, transfers, or gait.

Gait and Locomotion Training

In addition to the benefits stated above, gait or locomotion training is important in the patient's functional independence. Being able to ambulate functional distances will allow the patient more freedom in movement (ie, ability to walk from the bedroom to the dining room or bathroom), as well as allowing him or her to be a more social and productive member of the community. If gait is not possible, the ability of the patient to safely and independently use an appropriate assistive device (ie, w/c) will improve power and endurance while allowing the patient to be as functional as possible. Examples include w/c mobility training and gait training using the appropriate assistive device on level or uneven surfaces while progressively decreasing assistance, as appropriate.

Activities of Daily Living Training

All of the activities mentioned above must have the ultimate goal of facilitating improvements in the performance of ADLs to allow the patient the highest level of independence possible. Examples include training for activities such as dressing, grooming, bathing, transfers, and bed mobility.

CLINICAL PEARLS

The following are suggestions from the field for approaches that might help patients with degenerative diseases:

Focus 1: Parkinson's Disease

1. Rotation is important. Trunk rotation should be part of any physical therapy intervention for PD unless contraindicated due to spinal conditions or surgery or other conditions that contraindicate trunk rotation. Rotation decreases the tone of the axial musculature, thereby decreasing trunk rigidity, and opens a window that will allow the patient to perform movements that are more normal and functional. Rotation can be done supine in bed in the morning (lower trunk rotations) before the patient gets up, in sitting throughout the day, and in standing (as long as the patient is safe in this position). Rocking also decreases tone. The PTA may want to instruct the patient

to sit in a rocking chair in the morning while reading the paper or having coffee – not only does this help decrease axial tone, but it also assists in peristalsis that may decrease constipation.

2. Encourage the patient to participate in group exercises. Group exercises allow the patient to engage in social activities; talk to other individuals who may have a similar condition or situation; and improve flexibility, strength, and endurance.

3. Imagery may help. Incorporation of visual imagery may assist in motor performance, whether contraction or relaxation. Teaching the patient to visualize being "strong and stable like a tree" may assist in improving standing balance; also, visualization may assist in relaxation ("imagine that you are relaxing in your favorite place...").

4. Music and rhythm may help. Music often gives the individual a rhythmical beat that overrides the freezing episodes and can be used very effectively with walking or gait interventions.

Focus 2: Multiple Sclerosis

1. Encourage the patient to achieve optimum health and well being. Together with the goal of maintaining the strength of the unaffected muscles to compensate for loss of strength of other muscle groups, encourage the patient to maintain a high overall level of fitness. In this regard, allow the patient to take the responsibility for his or her health and well being by daily exercise, appropriate nutrition and hydration, following the medical advice provided by the physician, and maintaining a positive and optimistic mental outlook.

2. Watch out for fatigue and overheating. As mentioned earlier, one precaution for patients and clients with MS is fatigue and decreased tolerance to heat. Always consider the environment where the treatment occurs. Regulate the temperature as to minimize overheating, which will cause fatigue of the patient. Timing and sequencing of the treatment are also important. Encourage the patient to perform the more difficult and potentially more fatiguing activities early in the day and to conserve energy where possible.

3. Improve balance and coordination. An optimum level of balance and coordination decreases the risk of falls and prevents the development of secondary complications, which may be detrimental to the patient. Examples of exercise are provided above; it is suggested that these exercises are done with the incorporation of functional training that will improve the quality of life.

4. Normalize tone (decrease spasticity) before training for functional tasks. Performance of functional tasks will have a longer carryover if performed over the foundation of as normal a tone and pattern as possible. In this regard, abnormal tone must be decreased first to "open a window" by which the foundation of normal movement can occur. Use of stretching, relaxation, and tone-inhibiting postures are some examples of interventions that can decrease spasticity.

5. Compensate for impaired sensation by teaching the patient frequent skin checks for skin breakdown, using appropriate footwear when walking, and being cognizant of situations where lack of protective sensation may be dangerous (eg, cooking, taking a bath, or walking on uneven surfaces).

6. Adapt the environment and use appropriate orthotic appliances to protect the joint and improve function and safety. The patient's environment can be modified to assist in energy conservation and more efficient movement. Orthotic devices like an AFO may allow the patient to transfer and ambulate safer and more efficiently while protecting the joint from injury.

7. Discuss with the supervising PT the need to refer the patient to appropriate medical professionals as necessary. The patient may present with other signs and symptoms that can be better managed by other health care professionals. Referral to a neuropsychiatrist, speech therapist, or OT may assist the patient in improving function.

Focus 3: Amyotrophic Lateral Sclerosis

1. Optimize cardiopulmonary function. Maintenance of good cardiopulmonary health is very important in patients with ALS to avoid the rapid decline in functional level due to secondary complications arising from decreased oxygenation. Examples of interventions include diaphragmatic breathing exercises, assisted cough (as necessary), and postural exercises to maintain optimal trunk alignment, which is important in efficient breathing. More complex equipment and intervention may be necessary with some patients or with patients in the more advanced stages of the disease, and a referral to

a physician and a respiratory therapist may be appropriate.

2. Maximize functional performance. While this may be true when discussing the rehabilitation of all patients, maintenance of the highest functional performance is of utmost importance with patients and clients with ALS. Emphasis must be on the achievement or maintenance of the abilities to perform vital activities such as mobility in bed, transferring, locomotion, sitting and standing balance, and toileting and hygiene activities. Patients will benefit from a ROM and muscle-strengthening program to prevent contractures and to maintain and improve strength. A home program consisting of these exercises, done independently by the patient or assisted by the caregiver, is appropriate. The use of adaptive equipment may allow for performance of activities without assistance and should be considered. This equipment ranges from orthotic appliances to assist in ambulation or improve ROM to reacher sticks and dressing aids. Under the umbrella of adaptive equipment are personal care aids, which will also assist in optimizing function when used.

3. Discuss with the PT the options available to improve communication. As patients with ALS lose the ability to communicate verbally due to paralysis of the muscles of speech, alternative communication strategies may be considered. This may be in the form of a basic communication board or more complex computer equipment.

4. Optimum psychological health is important. Maintaining a positive mental outlook decreases stress, which is detrimental to the body's immune response. Examples of approaches to achieve good psychological health include daily exercise, participation in support groups, psychological consultation, and good nutrition, among others. It is important to remember that a potential reason for an observed decline in functional performance is depression. The PTA should communicate this finding to the PT.

CONCLUSION

Patients and clients with *degenerative diseases of the CNS* often access and could benefit from physical therapy services. Appropriate intervention is based on the identified functional limitations and impairments. An individualized treatment program developed by the PT can be effectively carried out by the PTA. A variety of treatment approaches have been presented in this chapter. Communication between the PT and the PTA is important to ensure that the patient receives care that is appropriate and evidence-based to optimize the patient's level of health and wellness.

CHAPTER QUESTIONS

1. What are the common signs and symptoms of PD, MS, and ALS?

2. What are common intervention strategies a PTA may use when working with patients with PD, MS, or ALS?

3. Why is rotation an important intervention when working with patients with PD?

4. What are two "clinical pearls" that can assist a PTA when working with patients with PD?

5. What precautions should you take during treatment sessions when working with a patient with MS?

6. What are four "clinical pearls" that can assist a PTA when working with patients with MS?

7. What interventions can you use to optimize the cardiopulmonary function of patients with ALS?

CASE STUDIES

For each of the following patient scenarios, identify the following:

a. Impairments and functional limitations presented.

b. Potential interventions that can be performed by the PTA to assist in improving the patient's functional performance.

Case #1: Parkinson's Disease

MG is a 72-year-old male who was diagnosed with PD 12 years ago. The client resides in an independent living facility with his wife. The environment provides the client with a wide spectrum of social interaction and cognitive challenges as well as good access to health care. MG is cognitively aware of his surroundings and the effects of his illness. He cites unsteadiness when walking and dressing, poor night vision, and occasional drooling as symptoms he experiences.

The client currently takes Sinemet and Mirapex. The subject reports that he experiences freezing episodes when his medications wear off. As a result, he and his wife carefully plan outings around peak medication times. The client reports increasing difficulty with ambulation and ADLs such as transfers, dressing, and bathing. The client also reports increased falls in the past several weeks. He is afraid that he might sustain severe injuries following a serious fall in the future.

The client presents with a stooped posture, rounded shoulders, and thoracic kyphosis. He ambulates to the department with a festinating gait. He also presents with pill-rolling tremor at rest. He transfers from the bed to the mat with minimal assistance. Functional mobility testing shows that the client is independent with bed mobility but requires minimal assistance to sit from the supine position. He requires minimal assist to perform sit to stand. Sitting balance is Good, while standing balance is Fair. ROM is within functional limits to all 4 extremities. Patient demonstrates weakness in his bilateral LEs. Patient demonstrates trunk rigidity. The patient scored a 17/28 in the Tinetti Balance and Gait tests, indicating risk for falls. The patient scored 6 inches in the Functional Reach test, and this also indicates a risk for falls. The Berg Balance test was also administered, and the patient scored a 38/56, also indicating a risk for falls.

Case #2: Multiple Sclerosis

P is a 45-year-old female who was diagnosed with MS 5 years ago. She currently works part-time as a telemarketer and has a phone and computer setup, which allows her to work at home. She reports progressive decline in functional ability in the past few years. She has had several periods of exacerbations and remissions since the diagnosis. She lives with her husband and a teenage daughter who both help her with her daily activities. Her current complaints include weakness of the LEs, fatigue, and bouts of vision disturbances (double vision). She reports lack of sleep at night due to leg cramps. The patient also mentions falling several times, usually during the night when she gets up to go to the bathroom.

The patient is able to ambulate independently at home, holding onto walls and furniture for support, as needed. In the community, she is able to ambulate short distances using a front-wheeled walker but fatigues easily. She uses a w/c as her primary mode of locomotion when outside.

ROM testing reveals tightness of bilateral hamstrings and calf muscles. Tone assessment using the modified Ashworth scale reveals a grade of 2 in the LEs. The patient demonstrates impaired UE and LE light touch and proprioception sensation, with the LEs more affected than the UEs.

Bed mobility, supine to sit, and transfers to the w/c are independent, but the patient performs these movements slowly. Sitting balance is Good for static and Fair+ to Good for dynamic. Balance in standing is Good static and Fair dynamic.

Patient scored a 16/28 in the Tinetti Balance and Gait Test and a 41/56 for the Berg Balance Test. Both of these tests indicate the patient's increased risk for falls.

Case #3: Amyotrophic Lateral Sclerosis

The patient is a 58-year-old male with a medical diagnosis of ALS. He reports that he was diagnosed with the condition 2 years ago. The patient is a retired truck driver and lives in a doublewide trailer with his girlfriend, who is his primary caregiver. The patient received home health supportive services: a nurse visits every month and a home health aide every other day to assist him with self-care activities.

The patient is still capable of speech communication, but his caregiver reports that the patient's speech is getting worse. The patient also reports difficulty in breathing at night and gets supplemental oxygen. During the time of the examination, the patient's vital signs are as follows: BP is 120/90, pulse is 88, and respiration is 20.

The patient is incontinent of bladder and has a foley catheter in place. Inspection of the skin reveals a slightly reddened sacral area.

He is able to move in bed with minimal assistance and use of the overhead trapeze bar. He requires minimal assistance to get up from supine to sit and to transfer from the bed to the w/c. The patient demonstrates poor sitting and standing balance. He is able to stand with minimal assist and take a few steps with assistance, but is unable to functionally ambulate. The patient uses the w/c as his primary mode of locomotion.

The patient demonstrates bilateral plantarflexion contractures and some tightness of both hamstrings. He has spasticity of both LEs (Grade 2 on the modified Ashworth Scale). Strength of both LEs and UEs is generally 3 to 3+/5. Patient demonstrates absent proprioception for both LEs and impaired light touch sensation bilaterally.

Suggested author answers are available at www.slackbooks.com/neuroquestions.

REFERENCES

1. Schenkman M, Cutson TM, Kichibhatla M, Chandler J, Pieper C. Reliability of impairment and physical performance measures with Parkinson's disease. *Physical Therapy.* 1997;77(1):19-27.

2. Melnick ME. Basal ganglia disorders: metabolic, hereditary, and genetic disorders in adults. In: Umphred DA, ed. *Neurological Rehabilitation.* 4th ed. St. Louis, Mo: Mosby; 2001:669-670.

3. Marsden CD. On-off phenomena in Parkinson's disease. In: Rinne UK, Klinger M, Stamm G, eds. *Parkinson's Disease: Current Progress, Problems, and Management.* Amsterdam, The Netherlands: Biomedical Press; 1990.

4. Koller WC, Glatt S, Vetere-Overfield B, Hassanein R. Falls and Parkinson's disease. *Clin Neuropharm.* 1989;12(2):98-105.

5. Aita JF. Why patients with Parkinson's disease fall. *JAMA.* 1982;247(4):515-516.

6. *New Parkinson's Drug Receives Marketing Clearance.* Mirapex is the first new Parkinson's drug cleared in U.S. this decade. http://www.nyschp.org/the_pharmacist/aug97/parkdrug.html. Accessed May 31, 2005.

7. Frankel D. Multiple sclerosis. In: Umphred DA, ed. *Neurological Rehabilitation.* 4th ed. St. Louis, Mo: Mosby; 2001:595-599.

8. National Multiple Sclerosis Society. The National MS Society's disease management consensus statement. http://www.nationalmssociety.org/Sourcebook-Early.asp. Accessed June 2, 2005.

9. Hallum A. Neuromuscular diseases. In: Umphred DA, ed. *Neurological Rehabilitation.* 4th ed. St. Louis, Mo: Mosby; 2001:377-378.

10. *Guide to Physical Therapist Practice*, 2nd ed. Alexandria, Va: American Physical Therapy Association; 2001.

11. Tinetti ME. Performance-oriented assessment of mobility problems in the elderly. *J Am Geriatr Soc.* 1986;34:119-126.

12. Berg K. Measuring balance in the elderly: validation of an instrument. *Physiother Canada.* 1989;41:304.

13. Duncan PW, et al. Functional reach: a new clinical measure of balance. *J Gerontol.* 1990;45:M192.

14. Podsiadlo D, Richardson S. The timed "up and go": a test of basic functional mobility for frail elderly persons. *J Am Geriatr Soc.* 1991;39:142.

15. Stebbins GT, Goetz. Factor structure of the Unified Parkinson's Disease Rating Scale: motor examination section. *Mov Disord.* 1998;13(4):633-636.

16. Kurtzke JF. A new scale for evaluating disability in multiple sclerosis. *Neurology.* 1955;5:580.

Chapter

13

CARDIOPULMONARY ISSUES ASSOCIATED WITH NEUROREHABILITATION PATIENTS

Christine R. Wilson, PT, PhD

KEY WORDS

aerobic exercise
asthma
breathing retraining
cardiac
chronic obstructive pulmonary disease (COPD)
congestive heart failure
cystic fibrosis
myocardial infarction
pulmonary
vascular

CHAPTER OBJECTIVES

- Describe the basic anatomy and physiology of the cardiovascular and pulmonary systems.

- Describe how neuromuscular pathologies can affect cardiovascular and pulmonary function.

- Describe common cardiovascular and pulmonary comorbidities seen in neurorehabilitation.

- Describe physical therapy examination, evaluation, and intervention tools and skills used in individuals with primary or secondary cardiovascular and pulmonary problems and which are appropriate for the PTA.

- Describe the signs and symptoms indicating that the PTA should instruct the patient to stop exercising.

INTRODUCTION

Movement is not possible unless the neuromuscular system receives adequate oxygenation and the waste product carbon dioxide is continuously removed. The cardiopulmonary system is responsible for carrying out this task: oxygen enters and carbon dioxide exits the body via the pulmonary system, and blood is pumped through the lungs and to the rest of the body by the cardiovascular system. Any problem within the *pulmonary* or *cardiac* systems resulting in inadequate oxygen delivery and/or inadequate carbon dioxide removal can contribute to functional movement difficulties within both the neuromuscular and musculoskeletal systems. Therefore, whenever a therapist is working with an individual in neurorehabilitation, the therapist needs to attend to pathological changes affecting the cardiovascular and pulmonary systems. These problems may interfere with movement capability and magnify the existing neuromuscular problems. The purposes of this chapter are to (1) review how neuromuscular pathologies can directly affect cardiac, vascular, and respiratory function; (2) discuss some of the major primary cardiovascular and pulmonary comorbidities, which may be seen in individuals in the neurorehabilitation setting; and (3) to introduce the examination, evaluation, and intervention tools and skills which may be used. The PTA may be asked to perform some functional exams subsequent to the initial evaluation and be responsible for delegated intervention. For these reasons, the PTA must have some understanding of the evaluation process.

BRIEF REVIEW OF ANATOMY AND PHYSIOLOGY OF CARDIOVASCULAR AND PULMONARY SYSTEMS

One of the main features shared by the *cardiovascular* and *pulmonary* systems is the pumping action that is required. The heart contracts about 80 times per min in order to pump blood through the pulmonary and systemic vessels. The ventilatory muscles and the thoraco-abdominal skeleton form the ventilatory pump, which moves air into and out of the lungs about 15 times per min. Air travels into the body from the nose and/or mouth through the pharynx, larynx, trachea, and progressively smaller airways (bronchi and bronchioles) until it reaches the alveolus. The alveolus is a thin-walled structure comprised of two cell types: thin cells that form the structure of the alveolus and surfactant producing cells. Surfactant is a soaplike substance that decreases the alveolar surface tension, allowing the ventilatory pump to generate smaller pressures to bring air into the lungs. Covered with pulmonary capillaries, the alveoli are the only places where the exchange of oxygen and carbon dioxide gases can occur. The accumulation of any fluid and/or mucous in an alveolus will interfere with gas exchange.

The four-chambered heart is comprised of atria, which receive blood, and ventricles, which pump blood out of the heart. The right side of the heart receives poorly oxygenated blood from the systemic circulation and pumps it through the pulmonary artery into the lungs. The left side of the heart receives well-oxygenated blood from the pulmonary veins and pumps it through the aorta into the systemic arteries, arterioles, and capillaries, which bring blood to the rest of the body. The heart receives its supply of well-oxygenated blood through coronary arteries, which branch off the aorta. The systemic circulation is regulated so that the brain will receive the same blood flow under conditions of rest or exercise.[1,2] If the exchange of oxygen or the pumping from the heart is compromised, the brain will still take the amount of blood it requires to function. As a result, some patients have insufficient oxygen delivered to skeletal muscles to allow proper functioning and, thus, fatigue quickly. The PTA needs to observe whether the patient has labored breathing during movement and whether that breathing is followed by complaints of being tired or whether the patient demonstrates signs of muscle fatigue.

NEUROMUSCULAR PATHOLOGIES AFFECTING CARDIOVASCULAR AND PULMONARY FUNCTION

Several types of neuromuscular pathologies are associated with direct effects on cardiovascular function. SCI can disrupt autonomic nerve fibers that regulate vasoconstriction and vasodilation. Normally, when an individual changes from a supine to an upright posture (sitting or standing), the vessels vasoconstrict to prevent blood from pooling in the legs. After some SCIs, this reflex is lost, and the individual can easily become hypotensive during positional changes. Hypotension means that the BP is low. This can cause dizziness due to inadequate cerebral blood flow and shortness of breath due to inadequate blood flow and gas exchange in the lungs. For this reason, patients may need frequent monitoring through use of a BP device. The PTA may be asked to perform this function during intervention sessions.

Adequate ventilatory pumping action requires (1) appropriate descending neural motor output from the brainstem respiratory control centers, (2) intact peripheral neuro-motor innervation of the ventilatory muscles, (3) adequate neurotransmitter release and binding at the junction between the end of the nerve and the muscle, and (4) ventilatory muscle contraction generating sufficient force. Problems in any of these areas can interfere with normal breathing. For example, an individual who has had a right cerebrovascular accident affecting the cerebral cortex and, thus, the motor innervation going to the muscles on the left side of the body may have decreased ventilatory movements of the left chest wall. This patient may have difficulty generating an adequate breath or a strong cough. Due to the bilateral innervation of the trunk and, thus, the chest wall muscles, an individual with a CVA may have bilateral involvement within the ventilatory system. Another individual with muscular dystrophy might need to use a mechanical ventilator because the ventilatory muscles are too weak to cause adequate ventilatory pumping movements due to degeneration of the muscles themselves (see Chapter 8). Any individual whose neuromuscular problem causes significant spinal curvature, such as kyphosis and/or scoliosis, will have additional difficulty generating adequate ventilatory pumping because the structural limitations affect the ability of the muscles to function adequately. Obviously, the cardiopulmonary problems discussed so far are secondary to existing pathology, and the disease process will affect the outcome of physical therapy. For this reason, the PT may delegate an intervention that incorporates breathing exercises during a functional activity that specifically focuses upon the functional limitations of the patient with CNS deficits.

PRIMARY CARDIOVASCULAR AND PULMONARY PATHOLOGIES

Cardiovascular Pathologies

The term *congestive heart failure* refers to a group of symptoms caused by inadequate ventricular pumping action, which can result from various pathologies.[3-5] Pumping ability can be decreased by damage to the heart muscle, caused by myocardial infarct (commonly called a heart attack) or cardiomyopathy, or valvular narrowing which impedes blood from leaving the ventricle. When left heart failure occurs, inadequate cardiac output (amount of blood leaving the heart per minute) can decrease blood flow to the brain and peripheral organs, causing light-headedness, dizziness, and hypotension. Since the left ventricle is unable to pump enough blood through the aorta, blood can back up into the lungs, causing pulmonary edema (fluid leaking from the pulmonary vessels into the alveoli). Pulmonary edema is associated with wheezing, a cough productive of white or pinkish (caused by the presence of red blood cells) frothy secretions, poor arterial oxygenation, and dyspnea (shortness of breath). Right heart failure causes blood to back up through the vena cavae into the venous system. This can cause visible distension of the jugular veins, swelling of the extremities, and fluid retention in the liver (causing hepatomegaly) and abdominal cavity (ascites). With the right heart not adequately pumping deoxygenated blood into the lungs, the individual will also display signs of shortness of breath. The PTA is not responsible for differentiating whether the shortness of breath is due to right or left heart failure, muscular problems, or anxiety. The PTA is responsible for recognizing the signs and symptoms and reporting it to the PT. If the PT is not available, the PTA should report this problem to the doctor and/or a nurse depending upon the specific clinical site.

Atherosclerosis can lead to narrowing of arterial vessels in many parts of the body, most commonly vessels supplying the brain, heart, and LEs.[3] Vessel narrowing can lead to ischemia (lack of adequate oxygen in the tissue) and, if ischemia is prolonged, infarction (death) of the tissue that is being deprived of the oxygen. Inadequate blood supply to the brain (due to head trauma or stroke) is discussed in other chapters of this text; therefore, this chapter will discuss pathologies involving the coronary vessels (which supply the heart) and the peripheral arteries (which supply the extremities).

When cardiac muscle is inadequately perfused (supplied) with blood, an individual may feel squeezing, tightness, or pain in the chest (angina) or pain in the jaw, back, or arm (especially the left). Other symptoms include nausea and heartburn.[4] Persons with diabetes or SCI whose cardiac sensory nerves are impaired may not experience pain or tightness when either cardiac ischemia or infarction is occurring. It is important to identify the onset of cardiac ischemia so that (1) the workload on the heart can be immediately decreased by stopping activity, and (2) the coronary blood flow can be increased by medication in order to prevent permanent damage to the cardiac muscle. Patients who have a history of cardiac ischemia frequently carry nitroglycerin medication with them to take when symptoms occur. The PTA is responsible for stopping intervention if it has been delegated to him or her. The PTA should call the PT or the physician before administering any medication unless instructed beforehand. The family members may be aware of the physician's recommendation and administer the medication if the PTA is in a home health environment.

The terms *arrhythmia* and *dysrhythmia* describe an irregular beating of the heart. This can be caused by cardiac ischemia or by damage to the specialized cells within the heart that transmit electrical impulses through the atria and ventricles. When an arrhythmia occurs, some individuals describe a fluttering or pounding sensation in the chest. Others may feel breathless, lightheaded, or dizzy, and some individuals may have no symptoms. If the arrhythmia causes a decrease in the cardiac output the individual may not be able to tolerate his or her usual level of activity and may complain of feeling tired. A change in the rhythm or strength of pulse can indicate the development of an arrhythmia. Monitoring pulse and BP before and after activity is a routine part of rehabilitation with any individual with activity intolerance. The therapist or PTA may need to monitor heart rate and BP several times during an intervention time period. This monitoring becomes a critical component of working with an individual with known cardiac or pulmonary disease.

Peripheral arterial disease involves narrowing or blockage of arterial vessels and predominantly affects the LEs. Inadequate blood flow usually occurs under conditions that require increased LE blood flow. For example, symptoms usually occur during some type of LE activity since blood flow must be increased to provide sufficient oxygen and nutrients to the contracting muscles. Individuals with peripheral arterial disease tend to report leg pain or discomfort after walking a certain distance. Once the patient stops walking, the pain or discomfort is relieved.

A deep vein thrombosis (DVT) is a blood clot that usually occurs in the LE, causing redness, swelling, warmth, and tenderness. This is a dangerous condition because a portion of the clot can break off and form an embolus, traveling through the venous system, into the heart, and lodge in a pulmonary vessel. Once it is wedged in a vessel within the lungs, it is called a pulmonary embolus. The embolus prevents blood from entering that portion of the lung, and may cause hypoxemia (decreased arterial oxygenation), breathlessness (dyspnea), rapid breathing, and chest pain. Since pulmonary emboli can be fatal, it is critical that any suspected DVTs are promptly evaluated by the doctor in order for anticoagulation therapy to be initiated. Individuals with DVTs should not participate in physical activity until laboratory blood tests of clotting indicate that anticoagulant therapy is effective and medical clearance has been obtained.

Pulmonary Pathologies

Chronic obstructive pulmonary disease (COPD) is one of the most common diseases in the United States.[5] Broadly categorized, COPD refers to asthma, bronchiectasis, chronic bronchitis, emphysema, and cystic fibrosis. However, the term COPD is usually used clinically to describe an individual with disease characteristic of emphysema, chronic bronchitis, or a combination of both. Emphysema is a disease caused by destruction of the elastic tissue of the lung.[5] This decreases the elastic recoil of the lung that causes expiratory air flow and results in the trapping of excess air in the lung (termed *hyperinflation*). The patient with emphysema may have an enlarged thorax (barrel chest), may use accessory muscles during resting breathing (especially sternocleidomastoid and upper trapezius), and may complain of dyspnea (breathing discomfort) at rest or during exercise. Chronic bronchitis is diagnosed clinically when an individual has had a productive cough (a cough which produces mucous) for 3 months per year for 2 years.[5] In addition to causing hyperinflation, this disease decreases oxygenation of arterial blood, which can cause the individual to become cyanotic, evidenced by bluish lips, mucous membranes, or conjunctiva.[3]

Asthma is a very common disease in both children and adults. It is characterized by inflammation which reverses spontaneously or with medication.[5,6] Individuals with asthma may alternate between periods of normal lung function and asthmatic episodes characterized by airway narrowing (caused by spasm of the smooth muscle surrounding the small airways), wheezing or coughing, and dyspnea. These episodes may be triggered by exposure to allergens, respiratory infections, cold environments, or exercise. The prevalence of asthma has increased,[5] and it is now recognized that asthma must be well controlled through medication and/or avoidance of events which trigger asthmatic episodes. When working with children, the parents should inform the PT that the child has asthma if it has been diagnosed. If the child does not have this medical diagnosis and the intervention has been delegated to the PTA, the PTA needs to identify whether the child is having breathing difficulty and immediately report these problems to the PT. If the patient is an adult, either the patient or the family can usually report if asthma has been diagnosed.

Bronchiectasis is characterized by abnormal dilation of 1 or more airways.[5] The disease can be acute or chronic, and the disease severity is usually determined by the number of airways affected. Inflammation is present in the affected airways, which can lead to an increase in the amount of mucous produced and trapping of the mucous in the dilated portion of the airway. This mucous will limit gas exchange. The patient may have difficulties even at rest, but the symptoms will become exaggerated during exercise.

Cystic fibrosis is a genetic disease, which is usually diagnosed in childhood. It affects exocrine glands of the body and results in overproduction and retention of mucous in the lungs and gastrointestinal tract. This causes hyperinflation, a chronically productive cough, and deficiencies in certain gastrointestinal enzymes, leading to decreased fat absorption by the gastrointestinal tract.[3-5] A PT may delegate the intervention of postural drainage to a PTA in order to assist the child in eliminating the excessive mucous within the lungs.

COMMON DISABILITIES, FUNCTIONAL LIMITATIONS, AND IMPAIRMENTS OF THE CARDIOPULMONARY SYSTEM

Physical activity requires the cardiovascular system to increase blood flow through the lungs and to the working muscle and requires the pulmonary system to increase the rate and depth of breathing in order to provide adequate gas exchange. Therefore, any decrement in cardiovascular and/or pulmonary system functioning will incrementally compound functional limitations as exercise intensity increases. Symptoms include breathlessness (dyspnea), fatigue, wheezing, chest pain, lightheadedness, and dizziness. Asthmatic individuals may develop a cough rather than the classic sign of wheezing. An individual undergoing cardiopulmonary stress may become cyanotic and have a rapid, shallow breathing pattern with increased accessory muscle usage and flaring of the nostrils. Headaches, disorientation, and confusion can occur if ventilation is inadequate. An individual may speak in short sentences, use only a few words, or speak rapidly because he cannot bring in enough air to speak in a usual fashion. As the individual decreases his daily activity level, activity tolerance decreases, and an individual with a chronic cardiovascular and/or pulmonary problem can lose both strength and endurance due to decreased skeletal muscle use.

EXAMINATION TOOLS, TESTS, AND MEASURES USED TO EVALUATE CARDIOVASCULAR AND PULMONARY FUNCTION

Physical examination of the cardiovascular and pulmonary system is divided into four categories: observation, palpation, percussion, and auscultation.[7] Observation refers to visual assessment of the individual, including assessment for cyanosis, edema, posture, accessory ventilatory muscle usage (evidenced by contraction of the sternocleidomastoid, upper trapezius, and/or abdominal muscles during resting breathing) and abnormal motions of the thorax and abdomen during resting breathing. Palpation includes palpation of the thorax for any areas of tenderness and palpating a pulse to assess heart rate and the thorax to assess respiratory rate. In addition, palpation of peripheral pulses in the LEs is performed to help determine if blood flow throughout the limb is normal. Percussion refers to tapping the thorax to determine the size of the heart, the level of the diaphragm, and the presence of excess air or fluid in the lungs. Auscultation refers to using a stethoscope to listen to the heart and lungs in order to determine if the heart sounds and breath sounds are normal or if there are any extra sounds, such as murmurs or wheezes. Sometimes, wheezing can be heard without using a stethoscope.

Pulmonary function tests (PFTs) are a series of tests that are commonly used by physicians to assess function of the respiratory system. Sometimes PFTs are performed before and after the patient inhales a bronchodilator medication to see if prescribing a medication might improve ventilation. The PFT measurements are reported in actual values and as percentages of the predicted value for that person based on height, sex, and age. Two commonly taken measurements are the total amount of air that can be exhaled (FVC) and the amount of air that can be exhaled (forced expiratory volume, FEV1) in 1 second. A normal FEV1/FVC ratio is about 0.80.[8] Pulmonary function tests can also include measurements of lung volumes, expiratory flow rates, and diffusing capacity (the ability of oxygen to diffuse from the alveolus into the pulmonary capillary). Lastly, inspiratory and expiratory (maximal inspiratory pressure [MIP] and maximal expiratory pressure [MEP]) muscle pressure measurements provide information about respiratory muscle strength.[9] The PTA may find any one or all of these measurements within the chart of a patient who has pulmonary problems either as a primary disease or secondary to a CNS problem.

Pulse oximetry can be used to give an approximation of oxygen saturation in the arterial blood.[10] A probe is usually placed on the finger or ear, and the monitor will provide an average saturation value, SpO$_2$. (The "p" indicates that the value is obtained using pulse oximetry.) Normal SpO$_2$ is at least 95%, which indicates that 95% of the hemoglobin sites are bound with oxygen. Pulse oximeters are used in many settings, from the intensive care unit to the outpatient or home setting. A PTA may be asked to monitor a patient's oxygen saturation value during an intervention session. The PT should identify the acceptable range of the S$_p$O$_2$ value as a treatment parameter for the PTA. If the oxygen saturation value drops below to lower limit, the PTA should stop the treatment and consult with the PT.

Exercise tolerance can be assessed in several ways. A stress test (also called an exercise tolerance test or graded exercise test) can be conducted by a physician to determine how much exercise an individual can tolerate and how the cardiovascular and pulmonary systems respond to exercise.[11,12] Stress tests are usually done on a treadmill or stationary cycle but can also be performed using an arm ergometer or a w/c. A 12-lead electrocardiogram (ECG) is monitored throughout the test so that any cardiac dysrhythmia or ischemia can be detected. In addition, BP readings are taken periodically throughout the test, and pulse oximetry is also used. The individual is asked periodically to rate how hard he is working using the Borg scale (also called the Rating of Perceived Exertion) or modified Borg scale.[13] Although the PTA is not responsible for measuring or interpreting any of the previous tests, the PTA may be asked to monitor patient responses that directly relate to the above-mentioned tests. The PT should identify the acceptable parameters during exercise. If the parameters are exceeded, the PTA should stop the intervention and consult with the PT. It is not the PTA's responsibility to determine why the value has changed.

PTs frequently use a 6- or 12-minute walk test (6MWT, 12MWT) to get baseline information on walking capability. This is a submaximal test where the individual is asked to walk as far as possible in the allotted time, and the outcome measure is the distance walked.[13] The individual may stop walking momentarily or take sitting breaks during the test, as necessary. These rests will be reflected in a shorter distance walked during the test. The reproducibility of this test is improved by having the individual take two practice tests and walk the same path within the same environment each time the test is taken.

INTERVENTION

Individuals with neurological conditions may have difficulty inspiring adequate air to clear secretions, generating an effective cough, or providing adequate gas exchange during increased activity. An intervention program designed for an individual participating in neurorehabilitation who has a concomitant cardiovascular and/or pulmonary condition may include interventions that specifically address those conditions. These interventions may include breathing exercise, coughing, airway clearance, strengthening and endurance training of inspiratory and/or expiratory muscles, chest wall mobility, and aerobic training.[9,13-16] Breathing exercises may involve encouraging the individual to move different areas of the chest wall during inspiration (eg, upper abdominal region [*diaphragmatic breathing*], lower ribs, middle chest wall, upper chest and sternum). By learning to move different areas of the chest wall, the individual may breathe more deeply, which may improve gas exchange. Other inspiratory breathing exercises include taking successive breaths of increasing depth and maintaining a maximal inspiration for several seconds. In the early postoperative period, incentive spirometers may be used with individuals to encourage deeper inspirations.[17] These disposable devices indicate the volume inspired with each breath, providing patients with a visual target that can be modified as inspiratory capacity improves. Individuals with obstructive lung diseases such as asthma and COPD may be encouraged to exhale gently through pursed lips, a technique known as pursed lip breathing. By preventing the smaller airways from collapsing prematurely, pursed lip breathing may improve the ability of the individual with obstructive lung disease to exhale more completely. Thus, the PTA may be asked to emphasize breathing alone or during exercise. Asking the patient to take a very slow deep breath and then to exhale through pursed lips affect both inhalation and expiration and, as a result, increase the patient's oxygenation process.

Coughing is a reflexive activity that prevents the inhalation of injurious particles or gases and expels excess secretions that are produced in the lungs. Individuals with weak coughs are less able to maintain healthy lungs. Persons with a lung disease causing excess secretion production (such as chronic bronchitis) are at an even higher risk for developing lung infections and may be taught to regularly cough voluntarily in order to prevent secretion accumulation in the lung. An effective cough requires a good inspiration; bringing the vocal folds together (closure of the glottis); strong contraction of the abdominal, intercostals, and pelvic floor muscles; and movement of the vocal folds away from each other. Cough strength may be improved by various movements during the expulsive phase, such as leaning forward, flexing the spine, pulling in the stomach, or using the hands or forearms to push the stomach inward.[9,13-16] Individuals who are not able to adequately contract the abdominal muscles [such as an individual who has a SCI] may be assisted in coughing by having another individual place a hand over the upper abdomen and push upward and inward during the expulsive phase. This assisted coughing maneuver is sometimes referred to as a *quad cough*. Care must be taken to ensure that the assisting individual's hand is below the xiphoid process in order to avoid injury. Sometimes, cough strength can be improved by coughing 2 or 3 times after one inspiration. Most individuals find that the strongest cough occurs in a sitting position, but this may vary. If a poor inspiration is the cause of a weak cough, techniques mentioned earlier to improve the depth of inspiration can be utilized. Weakness of the pelvic floor muscles may lead to urinary incontinence during a cough, a problem that is described by many older individuals. Strengthening of the pelvic floor muscles during functional activities may be indicated and may decrease the patient's fear of urinating in public when a voluntary or reflexive cough is produced. Some individuals are unable to voluntarily generate the vocal fold motions, which cause the explosive element of a cough. In this case, huffing is taught. Huffing involves a rapid, forceful exhalation and can be very effective in expelling secretions from the lung.

Individuals with lung diseases causing chronic or recurrent secretion production may be instructed to perform regular postural drainage. Postural drainage involves having the patient put him- or herself in a position that drains the congested region of the lung and voluntarily coughing to clear secretions after several minutes in the position. The patient may require the use of many positions if secretions are present throughout both lungs. Secretion movement may be facilitated by having another individual perform manual techniques such as percussion, vibration, or shaking over the congested lung region while the patient is in the position. Percussion involves tapping with a cupped hand on the chest wall throughout the respiratory cycle. Vibration and shaking are performed during expiration only, and require the assisting individual to make small and large oscillating movements, respectively. When manual techniques are used, the patient may only need to lie in a position for about 2 min before secretions move and can be expelled. Many of these techniques may be delegated to the PTA with the expectation that the patient's breathing and exercise tolerance will improve.

Individuals with neurological disorders may have weakness of the ventilatory muscles. Inspiratory muscle weakness may be associated with hypoxemia and/or hypercapnia, and expiratory muscle weakness may interfere with the ability to generate an effective cough. Strength is measured using a special dynamometer, which prevents the movement of air and measures the pressure generated during a maximal inspiratory or expiratory maneuver. Maximum inspiratory pressures are referred to as MIP, PImax, or MSIP (maximum static inspiratory pressure), and maximum expiratory pressures are referred to as MEP, PEmax or MSEP (maximum static expiratory pressure). These abbreviations are often found in the chart. If ventilatory pressures are low, muscle training can be instituted using a device that makes inspiration or expiration more difficult by having the individual move air through a smaller orifice (resistive loading) or by having the individual generate a certain pressure before air flow can occur (threshold loading device).[9]

A limited ability to move the chest wall might result in a stiff thorax that either cannot expand fully or requires the generation of more muscular force to expand. This problem is commonly found in patients with a chronic pulmonary disease as well as individuals following CNS injury. Therefore, maintaining or improving thoracic flexibility may be a critical component of a patient's overall improvement. Activities that emphasize rotation of the thoracolumbar spine help to maintain the width of the intercostal spaces. In addition, interventions that focus on maintaining full motion of the scapula, spine, head, and neck will assist in maintaining flexibility as well as relaxing accessory muscles, which may be chronically used to assist ventilation. These activities can be done in sidelying, sitting, or standing. Truck and head rotation during reaching is often delegated to the PTA. Emphasis should be placed on the success of the functional activity, which will automatically encourage rotation of the thoracolumbar spine. Having the patient reach toward the floor/ceiling, right/left, or forward/backward helps to mobilize the spine, thoracic cage, shoulder girdle muscles, and neck. Encouraging the patient to coordinate breathing with the activity will discourage breath holding. Putting both components into one functional activity may optimize the integration of the motor program into everyday life.

Most individuals participating in neurorehabilitation cannot maintain their premorbid activity level. This decrease in activity leads to a state of muscle deconditioning, when muscle fibers become less efficient and require more oxygen to support a given level of activity. Biopsies from LE muscles in individuals with either chronic obstructive pulmonary disease or congestive heart failure have shown that the number of oxidative (aerobic) enzymes is markedly decreased in these muscle fibers. Therefore, aerobic

(endurance) training activities can be included in some programs. An aerobic training program involves exercising a large muscle mass for extended periods of time in order to improve cardiorespiratory fitness. Walking and cycling are typical examples, but other types of activities can be incorporated into a training program as well (eg, w/c propulsion). When an aerobic training program begins at a very low level (eg, an interval program consisting of repeated bouts of slow walking for 60 seconds and resting for 30 seconds), the duration of the activity is gradually progressed in order to improve fitness. Although a PTA may be delegated a specific intervention protocol including breathing, aerobic training, and progressive resistive exercises, every patient's activity tolerance will be unique. With primary and/or secondary limitations within the cardiopulmonary system, the PT will often prescribe endurance training with repetitive practice, and the intervention may be delegated as long as the patient is stable. The PTA should be given clear instructions with respect to acceptable values of oxygen saturation, HR, and BP and signs and symptoms to watch for that indicate exercise intolerance.

CONCLUSION

Any individual in a neurorehabilitation program who has difficulty tolerating activity may be limited by a cardiac, vascular, or pulmonary problem that prevents adequate oxygen from being delivered to the working muscles. The PTA should look for the signs and symptoms associated with these problems in order to determine whether it is safe to continue with an intervention program or whether the intervention should be postponed until the PT (or another health professional) can evaluate the patient. As stated earlier, any shortness of breath, dizziness, complaints of muscle cramping, or chest discomfort might indicate that the individual is approaching or already has reached a level of physiological fatigue and that exercise needs to stop. The PTA's role is to recognize any of these behaviors and report them immediately to the PT. If the PTA has any question regarding the safety of a patient during exercise, the intervention should be stopped, the PT notified, and clearance made by the PT before resuming the functional exercise.

CHAPTER QUESTIONS

Regarding interactions between the cardiopulmonary and neuromuscular systems:

1. During an exercise session, how can a PTA monitor the cardiovascular and pulmonary response to exercise?

2. The appearance of which signs and/or symptoms indicate that the PTA should have the patient stop exercising and should report the signs and/or symptoms to the PT?

3. You are working with a patient who has chronic left heart failure. What signs and symptoms might indicate that the heart failure is progressing (getting worse)?

4. You ask a patient to give a strong cough, but the patient repeatedly produces a weak cough. What are some possible reasons why the patient cannot produce a strong cough?

5. You are working with a patient on his exercise program, and you hear that a patient's breathing is accompanied by a wheezing sound. What might be causing the wheezing? Will you take any action?

CASE STUDIES

Case #1

Patient is a 72-year-old male with moderately severe emphysema who has recently developed PD. The patient can ambulate independently but needs assistance moving from supine to a sitting position and standing from a seated position. He also becomes short of breath during these activities. The PT has delegated to the PTA an activity designed to increase trunk rotation, which is needed in order to move from supine to sidelying. The activity begins with the patient supine, knees bent, and shoulders abducted 90 degrees. The patient is asked to inhale and, as he gently exhales through pursed lips, let his knees gradually fall to the right to rest on the bed. He inhales and, as he is exhaling through pursed lips, moves his knees past the starting position, continuing the movement until his knees rest on the bed to the left. The PTA is asked to provide hands-on assistance to the patient, if necessary.

Questions

1. Why has the PT asked the PTA to do this activity, and why has the PT asked the PTA to include the breathing instructions with this activity?

2. Is the request within the domain of the PTA?

3. Would you take any baseline measurements before starting this activity?

4. How would you determine the patient's tolerance to the activity?

5. When would or why would the PTA ask the PT to reevaluate in order to change the interventions delegated?

Case #2:

This patient is a 66-year-old female who had a right cerebrovascular accident 4 weeks ago. Several days after the CVA, she was transferred to an extended care facility, where she developed bacterial pneumonia in the second week of her stay. She is able to resume physical therapy but still has a cough, which produces thin, clear secretions. She requires moderate assistance to stand up from a chair and to ambulate a few steps with a walker and has difficulty supporting weight on her left leg. The PT has delegated to the PTA a breathing exercise. The patient is lying on her right side with the left arm supported by a pillow. The PTA's hand is placed on the left lower chest wall and over the ribs. During inspiration, the patient is asked to focus on moving air into the left lung and to move her ribs up into the PTA's hand. The PTA may perform a quick stretch maneuver just before the patient begins to inspire in order to facilitate active expansion of the left lower chest during inspiration. The breathing exercise is then performed with the patient sitting and the PTA's hands on the right and left sides of the lower chest. After a deep inspiration, the patient is asked to give a strong cough.

Questions

1. Why has the PT asked the PTA to do this activity?

2. Is the request within the domain of the PTA?

3. Would you take any baseline measurements before starting this activity?

4. What might interfere with the patient's ability to do the activity?

5. When would or why would the PTA ask the PT to reevaluate in order to change the interventions delegated?

Suggested author answers are available at www.slackbooks.com/neuroquestions.

REFERENCES

1. Berne RM, Levy MN. *Cardiovascular Physiology.* 8th ed. St. Louis, Mo: Mosby; 2001.

2. Powers SK, Howley ET. *Exercise Physiology Theory and Application to Fitness and Performance.* 5th ed. Boston, Mass: McGraw Hill; 2004.

3. McCance KL, Huether SE. *Pathophysiology: The Biologic Basis for Disease in Adults and Children.* 4th ed. St. Louis, Mo: Mosby; 2002.

4. Goodman CC, Boissonnault WG, Fuller KS. *Pathology: Implications for the Physical Therapist.* 2nd ed. Philadelphia, Pa: WB Saunders; 2003.

5. Porth CM. *Pathophysiology-Concepts of Altered Health States.* 7th ed. Philadelphia, Pa: Lippincott Williams and Wilkins; 2005.

6. West JB. *Pulmonary Pathophysiology: The Essentials.* 5th ed. Baltimore, Md: Williams and Wilkins; 1998.

7. Bates B. *A Guide to Physical Examination and History Taking.* 5th ed. Philadelphia, Pa: JB Lippincott; 1991.

8. West JB. *Respiratory Physiology: The Essentials.* 5th ed. Baltimore, Md: Williams and Wilkins; 1995.

9. Irwin S, Tecklin JS. *Cardiopulmonary Physical Therapy: A Guide to Practice.* 4th ed. St. Louis, Mo: Mosby; 2004.

10. Paz JC, West MP. *Acute Care Handbook for Physical Therapists.* 2nd ed. Boston, Mass: Butterworth Heinemann; 2002.

11. American College of Sports Medicine. *ACSM's Resources for Clinical Exercise Physiology: Musculoskeletal, Neuromusular, Neoplastic, Immunologic, and Hematologic Conditions.* Philadelphia, Pa: Lippincott Williams and Wilkins; 2002.

12. Weisman IM, Zeballos RJ, eds. *Clinical Exercise Testing.* Basel, Switzerland: Karger; 2002.

13. DeTurk WE, Cahalin LP. *Cardiovascular and Pulmonary Physical Therapy: An Evidence-Based Approach.* New York, NY: McGraw-Hill; 2004.

14. Frownfelter D, Dean E, eds. *Principles and Practice of Cardiopulmonary Physical Therapy.* 3rd ed. St. Louis, Mo: Mosby; 1996.

15. Hillegass EA, Sadowsky HS. *Essentials of Cardiopulmonary Physical Therapy.* 2nd ed. Philadelphia, Pa: WB Saunders; 2001.

16. Pryor JA, Prasad SA, eds. *Physiotherapy for Respiratory and Cardiac Problems: Adults and Pediatrics.* 3rd ed. Edinburgh, Scatland: Churchill Livingstone; 2002.

17. Jones M, Moffatt F. *Cardiopulmonary Physiotherapy.* Oxford, England: BIOS Scientific Publishers Ltd; 2002.

Chapter

14

Complementary Therapies

Carol M. Davis, PT, EdD, MS, FAPTA

KEY WORDS

body work
ch'i
complementary therapies
energy work
holistic
mind work

CHAPTER OBJECTIVES

- Identification of the various types of complementary therapies.

- Differentiate traditional allopathic from holistic medicine.

- Identification of various complementary therapies used within a traditional physical therapy intervention program.

- Discuss appropriate roles of the PTA when taught or asked to use complementary therapies as part of intervention both within traditional and alternative environments.

INTRODUCTION

With the coming of the new millennium, the practice of health care has changed. Out of necessity, health care has shifted from almost exclusively identifying and eradicating disease to managing and preventing chronic illness. The quest for the "magic bullet" to cure infectious diseases has merged into the realization that we also need to lead healthier lives in order to prevent many chronic illnesses, particularly the premature debilitation of osteoarthritis, chronic pulmonary and cardiac disease, diabetes, and obesity. *Living healthier lives*, we have learned, usually requires lifestyle changes such as drinking adequate amounts of water; avoiding direct sunlight; avoiding toxins such as sugar, salt, caffeine, nicotine, alcohol, and red meat; eating healthy antioxidant foods, getting adequate rest (8 hours a night), and exercising 4 to 5 times a week. The better we live, the healthier we remain. There is no need to take a pill to prevent problems.

The face of rehabilitation in health care has changed, as well. The increasing prevalence of patients seeking complementary and alternative therapies for both acute and chronic illness[1,2] and the increasing number of health professionals practicing complementary and alternative therapies has influenced the practice of rehabilitation in a major way. PTAs will likely be practicing alongside other therapists using holistic therapies, and many PTAs will study various forms of complementary therapies to augment their practice with patients. When integrating a complementary therapy with traditional intervention, the PT and PTA need to ask: "What factors make the administration of that therapy *a part of rehabilitation*," rather than saying "yoga or T'ai chi." This chapter will answer that important question regarding justification of complementary therapies as part of physical therapy intervention.

HOLISTIC HEALTH

Complementary therapies are often termed *holistic*. What we mean by holistic therapies and holistic health is that the totality of a person is often incorporates four areas of need and function: the *physical* (traditionally the body and movement), the *intellectual* (the brain and mind functions), the *emotional* (feelings and needs), and the *spiritual* (the eternal questions that help us organize meaning – Who am I? Why have I lived? Why am I ill? What am I to do?)[3] How these four areas function while interrelating in the world refers to the social aspect of need and function. This *social* aspect becomes the fifth area to consider.

In rehabilitation, the focus is on helping patients correct disorders of function that are primarily physical, but both PTs and PTAs are strongly influenced by patients' intellectual, emotional, and spiritual needs, as well. The PT and PTA who practice holistically question the patient in such a way, most pointedly while taking the history, that illuminates problems and unmet needs in all five areas and then advocates to see that all those needs are addressed.[3]

Traditionally, fragmented care, in contrast to holistic care, is concerned only with the "part" of the person that falls under each professional's province. One result of this fragmentation is recognized when patients become labeled with their illness or disability, and therapists may answer the question: "Who are you seeing next?" with "'low back' at 1:30." In Eisenberg's[1] classic study from the early 1990s on the patterns of use of holistic therapies in the US, the increasing frequency of use of holistic therapies was, in part, reportedly due to patients' objections to the fragmentation and impersonal aspects of traditional health care. Astin's[2] later study found that people were turning to holistic and complementary therapies primarily because these approaches seemed more consistent with their ideas of health and healing.

COMPLEMENTARY AND ALTERNATIVE THERAPIES

In general, complementary and alternative therapies can be termed *holistic* and focus on using to advantage the inextricable link between mind and body. These therapies are administered in an effort to help a person regain health and stay healthy by facilitating the flow of that person's human energy or *ch'i*. Holistic theory posits that when human energy is balanced and flowing freely, it contributes to overall homeostasis, but when blocked, it interferes with health and renders the body and mind together vulnerable to pathogens and/or biochemical imbalance. The natural state of the human is to be in balance, to be healthy. Blocks to ch'i can occur from disruptions not just physically but in each of the four quadrants of function: physical, intellectual, emotional, and spiritual. Ideally, once a block to homeostasis of the ch'i occurs, a holistic practitioner would be able to detect that blockage and reverse it without the need for medications or major interventions. Evidence that people often heal themselves is the basis for the traditional double-blind placebo-based clinical trial.[4]

Complementary and alternative therapies are nontraditional interventions that can be administered either as a substitute to (alternative to) traditional allopathic therapies or in conjunction with (complementary with) traditional therapies. They can be classified as *systems, approaches, or techniques within approaches*.[5] Examples of health care *systems* include chiropractic, Ayurveda, traditional Chinese medicine, homeopathy, and naturopathy. Within systems are found *approaches* such as acupuncture, acupressure, and herbal therapies in traditional Chinese medicine. Even more basic is a *technique within an approach*, such as auricular acupuncture, found within the system of traditional Chinese medicine, and transcendental meditation and sesame seed oil massage, both found within the system of Ayurveda.[5] One of the first categorizations of holistic approaches was found in *The Chantilly Report of the NIH*,[6] which listed the following categories of alternative therapies.

Alternative Systems of Medical Practice

Seventy to 90% of all health care worldwide is considered an alternative system to western medical allopathic practice. Popular health care, community-based care, professionalized health care, traditional oriental medicine (including acupuncture and Ayurveda), homeopathy, anthroposophically extended medicine (elements of homeopathy and naturopathy), and naturopathic medicine[6] fall under the category of alternative medical practice.

Mind-Body Interventions

Psychotherapy, support groups, meditation, imagery, hypnosis, biofeedback, dance and music therapies, art therapy, prayer, mental healing, yoga, Ta'i chi, Qi gong, Alexander Technique, Feldenkrais Method, and Pilates are examples of mind-body interventions. Many interventions used by PTs and PTAs incorporate techniques drawn from the philosophies and techniques drawn from these approaches.[6,7]

Bioelectromagnetics Application to Medicine

Thermal applications of nonionizing radiation, radio frequency (RF) hyperthermia, laser and RF surgery, low energy laser, RF diathermy, nonthermal applications of nonionizing radiation for bone repair, magnets, and nerve stimulation fall within this classification.[6,7]

Manual Healing Methods

Among this group are touch; manipulation; osteopathy; chiropractic; massage therapy; Rolfing; soma therapy; neuromuscular therapy; and biofield or bioenergy therapeutics, which include healing touch, noncontact therapeutic touch, myofascial release (Barnes Method), craniosacral therapy, Reiki, Jin Shin Do, and manual lymph drainage. Specific Human Energy Nexus (SHEN) therapy, a biofield method of treating psychosomatic disorders by releasing repressed and suppressed debilitation emotions, also would be classified here.[6]

Pharmacological and Biological Treatments

Pharmacological and biological treatments are complementary medications and vaccines not accepted by allopathic medicine. Some of those alternative medications include the following:

- **Antineo-plastons**: peptide fractions originally derived from normal human blood and urine and thought to be a natural form of anticancer protection.
- **Cartilage products**.
- **Chelation therapy:** employing ethylene diamine tetra acetic acid (EDTA).
- **Immunoaugmentive therapy**: highly controversial, experimental form of cancer immunotherapy consisting of daily injections of processed blood products that are designed to rid the body of proteins that prevent the patient's immune system from detecting the cancer.
- **714-X**: a mixture of camphor and nitrogen designed to turn cancer cells deficient in nitrogen into normal cells.
- **Coley's toxins**: a mixture of killed cultures of bacteria designed to improve the immune systems of patients with cancer; this is no longer used in the United States but is used in China and Germany.

- **MTH-68**: a modified attenuated strain of the Newcastle disease virus of chickens, harmless to humans but shown in randomized controlled trials with placebo to exhibit promise for cancer patients.
- **Neural therapy:** injection of local anesthetics into autonomic ganglia, peripheral nerves, scars, glands, acupuncture points, and trigger points for pain control.
- **Apitherapy:** medicinal use of various products of the common honeybee for alleviating chronic pain, inflammation, and symptoms of neurological disease.
- **Iscador:** liquid extract from the mistletoe plant used to treat tumors.
- **Biologically guided chemotherapy**.[6]

Herbal Medicines

Herbal medical remedies rely on botanical knowledge of the effects of herbs on the body and mind. Most common are soy, St. John's Wort, Echinacea, ginko biloba, saw palmetto, arnica, and aloe.[6,7]

Diet and Nutrition

For the prevention of chronic disease, Dean Ornish's program, Pritikin-Plan, and Adkins plan are based on the philosophy that nutritional intake and, thus, diet are critical for not only maintenance of health but also prevention of common diseases.[6,7]

COMPLEMENTARY THERAPIES COMMONLY USED IN REHABILITATION

Energy medicine is another term given to holistic therapies used as complementary to traditional rehabilitation therapies such as neuromuscular facilitation, exercise, and work hardening. All medicine and all health care, traditional and holistic, can be seen as energetically based because we are influencing the flows of energy in each of our interventions, whether that flow of energy be found in blood flow, nerve flow, lymph flow, neurotransmitter flow, neuropeptide flow, steroid flow, hormone flow, the flow of thoughts, etc.[8] The goal of clinicians as facilitators of healing using complementary or holistic therapies is to help restore normal function, balance, and rhythm to the body systems so that the body can once again be in homeostasis and a state of healing or self regulation. As practitioners, therapists become transmitters of a healing energy that surrounds both the patient and the clinician. By way of intention, the energy is focused through the clinician into patients such that resonance is achieved.[8]

The second edition of *Complementary Therapies in Rehabilitation*[5] lists the following as approaches commonly used by therapists in rehabilitation settings.

Body Work

Therapeutic Massage

Therapeutic massage is an ancient healing array of practices of manual therapies that include stroking, tapping, stretching, shaking, vibrating rolling, rubbing, friction, clapping, gliding, kneading, percussion, and manipulation of tissue. This is practiced with the intent of altering the structure of the tissue and the consciousness of the recipient. It engages the musculo-skeletal, neurological, lymphatic, and circulatory systems.[9] Many traditional physical therapy techniques, although described according to neuro-musculo-skeletal research and science, could also be considered *body work*.

Craniosacral Therapy

This holistic manual therapy that energetically manipulates the flow of the cerebrospinal fluid within the craniosacral system promotes self-correction and healing throughout the entire body.[10]

Myofascial Release (Barnes Method)

Myofascial release is a holistic manual therapy that focuses on releasing inappropriate facial constrictions that distort tissue and the shape of the body. These restrictions can be found within the macrolevel of muscles and fascial layers down to the cellular level in such a way that flow or normal fascial and muscle gliding is restricted. Fascial tightness causes the body to lose its physiologic adaptive capacity and homeostasis is disrupted. It is believed that myofascial release uses energy through a piezoelectric effect to restore the length of the fascia by "releasing" primarily the polysaccharide layer of the fascia so that soft tissue is restored to its original shape.[11]

Complete Decongestive Therapy (Manual Lymph Drainage)

Manual lymphatic drainage is one component of a comprehensive lymphedema management program termed *complete decongestive therapy*. Within many European countries, this approach is considered traditional physical therapy intervention. Within the United States, lymph drainage is generally used with postsurgical cancer patients. Both molecular and energetic flows are affected. Complete decongestive therapy consists of skin care, lymphatic massage, and bandaging of the swollen limb, followed by active exercises.[12]

Rolfing or Structural Integration

Developed by Ida Rolf, this is a manual body-based therapy that mechanically and energetically changes the tissues of the body. The myofascial system is aligned so that gravity flows through the body tissues and supports upright posture and movement. In this way, structure and function are realigned to promote health and homeostasis. Deviations in posture and tissue restrictions serve to locate dysfunction. The therapy consists of 10 systematic and prescribed sessions of both structural integration and intense deep connective tissue manipulation in order to restore appropriate tissue length and upright posture.[13]

Mind and Body Work

T'ai Chi

Described as choreography of body and mind, T'ai chi is a form of movement exercise that has been shown by well-documented research studies to improve respiratory status, functional balance, and aerobic control.[14] Originally a martial art, T'ai chi movements are a response to an attacker. That attacker's own movement and, thus, his or her energy is used against that person by moving in such a way as to sidestep the attacker and throw him or her off balance. There are numerous forms of T'ai chi containing as many as 108 postures and movements. Family names are associated with different forms, such as Wu, Ch'en, Ch'uan and Chih. Each is distinctive but follows classic T'ai chi principles that are based on integrating the mind and body to facilitate the flow of energy in the movements.[14]

Biofeedback

Biofeedback is a process of electronically utilizing information from the patient's body to teach that person to recognize processes taking place inside his or her body, brain, nervous system, and muscles. Instruments reveal both conscious and unconscious actions that are occurring, and patients or clients are then instructed to use this sensory feedback information to change unwanted activity. In this way, people are able to learn how to control unwanted activity, such as muscle tension, BP, congestion of blood in the vessels of the brain that cause migraine headaches, etc.[15] Therapists use verbal, visual, and kinesthetic biofeedback through voice, demonstration, and manual contacts everyday and often do not recognize when one system is contradicting the other.

Yoga

There are many forms or approaches to yoga. The most commonly used in rehabilitation is hatha yoga. Yoga is derived from a Sanskrit verb meaning to unite, as in uniting the body, mind, and spirit. Classic yoga practice includes more than body movements and positions or asanas done with mindfulness and attention, especially to breathing. It is a broad philosophical model of health based on human experience. Hatha yoga is especially useful in rehabilitation to facilitate patients' attention to the importance of breathing and moving mindfully through a full ROM. Bringing the attention to the breath unites body and mind, and the meditative movement facilitates the spirit to be "in the now."[16]

Alexander Technique

Based on the study of his own habits of movement that interfered with function, F. M. Alexander developed a technique whereby the teacher helps the student organize the position of the head to the neck and back, redistributing muscle tone and opening up consciousness. Poor habits of movement are identified to the student by way of touch and direction, and the student is directed to change in ways that facilitate conscious control of movement, over-riding poor habits of motion. Choice is, thus, given to the student to move in ways that reinforce an "extended field of consciousness."[17]

Feldenkrais Method

Each person develops patterns of movement to maximize his or her basic needs when growing to maturity. Many of these highly individual patterns of movement are limited in skill, flexibility, and practice. Both mental and physical aspects are incorporated into these habitual patterns. Some movements optimize physical performance while others are inefficient ways of moving. Moshe Feldenkrais developed a method of movement that would assist people in functioning at a higher level. Efficient postural patterns and movements away from and back toward those postures are taught. Those patterns are performed with a minimal amount of effort accompanied by a well-developed kinesthetic sense of awareness. In this way, a person should easily recover from any movement or postural challenge or trauma. *Functional integration* is a one-on-one, hands-on approach, and *awareness through movement* is a verbally directed movement process that can be done in groups.[18]

Pilates

Joseph Pilates overcame his physical frailties by developing this exercise method that is performed on mats and on several types of apparatus that use springs to assist an injured individual in successful completion of movements that would be otherwise restricted. By altering spring tension or increasing the challenge of gravity, an individual can be assisted in strengthening toward functional movement. The Pilates environment consists of the Reformer, the Cadillac or trapeze table, the chair, the ladder barrel, and the mat. The focus of exercise is on strengthening the core or trunk so that the extremities can be supported in movement. Attention is given to the breath and the smoothness of movement.[19]

Energy Work

Reiki

Reiki is a Japanese word meaning universal life force that animates all living things. Reiki is the same as *ch'i*, *prana*, *pneuma*, or *ruah*. Reiki is a healing system that channels the universal life force through the practitioner's hands into the mind and body of the recipient, promoting energy balance, healing, and a state of well being within the physical, mental, emotional, social, and spiritual domains. Anyone can learn Reiki, but it must be transferred from a Reiki master to the student during the induction process called attunement. The learner opens up to channel the energy to another. Intentionality is critical to this process. Reiki practitioners focus attention of thought or concentration in a specific way in order to bring about a healing or balance by way of energy flow.[20]

Qi Gong

Qi gong is the foundational energy that underlies all energy techniques, including T'ai chi. This ancient Chinese medicine philosophy states that health and healing are dependent on a balance of vital energy, a still mind, and controlled emotions. Physical dysfunction results from disordered patterns of long-standing energy. To balance and restore energy flow, Qi gong uses exercises that include slow, controlled, nonimpact-type movements and postures that gain control over the COG. Qi gong integrates deep breathing, movement, and postures while stressing expansion of the BOS, trunk control, and improving rotation of the trunk and coordination of isolated extremity motions. The meditative component serves to make an individual more aware of his or her body, enhancing the ability to control muscle tension, posture, and movement and facilitating a peace of mind that leads to an overall sense of well being.[21]

Magnets

Often grouped with crystals, magnets are thought to be worthless in health and healing by most allopathic health practitioners. The research, as limited as it is, indicates that there may, indeed, be a healing effect of magnetic energy on the body and mind. Magnets exert their influence by way of a magnetic field emanating from them. Unipolar and bipolar refer to the presence of which poles (north or south) face the surface. Manufacturers claim one or the other is more therapeutically beneficial. In the literature, many claims are made that are not substantiated with good research. However, some studies with patients who are medically diagnosed with pain, wounds, and fibromyalgia indicate that magnets seem to offer a therapeutic affect. The literature must be studied with a careful eye in order to ascertain the true benefits of what strength of magnet and what polarity seemed to be most beneficial.[22] The therapeutic community needs to be aware of this research in order to advise patients who are seeking relief.

Acupuncture

Having been in existence as a therapeutic modality over 2000 years, acupuncture is 1 part of the system of traditional Chinese medicine. Its theory is based on the concept that the flow of ch'i can be influenced by mechanically and energetically stimulating acupuncture points that lie along pathways (or meridians) in order to restore balance and flow. Disease results in and from a deficiency of flow of ch'i. Acupuncture physicians study the signs that indicate an imbalance in one or both forms of ch'i, the yin and yang energy. These clinicians learn how to facilitate flow through needling the acupuncture points, direct stairways to the pathways of flow (or meridians).[23]

Therapeutic Touch

A manual therapy developed by Delores Kreiger, RN, PhD and Dora Kunz, therapeutic touch is considered a nursing intervention where the patient or client is not touched by the practitioner, but the energy field of that person is manually manipulated in such a way as to remove blocks and disturbances in it. In this way, noncontact therapeutic touch facilitates an improvement in energy flow in the environment around the patient such that the natural healing powers of the patient can be maximized. This holistic therapy is one of the few that have been taught in college curricula for credit because of Dr. Kreiger's position as an academic.[24]

THE ROLE OF THE PHYSICAL THERAPIST ASSISTANT IN THE USE OF COMPLEMENTARY AND ALTERNATIVE THERAPIES IN REHABILITATION

Each of these (and other) complementary therapies carries with it a learning process requiring that the person performing the therapy be schooled in the theory and practice of the technique. Some require extensive coursework followed by examination and certification. Others require learning of the technique, but do not require official certification. *When offered in a rehabilitation setting*, the PTA, acting within the scope of practice of an assistant to the PT, must work with the PT in instituting complementary therapies. For a PTA to be delegated the total responsibility of interventions using the following therapies, that PTA must be *licensed or certified* by agencies providing education in this modality: acupuncture, Reiki, manual lymphatic drainage, Alexander technique, Feldenkrais method, or Rolfing.

When offering modalities *that require certification* without the supervision of a PT, the PTA should step outside the boundaries of practice as a PTA and practice according to the stipulations of the license or certification that the complementary therapy offers. In other words, the PTA should perform as a certified or licensed complementary therapy practitioner but *not* as a PTA. And, for risk management purposes, a PTA should provide these therapies outside of traditional allopathic health care environments. Within an acute care, rehabilitation, or long-term care environment, the PTA will provide interventions delegated by the PT. For that reason, autonomy of practice by the PTA using any of these approaches would not be appropriate and would place the PTA's certification or license at risk. If the PT is licensed or certified to offer the above therapies, then the PTA can assist the PT according to the instructions of the PT in the rehabilitation setting. This is true of all of the complementary therapies described.

There is risk associated with the use of complementary therapies in traditional western medical management settings. For example, if a PT decides that a patient would benefit from yoga exercises and the PTA has been educated in the application of yoga as exercise, then the PTA is still required to work under the overall supervision of the PT even if the PTA knows more about yoga than the PT. Once a complementary therapy becomes part of the physical therapy program administered within the practice environment of the PT, the PT is still in charge of the process of patient care.

THE IMPORTANCE OF A GOOD COMMUNICATING RELATIONSHIP BETWEEN PHYSICAL THERAPIST AND PHYSICAL THERAPIST ASSISTANT

The optimal relationship between the PT and the PTA requires ongoing communication and decision making for the benefit of the patient or client. This does not change with the introduction of complementary and alternative therapies. The application of these energy–based techniques requires special education and development of the intention of the PT and PTA to be successful in utilizing them with patients and client. Ideally, the PT and PTA will learn, for example, myofascial release or pilates or craniosacral therapy together and, thus, be able both to benefit patients with these holistic methods as complementary to their rehabilitation process. Communication is critical to the effective partnership of the PT and PTA. However, in the rehabilitation setting when complementary therapies are offered to patients, whether it is magnets, myofascial release, therapeutic touch, or manual lymphatic drainage, the PTA must work under the specific supervision of the PT no matter how skilled he or she is in the application of these complementary therapies.

CONCLUSION

Holistic therapies have a great deal to offer in helping patients regain a higher quality of life and empowerment toward better health. At the least, these approaches offer energy-based methods that are often helpful when all traditional therapies have failed. At the most, holistic therapies require an interaction with patients that restores therapeutic presence to the application of physical therapy; they move both the PT and the PTA out of the business mode of the managed care administration of therapy and back into an emphasis on the whole person and empowerment. Sacrosanct in this process of administering complementary therapies is the mandated supervisory relationship of the PT and PTA. No matter how knowledgeable the assistant is in the administration of holistic therapies, the PT maintains supervisory control of the patient care process when practiced within western medical environments. Hopefully, empathic communication among the PT, the PTA, and the patient will round out the treatment so that the experience is fulfilling for each person.

CASE STUDIES

Case #1

Complementary Therapy in a Traditional Rehabilitation Setting
Mrs. J was referred to Dr. Hagen, DPT, for examination and evaluation of balance problems. Dr. Hagen was a staff PT in an outpatient neurorehabilitation center of a large teaching hospital.
Upon examination, Dr. Hagen determined that Mrs. J, who was in good health overall, had developed her unsteady gait after moving from her two-story home to an apartment where she no longer had any stairs to climb. As

a result of using the elevator and only walking on flat surfaces, her balance problems began from increasing weakness in her hips and knees. Examination using the Berg Balance Scale, including the forward reach and manual muscle testing, revealed that her problem was muscle weakness. She scored 3(-) in hip extensors, knee extensors, and ankle dorsiflexors bilaterally. No inner ear problems were noted, but she was experiencing some difficulty with her vision and her hearing.
Dr. Hagen consulted with PD, a PTA who worked with her in the neurorehab setting. Together, they devised an exercise program that included systematic strengthening of her pelvis and LEs and suggested participation in a group T'ai chi class taught by PD, the PTA, on Mondays, Wednesdays, and Fridays from 10:30AM to 12 noon.
PD had studied T'ai chi with a T'ai chi master and had gained skill to the extent that she was able to teach T'ai chi at the rehabilitation center, as a PTA under the supervision of the Director of Physical Therapy. The state in which they practiced allowed her to practice out of line of sight of the supervising PT, and her group met in a quiet common area near the main rehab gym. PD employed the assistance of several aids and family members as "spotters" for her patients during the group session.
Mrs. J recovered her strength very rapidly with exercises and T'ai chi. PD did a follow up assessment of her balance and reported that Mrs. J was functioning safely, and she felt she was ready for Dr. Hagen to do a final discharge evaluation. Mrs. J liked the T'ai chi group exercises so much that she enrolled in a wellness center group and continued with T'ai chi for several months.

Questions

1. Was an appropriate protocol used by both the PT and PTA with the delegation to the PTA of a group class that included the complementary approach referred as T'ai chi?

2. Once Mrs. J met the objectives of the traditional interventions as well as the functional balance activities of the T'ai chi, was it appropriate for the PTA to refer Mrs. J back for final examination and discharge, or could the PTA, as a T'ai chi instructor, do this independently?

Case #2

*Complementary Therapy Outside of the
Rehabilitation Setting*

Mr. K, a 65-year-old executive at a local bank, was evaluated by PT Connie W for beginning Parkinson' symptoms. Upon examination, Mr. K showed no involvement in his handwriting and moderate rigidity in his back and shoulders. He held his left arm in slightly more flexion at the elbow, and the fingers of his left hand were straight with slight MCP flexion. His head flexed forward 6 inches; his left arm showed diminished swing with gait, and his steps were shortened to a 12-inch stride. His turn-around time to the left was slower than the right, taking several more steps to complete. No shuffling gait was noted. No detectable tremor was found, but Mr. K reported that a slight tremor of his left hand was present upon awakening some mornings. He had full animation of his face, no seborrhea; his speech was clear and easily understood, but quiet. He reported no difficulty in self-care. He was quite concerned about how this diagnosis would affect his career at the bank, which included interaction with many powerful people who trusted him with their money. He was most anxious that he not show any sign of weakness or pathology.

Muscle strength was normal throughout. ROM in left shoulder flexion was slightly diminished to 150 degrees. Trunk rotation and cervical rotation were limited to two-thirds normal. With regard to balance, one-legged stance time was less than 10 seconds on either foot. He was able to stand from a chair 10 times in 30 seconds without using his arms to assist. He was able to pick up a pencil off the floor, but was unable to tandem stand.

Connie W, the PT, devised a therapeutic program composed of myofascial release, which she performed focusing on opening up the occipital ridge, the thoracic inlet, and pectoral areas and working to improve fascial length for trunk rotation and shoulder flexion. Exercises were designed to emphasize increasing fluidity in spine rotation and gait. In addition, she had Mr. K practicing one-legged stance and tandem stance at the sink at home and wanted him to start practicing yoga on a regular basis.

Estelle F, a PTA working with Connie W in the rehabilitation center, was also a certified Yoga instructor and had a part-time evening and weekend Yoga practice in a small storefront location quite near the rehabilitation center. Mr. K's PT knew that Estelle F, PTA, was also an excellent Yoga instructor, who specialized in assisting people with disabilities in assuming postures with supporting towels and who emphasized therapeutic breathing. She suggested to Mr. K that he enroll in her Yoga classes on Tuesday and Thursday evenings. Thus, Connie W, PT, would see Mr. K as an outpatient in the rehabilitation center on Mondays and Fridays, and Mr. K would take Yoga on Tuesday and Thursday evenings. This plan appealed to Mr. K, who sensed that he really must not be "all that disabled" if he could take Yoga as part of his physical therapy.

Estelle F, PTA, spoke with Connie W about Mr. K when he enrolled in her evening Yoga class. Connie W was able to share her examination and evaluation information on Mr. K with Estelle F and suggest an emphasis on trunk rotation and UE range in addition to yoga breathing exercises. Estelle F was able to supplement Mr. K's rehabilitation by implementing these suggestions in Mr. K's Yoga practice with much success.

Questions

1. Would the myofascial release techniques and the traditional exercises be considered physical therapy?

2. Would recommending yoga as a life activity be considered physical therapy, and should the PTA consider her class as part of the PT interventions designed by the PT? If so, how would the PT and PTA deal with the concept of supervision? If not, why would the PT recommend the individual enroll in the yoga class?

3. Once the individual completed the intervention aspect of the traditional PT program and continued with the yoga, would it still be considered physical therapy?

Suggested author answers are available at www.slackbooks.com/neuroquestions.

REFERENCES

1. Eisenberg DM. Unconventional medicine in the United States: prevalence, costs, and patterns of use. *N Engl J Med.* 1993;328:4.

2. Astin JA. Why patients use alternative medicine: results of a national study. *JAMA.* 1998;279:1548-1553.

3. Davis CM. *Patient Practitioner Interaction: An Experiential Manual for Developing the Art of Health Care.* 3rd ed. Thorofare, NJ: Slack Incorporated; 1998.

4. Davis CM. Complementary therapies in rehabilitation. In: Gonzalez EG, Myers SM, Edelstein JE, et al, eds. *Downey and Darling's Physiological Basis of Rehabilitation Medicine.* 3rd ed. Boston, Mass: Butterworth–Heinemann; 2001:777-793.

5. Davis CM. *Complementary Therapies in Rehabilitation: Evidence for Efficacy in Therapy, Prevention, and Wellness.* Thorofare, NJ: SLACK Incorporated; 2004.

6. *Alternative Medicine: Expanding Medical Horizons.* The Chantilly, Virginia workshop report on alternative medical systems and practices in the United States to the National Institutes of Health. Pittsburgh, Pa: Superintendent of Documents; 1992.

7. Spencer JW, Jacobs JJ. *Complementary/Alternative Medicine: An Evidence-Based Approach.* 2nd ed. St. Louis, Mo: Mosby, 2002.

8. Oschman JL. *Energy Medicine: The Scientific Basis.* New York, NY: Churchill-Livingstone; 2000.

9. Kahn J. Therapeutic massage and rehabilitation. In: Davis CM. *Complementary Therapies in Rehabilitation: Evidence for Efficacy in Therapy, Prevention, and Wellness.* Thorofare, NJ: SLACK Incorporated; 2004:27-44.

10. Wahl DG. Craniosacral therapy. In: Davis CM. *Complementary Therapies in Rehabilitation: Evidence for Efficacy in Therapy, Prevention and Wellness.* Thorofare, NJ: SLACK Incorporated; 2004:45-58.

11. Barnes JF. Myofascial release: the missing link in traditional treatment. In: Davis CM. *Complementary Therapies in Rehabilitation: Evidence for Efficacy in Therapy, Prevention, and Wellness.* Thorofare, NJ: SLACK Incorporated; 2004:59-81.

12. Funk B. Complete decongestive therapy. In: Davis CM. *Complementary Therapies in Rehabilitation: Evidence for Efficacy in Therapy, Prevention, and Wellness.* Thorofare, NJ: SLACK Incorporated; 2004:82-97.

13. Deutsch J. The Ida Rolf method of structural integration. In: Davis CM. *Complementary Therapies in Rehabilitation: Evidence for Efficacy in Therapy, Prevention, and Wellness.* Thorofare, NJ: SLACK Incorporated; 2004:100-105.

14. Bottomley JM. T'ai chi: choreography of body and mind. In: Davis CM. *Complementary Therapies in Rehabilitation: Evidence for Efficacy in Therapy, Prevention, and Wellness.* Thorofare, NJ: SLACK Incorporated; 2004:109-130.

15. Bottomley JM. Biofeedback: connecting the body and mind. In: Davis CM. *Complementary Therapies in Rehabilitation: Evidence for Efficacy in Therapy, Prevention, and Wellness.* Thorofare, NJ: Slack Incorporated; 2004:131-155.

16. Taylor MJ. Yoga therapeutics: an ancient practice in a 21st century setting. In: Davis CM. *Complementary Therapies in Rehabilitation: Evidence for Efficacy in Therapy, Prevention, and Wellness.* Thorofare, NJ: SLACK Incorporated; 2004:157-178.

17. Zuck D. The Alexander technique. In: Davis CM. *Complementary Therapies in Rehabilitation: Evidence for Efficacy in Therapy, Prevention, and Wellness.* Thorofare, NJ: SLACK Incorporated; 2004:179-199.

18. Stephens J, Miller TM. Feldenkrais method in rehabilitation: using functional integration and awareness through movement to explore new possibilities. In: Davis CM. *Complementary Therapies in Rehabilitation: Evidence for Efficacy in Therapy, Prevention, and Wellness.* Thorofare, NJ: SLACK Incorporated; 2004:201-218.

19. Anderson B. Pilates rehabilitation. In: Davis CM. *Complementary Therapies in Rehabilitation: Evidence for Efficacy in Therapy, Prevention, and Wellness.* Thorofare, NJ: SLACK Incorporated; 2004:219-231.

20. Singg S. Reiki: an alternative and complementary healing therapy. In: Davis CM. *Complementary Therapies in Rehabilitation: Evidence for Efficacy in Therapy, Prevention, and Wellness.* Thorofare, NJ: SLACK Incorporated; 2004:236-252.

21. Bottomley JM. Qi gong for health and healing. In: Davis CM. *Complementary Therapies in Rehabilitation: Evidence for Efficacy in Therapy, Prevention, and Wellness.* Thorofare, NJ: SLACK Incorporated; 2004:253-282.

22. Spielholz NI. Magnets: what is the evidence of efficacy? In: Davis CM. *Complementary Therapies in Rehabilitation: Evidence for Efficacy in Therapy, Prevention, and Wellness.* Thorofare, NJ: SLACK Incorporated; 2004:283-306.

23. LaRiccia PJ, Galantino ML. Acupuncture theory and acupuncture: like therapeutics in physical therapy. In: Davis CM. *Complementary Therapies in Rehabilitation: Evidence for Efficacy in Therapy, Prevention, and Wellness.* Thorofare, NJ: SLACK Incorporated; 2004:307-320.

24. Anderson EZ. Therapeutic touch. In: Davis CM. *Complementary Therapies in Rehabilitation: Evidence for Efficacy in Therapy, Prevention, and Wellness.* Thorofare, NJ: SLACK Incorporated; 2004:321-331.

GLOSSARY

Constance "Connie" Carlson, PT, MS Ed

acceptance: The act of accepting. In the five stages of dying according to Dr. Elisabeth Kübler-Ross, the final stage. Individuals who reach this stage come to terms with impending death and await the end with quiet expectation.

adaptation: Adjustment of an organism to a change in internal or external conditions or circumstances.

adjustment: The ongoing process of responding to the world with a positive adaptive response that allows the person and significant others to grow and mature in regard to all aspects of life.

aerobic exercise: Exercise of sufficient intensity, duration, and frequency that improves the efficiency of oxygen consumption during activity or work. Endurance-type exercise that relies on oxidative metabolism as the major source of energy production.

affective disorder: A disorder marked by a disturbance of mood accompanied by a full or partial manic or depressive syndrome that is not caused by any other physical or mental disorder.

amyotrophic lateral sclerosis: A degenerative disease caused by degeneration of the motor neurons of the spinal cord, medulla, and cortex. Symptoms include muscular weakness and atrophy with spasticity and hyperreflexia.

anger: The basic emotion of extreme displeasure or exasperation in reaction to a person, a situation, or an object. Anger is instrumental in mobilizing and enhancing our ability to respond to adverse situations; for that reason, it may be essential to survival in some situations.

anosognosia: The apparent denial or unawareness of one's own neurological defect.

anoxic brain injury: A type of brain injury where the damage is caused by the brain being deprived of all oxygen for a time.

anxiety: A vague feeling of apprehension, worry, uneasiness, or dread, the source of which is often nonspecific or unknown to the individual. Anxiety is the normal reaction to anything that threatens one's body, lifestyle, values, or loved ones. Excess anxiety interferes with efficient functioning of the individual.

aphasia: Absence or impairment of the ability to communicate through speech, writing, or signs because of brain dysfunction.

apraxia: Inability to perform purposeful movements although there is no sensory or motor impairment. Inability to motor plan, manipulate objects, or use objects properly.

assertiveness: The state or quality of being assertive, which is characterized by self-confidence, determination, and boldness in asserting opinions or otherwise make one's presence or influence felt.

asthma: A reversible obstructive lung disease caused by increased reaction of the airways to various stimuli. It is a chronic inflammatory condition with acute exacerbations.

athetosis: From the Greek origin of the word: "without posture;" a dyskinetic condition that includes inadequate timing, force, accuracy, and coordination of movement in the limbs and trunk.

avoidance: Psychological coping strategy in which the source of stress is ignored or avoided.

autonomic dysreflexia or hyperreflexia: A condition commonly seen in patients with injury above the T6 level of the spinal cord. It is caused by massive sympathetic discharge of stimuli from the autonomic nervous system. Symptoms include sudden hypertension, bradycardia, sweating, severe headache, and gooseflesh.

balance: The ability to maintain a functional posture through motor actions that distribute weight around the body's COG, both statically and dynamically.

balance examination: Assessment of balance.

belief: A state or habit of mind in which trust, confidence, or reliance is placed in some person or thing. Something believed; a statement or body of statements held by the advocates of any class of views.

body-weight support during gait training: A technique used in rehabilitation of individuals with CVA, BI, or SCI in which a portion of the patient's weight (trunk and proximal legs) is supported by a harness while the person gait trains on a treadmill or over land. The harness supports the weight so that the person may practice the task of walking with a low risk for falling and reduced gait deviations.

body work: Body work is an umbrella term for the many techniques, both ancient and modern, that promote relaxation and treatment of ailments (especially those of the musculoskeletal system) through lessons in proper movement, postural reeducation, exercise, massage, and other forms of bodily manipulation.

breathing retraining: Techniques used to teach a person how to improve his or her breathing patterns, breathe more deeply, and exhale more completely.

cardiac: Pertaining to the heart.

cerebral palsy (CP): A diagnostic term applied principally to a history of anoxia for a variety of reasons shortly before, during, or after the birth process, and up to 2 years of age. The same conditions or experiences are often labeled with alternate diagnostic terms that vary with the geographical area and the clinic policy.

cerebrovascular accident (CVA): A general term most commonly applied to cerebrovascular conditions that accompany either ischemia (loss of blood flow to the brain due to an embolus or thrombus), hemorrhage into the brain, or rupture of an extracerebral artery causing subarachnoid hemorrhage.

ch'i: There is a constant flow of energy called Qi (pronounced Chi) in Chinese, Ki in Japanese and Prana in Ayurveda. This energy has positive and negative constituents called Yang and Yin respectively. In a normal person, these two factors are in balance. Whenever there is obstruction to the flow of energy, deficiency or excess of energy in a particular organ, or there is imbalance of positive and negative factors, the person becomes ill.

chronic obstructive pulmonary disease (COPD): A term that refers to a number of disorders that affect movement of air in and out of the lungs, particularly within the small airways. The most important of these disorders are obstructive bronchitis, emphysema, and chronic unremitting asthma. Also called *chronic obstructive lung disease.*

cognition: Mental processes such as awareness, recognizing, learning, memory, thinking, problem solving, reasoning, judgment, intuition, insight, perceiving, feeling, and sensing. The act or process of knowing.

coma: A complete paralysis of cerebral function; a state of unresponsiveness. Patients in coma do not obey commands, speak, or open eyes and cannot be aroused by external stimuli. Defined clinically as an inability to follow a one-step command consistently; Glasgow Coma Scale of 7 or less.

complementary therapies/medicine: Complementary medicine is usually not taught or used in Western medical schools or hospitals. Complementary medicine includes a large number of practices and systems of health care that, for a variety of cultural, social, economic, or scientific reasons, have not been adopted by mainstream Western medicine. Complementary medicine is different from alternative medicine. Whereas complementary medicine is used together with conventional medicine, alternative medicine is used in place of conventional medicine.

concomitant: Accessory; taking place at the same time.

congestive heart failure: A condition in which the heart is unable to pump sufficient blood to supply the body's needs. Backup of blood into the pulmonary veins and high pressure in the pulmonary capillaries lead to subsequent pulmonary congestion and pulmonary hypertension. Failure may occur on both sides of the heart or may predominantly affect one side or the other.

constraint-induced movement therapy: A rehabilitation strategy following brain damage (from a CVA or TBI) in which the uninvolved extremity is constrained so that it cannot be used, requiring the patient to use the involved limb for several hours a day, multiple days a week, for several weeks.

contralateral: Originating in or affecting the opposite side of the body, as opposed to homolateral and ipsilateral.

contre-coup injury: An injury to the brain located on the side opposite that of the primary injury, as when a blow to the back of the head forces the frontal and temporal lobes against the irregular bones of the anterior portion of the cranial vault.

coping: The process through which individuals deal with the variety of social and environmental factors encountered in life.

coup injury: Injury to the brain at the site of the impact.

crede: For emptying a flaccid bladder, the method of applying pressure over the symphysis pubis to expel the urine periodically. This technique is sometimes used therapeutically to initiate voiding in bladder retention for person with paralysis following SCI.

crisis: An unstable period in a person's life characterized by inability to adapt to change resulting from a precipitating event.

culture: The body of customary beliefs, social forms, and material traits constituting a distinct complex of tradition of a racial, religious, or social group. A complex of typical behavior or standardized social characteristics peculiar to a specific group, occupation or profession, sex, age, grade, or social class.

cystic fibrosis: An inherited disorder of sodium and chloride ion transport in the exocrine glands affecting the hepatic, digestive, male reproductive, and respiratory systems. The basic defect predisposes to chronic bacterial airway infections leading almost all persons to develop progressive loss of pulmonary function.

degenerative disease of the CNS: Disease of a component(s) of the central nervous system in which the individual's condition gradually deteriorates.

denial: Refusal to admit the reality or to acknowledge the presence or existence of something; keeping of anxiety-producing realities from conscious awareness. This is a defense mechanism.

dependence: A form of behavior that suggests inability to make decisions. A state of reliance on another.

depression: A mental disorder marked by altered mood nearly every day. There is a marked loss of interest in all usually pleasurable outlets such as food, sex, work, friends, hobbies, or entertainment.

development: The changes that occur across an individual's lifespan from birth until death.

developmental coordination disorder: A term used to describe a childhood disorder characterized by poor coordination and clumsiness. Uncoordinated movement is an abnormality of muscle control or an inability to finely coordinate movements, resulting in a jerky, unsteady, to-and-fro motion of the trunk or the extremities.

developmental delay: The failure to reach expected age-specific performance in one or more areas of development (eg, motor, sensory-perceptual, intellectual). A wide range of childhood disorders and environmental situations in which a child is unable to accomplish the developmental tasks typical of his or her chronological age.

developmental disabilities: A physical or mental handicap or combination of the two that becomes evident before age 22, is likely to continue indefinitely, and results in significant functional limitation in major areas of life.

diffuse axonal shearing: Term referring to the neuronal damage associated with traumatic rotational acceleration of the brain during unrestricted movement. A spreading force applied parallel to the planes of the axons but opposite in direction to whatever force was present.

diplegia: Term used to describe paralysis of similar extremities on both sides of the body. In CP, excessive stiffness usually in all extremities, but greater stiffness in the legs than in the arms.

disablement: A concept referring to the variety of impact that disease(s) and pathology(ies) have on the functioning of body systems, on human performance, and on human functioning in societal roles, with a focus on what the individual is unable to achieve.

disengagement: Any withdrawal from participation in customary social activity or activities that have personal meaning.

Down syndrome: A chromosomal abnormality, usually due to an extra copy of the 21st chromosome. This syndrome usually, although not always, results in decreased muscle tone at birth, asymmetrical or odd shaped skull, joint hyperflexibility, upward slanting eyes (unusual for ethnic group), small mouth with protruding tongue, broad short hands, delayed mental and social skills, and a heart murmur.

dynamic systems theory: A theory of movement organization in which the order and pattern of movement performed to accomplish a goal comes from the interaction of multiple, nonhierarchical subsystems.

dysfunctional: Term related to an abnormal, inadequate, or impaired action or function.

dysphagia: Inability to swallow or difficulty in swallowing.

dysphasia: Impairment of speech resulting from a brain lesion.

empowerment: To enable.

enablement: A concept referring to how disease and pathology impact the functioning of body systems, human performance and functioning, and societal roles, with a focus on what the individual is able to achieve.

energy work: Energy work is a general term for modalities that are based on the idea that the human body consists of energy fields that can be stimulated through various techniques in order to promote wellness. The concept of energy fields as a vital life force can be traced back to the oldest medical systems and is known as Qi in China, Ki in Japan, and Prana in India. Some energy modalities, such as *acupuncture* and *shiatsu*, have their roots in ancient medicine, while others, such as *therapeutic touch* and *polarity therapy*, are a contemporary and eclectic interpretation of one or more ancient practices. However, the underlying basis of all of these modalities is the idea of energy flow in the body.

engagement: In the behavioral sciences, a term often used to denote active involvement in everyday activities that have personal meaning.

extrinsic feedback: Feedback or information that is given by an outside or external source.

facilitation: The hastening of an action or process; especially the addition of the energy of a nerve impulse to that of other impulses activated at the same time. In neuromuscular rehabilitation, a generic term referring to various techniques that elicit muscular contraction through reflex activation.

family-centered care: An approach to the planning, delivery, and evaluation of health care that is governed by mutually beneficial partnerships among the health care providers, patients, and families. Family-centered care applies to patients of all ages, and it may be practiced in any health care setting.

functional training: The education and training of patients/clients in ADLs and instrumental ADLs that are intended to improve the ability to perform physical actions, tasks, or activities in an efficient, typically expected, or competent manner.

genetic disorders: A medical disorder caused by a mutation or change in a gene.

Glasgow Coma Scale: A scale for evaluating and quantifying the degree of coma by determining the best motor, verbal, and eye-opening responses to standardized stimuli. Coma is diagnosed by the absence of motor, eye-opening, and verbal responses. A score of 7 or less indicates coma; 9 or greater excludes the diagnosis of coma.

handling techniques: In this context, refers to techniques of physical contact with the patient's body to guide directly the movement and postural adaptation to a more normal pattern; usually refers to functional movement patterns used in daily care.

hemiparesis: Weakness or incomplete paralysis on one side of the body.

hemiplegia: Paralysis of one side of the body.

hemorrhagic stroke: Term used to describe a CVA in which a blood vessel in the brain ruptures causing loss of circulation to an area of the brain and compression of surrounding brain tissue; this causes injury and possible death to the nerve cells.

helplessness: Psychological state characterized by a sense of powerlessness or the belief that one is not capable of meeting an environmental demand competently.

holistic: A concept in which understanding is gained by examination of all parts working as a whole; a model or approach to health care that considers all internal and external influences during the process.

homonymous hemianopia: Loss of the same side of the field of vision in both eyes.

hope: The expectation that something desired will occur.

hostility: In psychiatry, the manifestation of anger, animosity, or antagonism in a situation in which such a reaction is unwarranted. Hostility may be directed toward oneself, others, or inanimate objects. It is usually a symptom of depression.

hypoxic brain injury: A type of brain injury where the damage is caused by an oxygen deficiency or a decreased concentration of oxygen in the blood in the brain.

impairment: A loss or abnormality of anatomical, physiological, mental, or psychological structure or function.

impairment training: Interventions that are system specific and focus on improving or eliminating the impairment.

infarct: An area of tissue in an organ or part that undergoes necrosis following cessation of the blood supply. This may result from occlusion or stenosis of the supplying artery or from occlusion of the vein that drains the tissue.

inhibition: The repression or restraint of a function or process. In neuromuscular rehabilitation, a generic term referring to various techniques that deter muscular contraction.

innate motor behaviors: Motor behaviors that are present at birth such as sucking, swallowing, plantar or palmar grasp, flexor withdrawal, and tonic labyrinthine reflex. Previously, these motor behaviors were referred to as primitive reflexes.

intrinsic feedback: Feedback that comes to an individual through his or her various sensory systems because of the desired movement.

ipsilateral: On the same side; affecting the same side of the body. The opposite of contralateral.

ischemic stroke: A CVA caused by a local deficiency of blood supply in a blood vessel due to obstruction.

lacunar infarction: Term used to describe small CVAs that have occurred deep in the brain and leave small crescent-shaped cavities where the nerve cells have died.

learning disability: A disorder in one or more of the basic physiological processes involved in understanding or using spoken or written language. This may be manifested in disorders of listening, thinking, talking, reading, writing, spelling, or doing arithmetic. They include conditions that have been referred to as, for example, perceptual handicaps, brain injury, minimal brain dysfunction, dyslexia, and developmental aphasia. They do not include learning problems that are primarily caused by visual, hearing, or motor handicaps, mental retardation or emotional disturbance, or environmental disadvantage.

learned nonuse: A phenomenon observed when monkeys had sensory input to one extremity surgically severed, and even though there was nothing wrong with the motor components of the limb, the monkeys quit attempting to use the affected limb after a short time. When the animal successfully used compensatory techniques with the unaffected limb, the strategy reinforced the nonuse.

locomotion: The ability to move from one place to another.

magical thinking: The belief that one's thoughts, words, or actions will produce an outcome that defies normal laws of cause and effect; the belief that one's words have the power to make things happen. For example, a client may believe his or her thoughts can cause earthquakes.

maladaptive: Marked by poor or inadequate adaptation.

mental retardation: A term designating below-normal intellectual function that has its cause or onset during the developmental period and usually in the first 2 years after birth. The causes may be, but do not have to be, genetic, Rubella in first trimester, intrauterine trauma, or infection. This term is falling out of favor; the preferred terminology is developmental delay.

mind work: The altering of the body energy by changing the way one thinks. Specifically, moving thought from the linear left brain and focusing attention down into the body in order to feel what is happening throughout the body or to concentrate on different parts of the body. Also known as "mindfulness" attention. An example of mind work is when, in most complementary therapies, people are asked to focus their concentration on their breath. Getting out of the linear, analytical left brain and into the body, or breath, so that the energy can flow more easily.

mitochondrial disease: Diseases that result from failures of the mitochondria that are responsible for creating more than 90% of the energy needed by the body to sustain life and support growth. These diseases appear to cause the most damage to cells of the brain, heart, liver, skeletal muscles, kidney, and endocrine and respiratory systems. Depending upon which cells are affected, symptoms may include loss of motor control, muscle weakness and pain, gastrointestinal disorders, swallowing difficulties, poor growth, cardiac disease, liver disease, diabetes, respiratory complications, seizures, visual or hearing problems, lactic acidosis, developmental delays, and susceptibility to infection.

motor control: The ability of the CNS to control or direct the neuromotor system in purposeful movement and postural adjustment by selective allocation of muscle tension across appropriate joint segments.

motor development: Growth and change in the ability to perform physical activities, such as sitting up, coming to standing, walking, skipping, running, and throwing.

motor learning: The acquisition of skilled movement based on previous experience. A set of processes associated with practice or experience and leading to relatively permanent changes in the capability for producing skilled action. See *stages of motor learning*.

motor program: A specific neural circuit or the neural connections that are stereotyped, hard wired, and store the rules for generating movements such as stepping.

multiple sclerosis (MS): A degenerative, chronic disease of the white matter of the CNS characterized by inflammation, demyelination, and the development of hardened plaques. The symptoms and signs are numerous; the course is erratic; its etiology appears to be autoimmune.

muscular dystrophy (MD): The largest and most common group of progressive neuromuscular disorders of childhood that are genetic in origin. MD is characterized by ongoing symmetric muscle wasting without neural or sensory deficits.

myocardial infarction: A condition caused by partial or complete occlusion of one or more of the coronary arteries with resultant necrosis of myocardial tissue. Also known as a heart attack or coronary.

neuroplasticity: Anatomical and electrophysiological adaptive changes in the brain allowing one to learn or relearn functions previously lost due to cellular death at any age and in response to demands from the internal and external environments.

neuromechanism: A neurological system whose component parts work together to produce CNS functioning.

neuromuscular examination: A comprehensive screening and specific testing process of the nervous and muscular systems and their interaction, leading to diagnostic classification or, as appropriate, referral to another practitioner.

neurorehabilitation: Rehabilitation of individuals with disease, pathology, or trauma affecting the CNS or peripheral nervous system.

osteogenesis imperfecta (OI): A congenital condition of abnormal fragility of the bones caused by defects in the amount or structure of type 1 collagen. The three classic symptoms of OI include fragile bones, early hearing loss, and whites of the eyes that appear bluish. Not all people with OI have hearing loss or blue sclera, but all will have fragile bones. Not all people with OI develop fractures.

paraplegia: Term used to describe paralysis affecting the lower portion of the trunk and legs. The impairment or loss of motor and/or sensory function in the thoracic, lumbar, or sacral (but not cervical) segments of the spinal cord, secondary to damage of neural elements within the spinal canal.

Parkinson's disease (PD); parkinsonism: A degenerative disease of the substantia nigra; cause is unknown for idiopathic parkinsonism; disease is characterized by slow movements, rigidity, a resting tremor, and postural instability.

persistent vegetative state: A long-standing condition (a year or more) in which the patient utters no words and does not follow commands or make any response that is meaningful. The transition of a person from a state of "coma" to one of "vegetative behaviors" reflects subtle changes over a period of several weeks from a condition of no response to the internal or external environment (except reflexively) to a state of wakefulness but with no indication of awareness (cortical function). A patient in this state may have a range of biological responses at the sub-cortical

pervasive developmental disorder: A diagnostic term used to describe a neurological disorder that affects a child's ability to communicate, understand language, plan, and relate to others. The disorder is not the same as autism (autistic disorder), but there are similarities of behaviors between the two diagnoses.

physical therapist assistant (PTA): An individual who is a graduate of an accredited PTA education program, is licensed or certified, and assists the PT in the provision of physical therapy. The PTA performs physical therapy interventions, tests and measures, and related tasks that have been selected and delegated by the supervising PT.

physical therapy diagnosis: The process and result of evaluating physical therapy examination data and determining the label(s) that identifies the impact of a condition on function at the system level and whole person level.

physical therapy examination: A comprehensive screening and specific testing process completed by a PT and leading to diagnostic classification or, as appropriate, to a referral to another practitioner.

physical therapy intervention: The purposeful interaction of the PT or PTA with the patient/client and, when appropriate, with other individuals involved in patient/client care, using various physical therapy procedures and techniques to produce changes in the condition.

practice context: The context or way a therapist chooses to teach a motor activity.

practice schedule: The frequency at which a patient practices a motor task; the schedule for practice of a task or activity.

premorbid: Prior to the development of the disease.

prognosis: The determination of the level of optimal improvement that might be achieved by the patient/client, and the time needed to achieve that level.

pulmonary: Pertaining to or involving the lungs.

pusher syndrome: A clinical disorder following left or right brain damage in which patients actively push away from the nonhemiparetic side, leading to a loss of postural balance. The mechanism underlying this disorder and its related anatomy has only recently been identified. Investigation of patients with severe pushing behavior has shown that perception of body posture in relation to gravity is altered. The patients experience their bodies as oriented "upright" when the body actually is tilted to the side of the brain lesion (to the ipsilesional side). In contrast, patients with pusher syndrome show no disturbed processing of visual and vestibular inputs determining visual vertical.

quadriplegia: Term used to describe paralysis in all four extremities; often used when describing the movement dysfunction in individuals following cervical neck SCI or those with a form of CP.

quality of life: The degree of satisfaction that an individual has regarding a particular style of life. Concept defined by an individual's perceptions of overall satisfaction with his or her living circumstances, including physical status and abilities, psychological well-being, social interactions, and economic conditions.

Rancho Los Amigos Levels of Cognitive Function: A scale widely used to classify a neurological patient's level of cognitive dysfunction according to behavior. This scale provides eight levels with descriptors.

role-playing: The assignment and acting out of a role in a treatment setting to provide individuals an opportunity for people to see themselves as others see them. It is also used to teach skills a person will need when interacting with others.

sacral sparing: A term used to describe partial or complete preservation of motor function, sensory function, or both in the S4 and S5 spinal segments of the spinal cord following a SCI. Presence of sacral sparing indicates an incomplete SCI.

sensory retraining or sensory training: General term for therapy aimed at enabling a person to regain contact with his or her environment; includes body-awareness activities and sensory activities using objects.

sensory testing: Evaluation of the sensory system.

shock: A sudden or violent disturbance in the mental or emotional faculties. Something that causes outrage, horror, stupefaction, disturbance, or agitation in a person.

shoulder pain after stroke: A frequent complication following a CVA, which can cause psychoemotional distress and limit function. There is no single cause for this disorder, but it is theorized to be caused by muscle imbalance, adhesive capsulitis, joint subluxation, nerve damage, and/or reflex sympathetic dystrophy.

spiritual: Term used to describe or relating to the moral feelings or states of the soul as distinguished from the external actions.

spirituality: That aspect of human thought and communication that focuses upon the belief that man has more that a physical body and that aspect does or may join a universal energy that has a higher power source than any one individual. This may or may not have a direct connection with formal religion.

spondylosis: The breaking down of a vertebral structure.

stages of motor learning: A theory of motor learning related to the stages of learning a new skill. These stages are known as the cognitive/acquisition stage, associative/refinement stage, andautonomous/retention stage.

stroke: A synonym to cerebrovascular accident (CVA).

systems model: A conceptual representation that incorporates a set of major functional divisions or systems within the CNS, which interlock and interrelate to create the functional whole. Although each division may be considered a whole in and of itself, with multiple subsystems interlocking to form its entire division, each major component or division influences and is influenced by all others, and thus, the totality of the CNS is based on the summation of interactions, not individual function.

tetraplegia: Term used to describe paralysis in all four extremities and the trunk. Impairment or loss of motor and/or sensory function in the cervical segments of the spinal cord due to damage of neural elements within the spinal canal. Current preferred term to quadriplegia.

therapeutic exercise: The systematic performance or execution of planned physical movements, postures, or activities intended to enable the patient/client to remediate or prevent impairments, enhance function, reduce risk, optimize overall health, and/or enhance fitness and well-being.

transient ischemic attack (TIA): A temporary interference with blood supply to the brain. The symptoms may last for only a few moments or for several hours. After the attack, no evidence of residual brain damage or neurological damage remains. Not all individuals who experience a TIA will, within the predictable future, develop an ischemic stroke or CVA.

trauma: A physical injury or wound caused by external force or violence. An emotional or psychological shock that may produce disordered feelings or behavior.

traumatic brain injury (TBI): A term used to describe brain damage caused by trauma (an external force or violence).

triplegia: Term used to describe paralysis or paresis of one side of the body and one extremity on the other side of the body; paralysis of three limbs.

unilateral neglect: The state in which an individual is perceptually unaware of and inattentive to one side of the body and the immediate unilateral area that the patient visualizes.

vascular: Pertaining to or composed of blood vessels.

REFERENCES

1. Aarogya.com. Available at: http://www.aarogya.com/Complementary/Bodywork/index.asp. Accessed November 19, 2005.

2. Alternative Medicine Foundation. Available at: http://www.amfoundation.org/energywork.htm. Accessed November 19, 2005.

3. American Physical Therapy Association. Guide to physical therapy practice. 2nd ed. J Am Phys Assoc. 2001;81(1).

4. Blanton S, Wolf SL. An application of upper-extremity constraint-induced movement therapy in a patient with subacute stroke. *Phys Ther.* 1999;79:847-853.

5. Bottomley JM. Quick Reference Dictionary for Physical Therapists. 2nd ed. Thorofare, NJ: SLACK Incorporated; 2003.

6. Goodman CC, Boissonnault WG, Fuller KS. Pathology: Implications for the Physical Therapist. 2nd ed. Philadelphia, Pa: Saunders; 2003.

7. Gove PB, ed. Webster's Third New International Dictionary of the English Language, Unabridged. Springfield, Mass: Merriam-Webster Inc; 1986.

8. Institute for family centered care. Family-centered care: questions and answers. Available at: http://www.familycenteredcare.org/pdf/fcc_qa.pdf. Accessed November 19, 2005.

9. Karnath HO, Broetz D. Understanding and treating "pusher syndrome." J of Am Phys Assoc. 2003;83(12). Available at: http://www.ptjournal.org/PTJournal/Dec2003/v83n12p1119.cfm. Accessed November 20, 2005.

10. NICHCY, the National Dissemination Center for Children with Disabilities. Available at: http://www.nichcy.org/pubs/factshe/fs1txt.htm. Accessed November 19, 2005.

11. National Library of Medicine and National Institutes of Health. Medline Plus Medical Encyclopedia. Available at: http://www.nlm.nih.gov/medlineplus/encyclopedia.html. Accessed November 19, 2005.

12. Philpot DJ. Special Education Glossary. Available at: http://www.dphilpotlaw.com/html/glossary.html. Accessed November 19, 2005.

13. Shumway-Cook A, Woollacott MH. Motor Control: Theory and Practical Applications. 2nd ed. Philadelphia, Pa: Lippincott Williams and Wilkins; 2001.

14. Umphred DA, ed. Neurological Rehabilitation. 4th ed. St. Louis, Mo: Mosby Inc; 2001.

15. United Mitochondrial Disease Foundation. What is mitochondrial disease? Available at: http://www.umdf.org/mito_info/whatismito.aspx. Accessed November 19, 2005.

16. While you are waiting. About brain injury: a glossary of terms. Available at: http://www.biausa.org/Pages/definitions.html. Accessed November 19, 2005.

17. Zollman C, Vickers A. ABCs of complementary medicine: what is complementary medicine? BMJ. 1999;319:693-696.

INDEX